Biosurveillance

Methods and Case Studies

Biosurveillance

Methods and Case Studies

Edited by

Taha Kass-Hout

Xiaohui Zhang

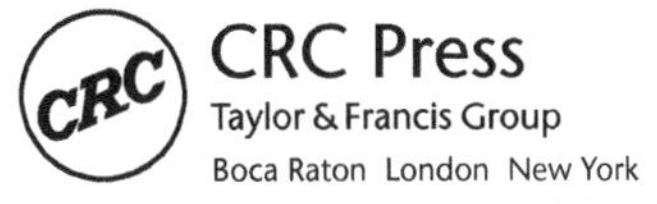

CRC Press is an imprint of the
Taylor & Francis Group, an **informa** business
A CHAPMAN & HALL BOOK

CRC Press
Taylor & Francis Group
6000 Broken Sound Parkway NW, Suite 300
Boca Raton, FL 33487-2742

First issued in paperback 2019

ISBN-13: 978-1-4398-0046-1 (hbk)
ISBN-13: 978-0-367-38341-1 (pbk)

Visit the Taylor & Francis Web site at
http://www.taylorandfrancis.com

and the CRC Press Web site at
http://www.crcpress.com

Contents

Foreword

There is no more exciting, challenging, and sometimes frustrating discipline of public health than the management of surveillance and investigation information in support of action to protect health and mitigate adverse events. While having its roots in 21st-century infectious disease threats to health on a grand scale, biosurveillance has come to encompass a broader scope of the science and practice of managing population health-related data and information so that effective action can be taken to mitigate adverse health effects from urgent threats. This expansive scope is reflected in the diverse collection of reports and perspectives brought together in this text, *Biosurveillance.*

History provides many examples of leaps forward in the practice of monitoring health-related factors in populations.* The observational methods developed by the Greeks and applied to human health by Hippocrates set the stage for the science of epidemiology. The development of systems of health care and codification of health events established the basic building blocks for public health surveillance. European experiences analyzing systematic health data, starting with mortality statistics in the 17th century, established the roots of Western public health practice and demonstrated the value of surveillance data. Perhaps the best-known example of this applied value was from John Snow, the British physician who analyzed the geographic distribution of cholera cases in London in 1854 and showed an association with a specific water distribution system. The removal of the Broad Street pump handle reduced the incidence of cholera and created the momentum for public health surveillance and investigation to contribute directly to population interventions that improve health. Personal computer tools like Epi Info™ developed in the 1980s allowed another leap for public health surveillance and investigation, making possible systematic collection methods, data management, and more adaptable analyses that accelerated the cycle from collection to application. More recent Internet technologies and methods, many described in this text, have allowed for more standardized data collections, a wider reach for collection, distributed and layered analyses, and timely sharing of data and findings. We have great hopes that the widespread implementation of electronic health records in the United States will lead to another leap forward for public health and the advancing practice of biosurveillance.

The excitement, challenge, and frustrations of biosurveillance are products of our health care systems, prompting the evolution of codification standards for disease, injuries, and their associated risk factors; advances in information

* Thacker, S.B. Historical development. In Teutsch S.M., Churchill R.E., eds., *Principles and Practice of Public Health Surveillance.* New York: Oxford University Press; 2000:253–86.

technology; and social perceptions of health vulnerability and the net benefit of health information exchange. Because these factors churn inexorably, our biosurveillance capability is incomplete and continually in flux. These tensions are a reflection of the immaturity of the disciplines of biosurveillance and knowledge management for population health. These tensions also create a tremendous opportunity for new leaps forward in our capability to improve awareness and decision making among all those with a role in our health enterprise, from world and country leaders all the way to the individuals who make personal and population health-affecting decisions every day. Robust and diverse interests are needed in the field to leverage creative opportunities, identify and focus on the most promising approaches, and translate them for wider application. More attention, more perspective, and more excitement will all generate more momentum to advance the field. This text compiled and edited by Drs. Kass-Hout and Zhang provides an important venue for the sharing of ideas and engagement of health scientists and practitioners that will be needed to ensure progress.

Daniel M. Sosin, MD, MPH
Acting Director, Office of Public Health Preparedness and Response
Centers for Disease Control and Prevention

Acknowledgments

We express our gratitude to all contributing authors who made this book possible and purposeful. Without their extensive offerings of their expertise, knowledge, wisdom, practical guidance, and lessons learned, the enhancement of biosurveillance research and practice would have been less realized. The authors and editors have taken time from demanding responsibilities to reflect on the principles and methods they have learned over many years of research, planning, implementing, and assessing biosurveillance-related projects and programs. Their gifts to enhancing the field of biosurveillance are deeply appreciated.

Dr. Barbara Massoudi provided invaluable advice, early encouragement, and support. She has shaped the concepts, insights, and useful suggestions on the scope and focus of this text. We are grateful for her contributions.

A significant credit goes to Dorothy Chiu for her wonderful work in revising, editing, and offering her constructive ideas on all the chapters. The project's undertaking would not have been feasible without her technical and communication proficiencies.

David Grubbs and Amber Donley at Chapman & Hall/CRC, Taylor and Francis Group, have been instrumental in the shaping, production, and refinement of several drafts of the book. They were committed to the fruition of this work, and are the channel through which the message of the book is disseminated.

We now acknowledge you, the reader, for undertaking the task of reading this book and reaping from it lessons and insights to apply in your work for a lifetime.

Finally, this book is dedicated to Dr. Ralph Frankowski.

Taha A. Kass-Hout, MD, MS, and Xiaohui Zhang, PhD

The Editors

Dr. Taha A. Kass-Hout has more than 14 years of experience in health, public health, and informatics, and has led research and development initiatives, critical assessment of new and emerging health IT technologies, and development of new capabilities and solutions in health and public health for federal, state, commercial, and international health organizations. In 2005, Taha served as a senior medical advisor to the United States' Nationwide Health Information Network (NHIN) Prototype. During the response to the 2003 SARS outbreak, Taha led the U.S. informatics and information task at the U.S. National Center for Infectious Diseases at the Centers for Disease Control and Prevention (CDC).

Taha holds memberships in several professional national and international societies, has published in several peer-reviewed journals, presented at numerous national and international forums, and has been an invited guest speaker at various health and policy events. Taha holds a doctor of medicine degree and a master of science degree in biostatistics, and has had clinical training at Harvard's Beth Israel Deaconess Medical Center and the University of Texas Health Sciences Center at Houston. *Contact information*: Taha A. Kass-Hout, MD, 932 Perimeter Walk, Atlanta, Georgia, U.S.A.; phone: (404) 487-8615; e-mail: kasshout@gmail.com.

Dr. Xiaohui Zhang serves as president of the International Public Health Institute, a nonprofit organization. With more than 20 years experience, Dr. Zhang has dedicated himself to the application of information technology and decision-making techniques to health care management, public health, and ecosystem protection.

Dr. Zhang has led the scientific effort in the development of infectious disease surveillance systems, disease outbreak early detection and early warning systems, information systems supporting organized population-based screenings (such as for newborns and cancer), public health emergency preparedness and response systems, and information systems for supporting comprehensive health care management for children enrolled in Medicaid. The surveillance systems have been deployed in 13 states and two major cities in the United States.

After the SARS outbreak in 2003, Dr. Zhang frequently traveled to China and Hong Kong, working with the public health agencies in China and Hong Kong to help in the planning and architecture of disease surveillance systems and to improve global public health capacity. In support of the 2004 Asian tsunami relief efforts, Dr. Zhang led volunteers to make available Web-based reporting tools for injury registry, disease case, and environmental event reporting. After the 2008 Sichuan earthquake in China, Dr. Zhang facilitated international technical support for the disaster relief.

Dr. Zhang holds a PhD in resource management, focusing on high performance modeling and simulation, and an MS degree in systems engineering, both from the University of Arizona. He has authored more than 40 publications in the areas of information technology, disease surveillance, decision-making support, operational research, environmental modeling, artificial intelligence, simulation, and electrical engineering. *Contact information*: Dr. Xiaohui Zhang, International Public Health Institute, 4400 E Broadway Blvd, #705, Tucson, Arizona 85711, U.S.A.; phone: (520) 202-3823; fax: (520) 202-3340; e-mail: zhang.iphi@gmail.com.

Introduction

Since the dawn of our collective memory, plague and contagious disease have been frightening, unseen, implacable enemies. It is not surprising that efforts to understand contagious illness extend back nearly as far as the written word. Hippocrates, the father of the western medical tradition, observed patterns of illness associated with temporal, geographic, and environmental conditions. The Persian physician Avicenna, in the 11th century, further speculated on the nature of contagion and disease spread, proposed the use of syndrome definitions for diagnosing diseases, and introduced the practice of quarantining. As the bubonic plague ravaged Europe and the Middle East in the 14th century, Islamic scholars advanced theories of tiny, unseen entities spreading the illness through contact, and by the 16th century, the germ theory of disease was taking root in Western Europe. John Graunt's analysis of mortality rolls in the aftermath of the Great Plague of 1666 pioneered the use of statistical analysis for understanding the behavior of contagious disease. For most modern epidemiologists, the turning point was Dr. John Snow's analysis of the Broad Street cholera outbreak of 1854, which combined statistical and spatial analysis, allowing for the localization of the source of infection and management of the outbreak. The lesson became clear: the sooner an outbreak was identified and localized, the greater the probability to contain and lessen the effects of the outbreak.

At the beginning of the 21st century, the shadow of a pandemic still casts fear across our modern generation. Several factors have conspired to increase the potential destructive power of epidemics. Both human and animal populations are densely packed in artificial environments. Pathogens have developed resistance to established treatments, and the anthrax attacks of 2001 have illustrated that deliberate propagation of an infectious disease is a real threat in the modern age. The geographic barriers that have provided protection in the past have been bypassed. The geographical isolation between plants and animals has been gradually broken by the intentional or natural transport of organisms caused by human travel, tourism, or trade. Foods and materials we use may come from anywhere around the globe. The acceleration of transportation has increased the speed and reach of a disease. Steam-powered transport made it possible for the 1918 influenza pandemic to cross oceans within weeks. As evidenced by the SARS outbreak of 2003, an infection may now travel from continent to continent in a matter of hours. A pathogen does not respect geographic or national boundaries. It is a global threat that all nations of the world need to face.

Although technology has contributed to the speed and distance with which disease can spread, it also provides the key for meeting current and future epidemic threats. One of the most exciting innovations in public health is the development of automated biosurveillance systems that can churn through vast amounts of health-related data to support early identification, situation awareness, and response management for epidemiologists and public health officials. The aim of this book is to capture the story of these modern-day pioneers who are walking in John Snow's footsteps, and to portray the current state of the art in biosurveillance, where some of the most promising aspects of modern information technology can be applied to this age-old challenge of combating the spread of disease and illness.

Despite the excitement that has greeted the initial generation of biosurveillance systems, several difficult challenges remain. As this book illustrates, biosurveillance operates in a complex, multidimensional problem space, and can be viewed from many different perspectives. Perhaps no single factor will affect the design of a biosurveillance system more than the data it uses. There is a tension between the most reliable sources of data (such as confirmed laboratory results) and the syndromic approaches that offer an earlier opportunity for detection (emergency department [ED] chief complaints, or over-the-counter sales). Animal data, vital statistics, and environmental data may identify the type of endemic relationships that Hippocrates first documented. Collecting and aggregating data from multiple sites raise issues of data granularity, quality, latency, and underlying meaning. Experience in developing detection algorithms has shown this to be a formidable undertaking, given the effort needed to obtain or create data sets for calibration, as well as tuning algorithms to reduce the false alarm rate.

Experience from fielding the first generation of biosurveillance systems has shown a host of operational issues that need to be addressed for a successful system. One of the most frequently noted shortcomings was that the role of humans (epidemiologists, public health officials, and the system developers themselves) was not well defined, as these systems primarily focused on automation. How were alerts to be validated and communicated? How could the system better support multiple organizations at the local, state/province, national, and even global level? What elements from the "information storm" are most important to convey accurate situation awareness at these different levels? How can such a system support different communities of interest, such as respiratory or foodborne illnesses, and different types of users? How easily can the system incorporate new data sources, and identify new types of threats? Practical considerations, particularly cost, are also important. Some existing systems are proving too costly to operate and maintain, let alone expand to incorporate more data sources. Quantifying the added value provided by a biosurveillance system will be necessary for increasing public investments to support them and making widespread deployment of these systems a reality.

Innovators today are pushing the envelope as to what we would consider a biosurveillance system. Some are taking advantage of new technologies such as Web-crawling, remote sensing, and SMS texting to provide flexible, lower-cost input channels for surveillance. Others are adopting a "system of systems" approach, where a given system will need to reason based on its own raw data as well as conclusions from other automated systems. The scope of these systems is also expanding from early detection to support the entire outbreak and management cycle. For Dr. Snow, this was easy, as he only needed to remove the handle of the water pump that was dispensing the contaminated water. For all of us in the global health community, this is a challenge we dare not ignore.

I have tried to organize this book practically, following natural sequence from theory to application. The initial chapters of the book build a foundation of knowledge for the reader. Later chapters contain more applied case studies written by experts from the field relating their practical experience within their professional domain. I would like to thank all of the authors in this volume for sharing their insights, as well as their candid appraisals of lessons learned and unresolved issues that will help chart the future of biosurveillance. I would also like to thank the many dedicated experts and pioneers in the public health community who, although they may not be listed as authors in this collection, made indispensible contributions to our understanding of biosurveillance. I am also grateful to the many organizations and companies that have supported my involvement with biosurveillance over the years, including the U.S. Centers for Disease Control and Prevention (CDC), Innovative Support to Emergencies, Diseases, and Disasters (InSTEDD), the Rockefeller Foundation, and Google.org.

Taha A. Kass-Hout, MD, MS
(with contributions from Walton J. Page, Jr.)

1

Timeliness of Data Sources

Lynne Dailey, PhD, MPH, BSc
Edith Cowan University
Perth, Western Australia

CONTENTS

1.1 Introduction

Successful outbreak detection requires the accurate identification of the moment when the number of cases has exceeded the number of expected for a certain period or geographic region (Lemay et al. 2008). New surveillance methods are being developed and tested to improve the timeliness of disease outbreak detection. One promising set of approaches is known as *biosurveillance,* wherein various information preceding firm clinical diagnoses of health events is captured early and rapidly from existing, usually electronic, data sources, and analyzed frequently to detect signals that might indicate an outbreak (Hopkins et al. 2003).

Researchers have studied many alternative data sources for biosurveillance, including sales of over-the-counter (OTC) pharmaceuticals (Davies and Finch 2003; Hogan et al. 2003; Najmi and Magruder 2004), emergency department visits (Lazarus et al. 2002; Lewis et al. 2002; Tsui et al. 2002), ambulance dispatches (Mostashari et al. 2003), and nurse hotline calls (Rodman, Frost, and Jakubowski 1998). Data sources used for comparison include reportable disease cases (Lewis et al. 2002; Mostashari et al. 2003;

Rodman, Frost, and Jakubowski 1998), hospital admissions (Davies and Finch 2003; Hogan et al. 2003; Lazarus et al. 2002), and clinical visits—in particular, those of certain syndromic categories and deaths (Lazarus et al. 2001; Tsui et al. 2002).

For biosurveillance, the usefulness of a signal is highly dependent on how early the warning is received. The performance of a biosurveillance system can be measured by three indices for the alarms generated: sensitivity, specificity, and timeliness (Buckeridge et al. 2005; Mandl et al. 2004).

In the context of biosurveillance, timeliness is the period between the occurrence of an event, such as an outbreak, and its detection (Wagner, Moore, and Aryel 2006). Timeliness does not have a well-established definition represented by a mathematical equation (Stoto et al. 2005). However, researchers generally define timeliness as the difference between the time of an event and that of the reference standard for that event. In the literature, timeliness has been used interchangeably with the terms "earliness" and "time lead" (Hogan et al. 2003; Magruder 2003).

Timeliness has been characterized through various methods of different levels of complexity. These methods are peak comparison, aberration detection comparison, and correlation (see Figure 1.1).

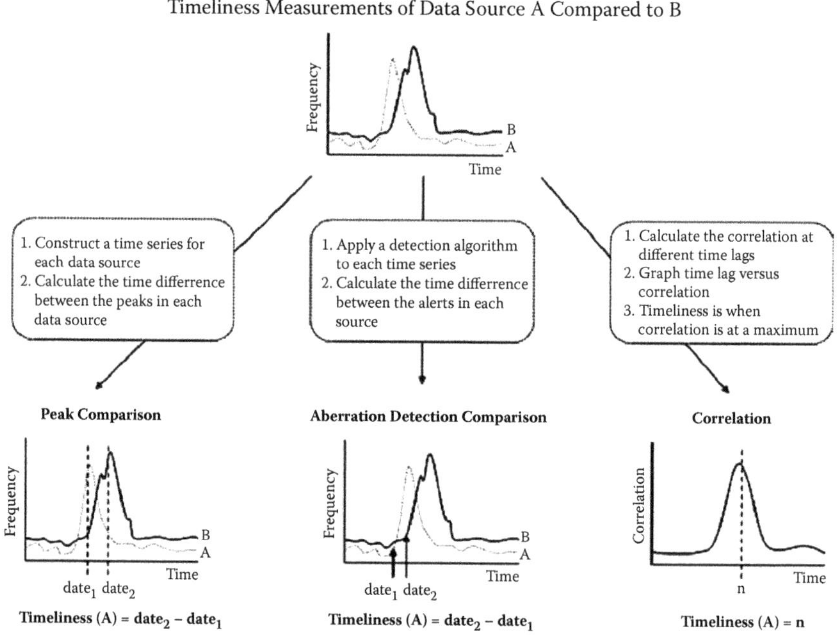

FIGURE 1.1
Three methods for determining the timeliness of data source A compared to data source B. (From Dailey, Watkins, and Plant 2007. Timeliness of data sources used for influenza surveillance. *J Am Med Inform Assoc* 14: 626–31.)

The following sections outline the methods for describing timeliness, provide examples from the literature, and identify the strengths and limitations. Many of the case studies presented are based on the surveillance of influenza. This disease has been used as a model infection for studies on respiratory syndrome and provides regular outbreaks to study.

1.2 Peak Comparison

Peak comparison involves calculating the temporal distance between the peaks or maximal values observed in data sources, and considers them in relation to one another (see Box 1.1).

Peak comparison has been used to measure the time difference between two data sources (Davies and Finch 2003; Lenaway and Ambler 1995; Proctor, Blair, and Davis 1998; Welliver et al. 1979). Welliver and colleagues (1979) compared the weekly percentage change in nonprescription cold remedy sales in a Los Angeles supermarket chain to the proportion of positive influenza isolates from children presenting to a pediatric hospital. They found that sales of nonprescription cold remedies peaked 7 days earlier than the peak in virus isolation in one season (Welliver et al. 1979). It is unknown whether this time difference would exist today if the study were repeated using modern laboratory methods.

Lenaway and Ambler (1995) analyzed a school-based influenza surveillance system that included 44 schools in a Colorado county. This study compared five influenza seasons and found varied results. In two of the 5 years, absenteeism surveillance peaked 7 days earlier than sentinel surveillance. For the other 3 years, there was no time difference between peaks (Lenaway and Ambler 1995). Hence, over the 5-year period, the peak in school-based absenteeism occurred on average 2.8 days earlier than the peak in ILI sentinel influenza surveillance.

One study investigated retrospective peaks associated with the 1993 Milwaukee *Cryptosporidiosis* outbreak (Proctor, Blair, and Davis 1998). The first data source to peak was turbidity measurements of the water treatment plant's effluent. This source was used as the reference for calculating timeliness (see Table 1.1).

Customer complaints and rates of diarrhea among nursing home residents were the most timely data sources with lags of 2 and 11 days, respectively. The peak in emergency department presentations relating to gastrointestinal illness and laboratory-confirmed cases of *Cryptosporidium* followed 15 days beyond the reference date. Surrogate morbidity peaks based on telephone surveys (35 days) and school absenteeism (64 days) were the least timely. In a real-time surveillance system, data sources are only timely if the information

BOX 1: HOW TO CALCULATE TIMELINESS—PEAK COMPARISON

1. Construct a time series for each data source
   a. Plot the frequency (number of cases) on the y-axis
   b. Plot time on the x-axis. Time can be recorded by day, date, month, etc.

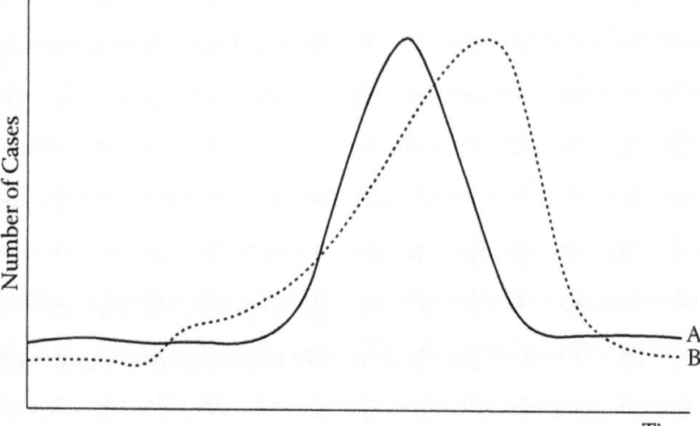

2. Identify the peak of each time series

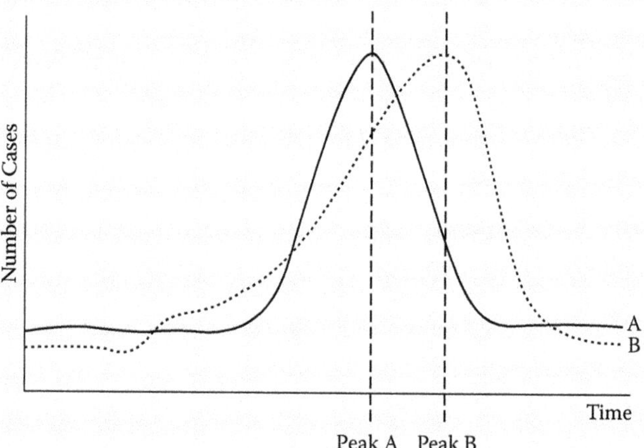

3. Calculate the time difference between the peaks in each data source
   a. Timeliness A = day (peak B) – day (peak A)

TABLE 1.1

Data Source Timeliness Relative to the Peak in Water Treatment Plant Turbidity Measurements Associated with the 1993 Milwaukee *Cryptosporidium* Outbreak

Data source	Timeliness relative to peak in water treatment plant
Consumer complaint logs	2 days
Nursing home diarrheal rates	11 days
Laboratory confirmed cases of *Cryptosporidium*	15 days
Gastrointestinal-related emergency department visits	15 days
Resident telephone survey	35 days
School absentee logs	64 days

Source: Proctor, Blair, and Davis 1998. Surveillance data for waterborne illness detection: an assessment following a massive waterborne outbreak of *Cryptosporidium* infection. *Epidemiol Infect* 120: 43–54.

is available for analysis and action. The authors noted that the dates used to construct the peaks did not correspond to the dates that the data were actually available for analysis.

Benefits of the Peak Comparison Method:

- The method can be used to assess preexisting data sources with known outbreaks.
- The method can be used as a preliminary measure to determine the relationship between data sources.
- The method can be used to indicate temporal trends.

Limitations of the Peak Comparison Method:

- The method cannot be used prospectively as peaks can only be identified retrospectively.
- Peak comparison may lead to the wrong conclusion regarding the timeliness of one data source to another. For example, as shown in Figure 1.2, data source A had an earlier peak than data source B.
- Its capacity for outbreak detection is limited. Comparing the peaks between two time series does not address the question of when an outbreak could potentially be detected. Algorithmic detection is required to test a source's potential for outbreak detection via alert comparison.

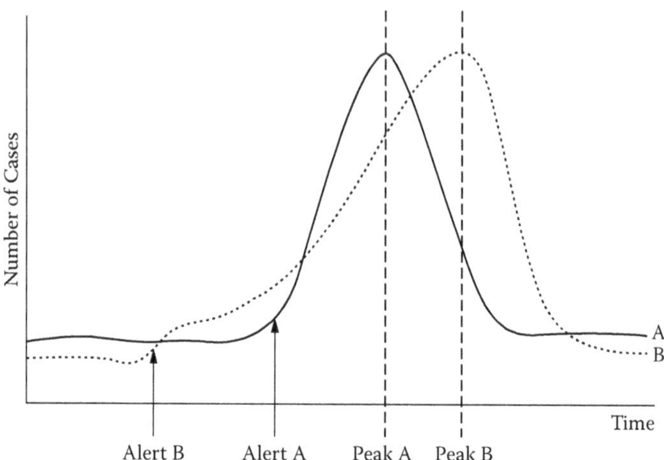

FIGURE 1.2
Example of later peak and earlier alert in two data sources.

1.3. Aberration Detection

Biosurveillance algorithms typically operate in a binary fashion: on any given day they either alert or they do not. An alert indicates that the data being monitored has exceeded a threshold during an outbreak period. Operating in this way, the performance of a detection algorithm in the context of a particular data source can be characterized according to its timeliness (see Box 1.2) (Buckeridge et al. 2005).

Aberration detection involves comparing the date of alert generated by an algorithm based on one data source against the date of alert in another. This method can be based on a simple threshold where an alert is generated when the time series exceeds a specific value (Davies and Finch 2003; Irvin, Nouhan, and Rice 2003; Quenel et al. 1994). Historically, thresholds have been based on two or three standard deviations above the mean (Irvin, Nouhan, and Rice 2003), or arbitrary sales thresholds for OTC pharmaceuticals (Davies and Finch 2003). This method is simple and able to detect shifts in excess of the specified threshold rapidly (Lawson and Kleinman 2005). However, it does not account for temporal features in the data, such as day-of-week effects or seasonality.

More complex algorithms have been applied to influenza outbreaks and include moving averages (Hogan et al. 2003; Ritzwoller et al. 2005), the scan statistic and its variations (Ritzwoller et al. 2005; Yuan, Love, and Wilson 2004), and the cumulative sum (CUSUM) (Heffernan et al. 2004; Ivanov et al. 2003). Moving averages and CUSUMs are based on quality-control methods that set an upper and lower control limit or threshold (Wong and Moore

BOX 2: HOW TO CALCULATE TIMELINESS—ABERRATION DETECTION

1. Construct a time series for each data source
   b. Plot the frequency (number of cases) on the y-axis
   c. Plot time on the x-axis. Time can be recorded by day, date, month, etc.

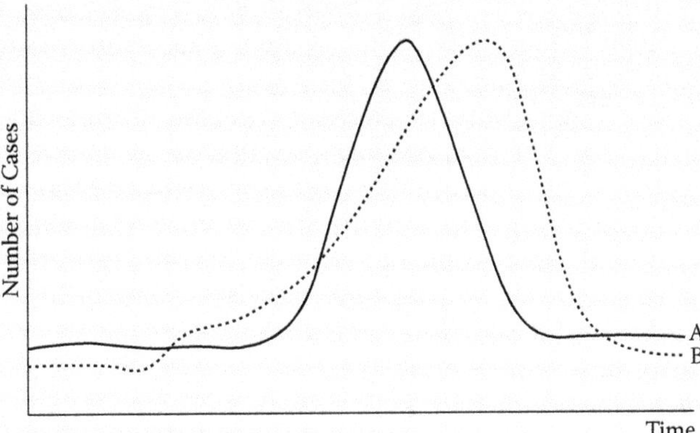

2. Apply a detection algorithm to each time series
3. Identify the first date of alert in each time series

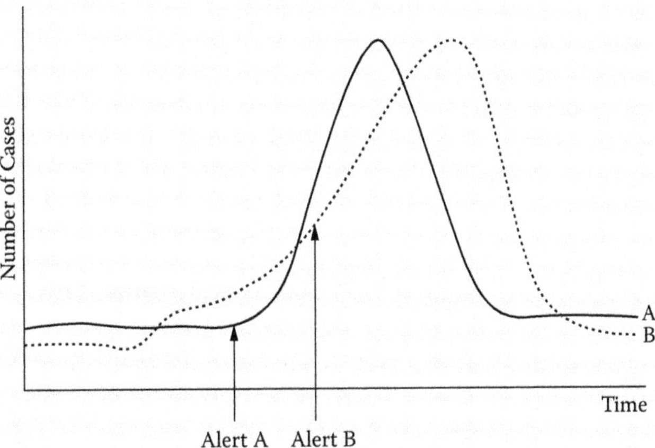

4. Calculate the time difference between the alerts in each data source
   d. Timeliness A = day (alert B) – day (alert A)

2006). The moving average calculates the mean of the previous values and compares it to the current value. Data closer in time to the current day can be given more weight than data farther in the past, as is the case with an exponentially weighted moving average (EWMA). Moving average charts are more sensitive than thresholds at detecting small shifts in the process average (SAS 2005). However, predictions become accustomed to increasing counts during the early stages of an outbreak, and this increases the time to alert (Wong and Moore 2006). This problem is the prime motivation for using the CUSUM approach.

The CUSUM method involves calculating the cumulative sum over time of the differences between observed counts and a reference value that represents the in-control mean (O'Brien and Christie 1997). As the algorithm is based on the accumulation of differences, the CUSUM detects an aberration very quickly and is able to detect small shifts from the mean (O'Brien and Christie 1997; Wong and Moore 2006). However, the algorithm will signal a false alert if deviations in the underlying process that are not associated with an outbreak occur, such as a steady rise in the mean (Moore et al. 2002).

Spatial scan statistics are used to detect geographical disease clusters of high or low incidence, and evaluate their statistical significance using likelihood-ratio tests (Kulldorff 1997). This algorithm identifies a significant excess of cases within a moving cylindrical window over a defined spatial region and is able to adjust for multiple hypothesis testing (Kulldorff 1999). It differs from the other algorithms described, as it is able to detect spatial as well as temporal clusters.

The comparison of alerts generated by aberration detection algorithms has been used to measure the time difference between two data sources. An English study applied the peak comparison method and thresholds for comparing OTC sales of cough/cold remedies to emergency department admission data (Davies and Finch 2003). Analyses demonstrated that peak sales both preceded and lagged the peak in admissions over the years investigated. However, increases above a defined threshold of OTC sales occurred 14 days before the peak in emergency department admissions in all 3 years of the study (Davies and Finch 2003).

Quenel and colleagues (1994) applied thresholds to determine the date of alert for various health service–based indicators from hospitals and absenteeism records. The threshold above which an alert was declared was defined as the upper limit of the 95% confidence interval of the weekly average calculated from nonepidemic weeks. An epidemic week occurred when 1% of specimens were positive for influenza A. The health service–based indicators increased before virological confirmation over the 5-year period. The emergency visit indicator was the earliest (average 11.2 days, range 7–28 days before virological confirmation) followed by sick-leave reports collected by general practitioners (average 8.4 days, range 7–21 days) (Quenel et al. 1994).

The timeliness of algorithmic alerts from an emergency department surveillance system based on chief complaint data was compared to the date of the influenza season peak identified by the Centers for Disease Control and Prevention (CDC) (Irvin, Nouhan, and Rice 2003). An alert was defined as a value that exceeded two standard deviations greater than the historical constant mean on two of three consecutive days. For the influenza season investigated, emergency department chief complaints alerted 14 days earlier than the peak in CDC influenza reports.

The use of emergency department medical records for the early detection of influenza-like illness (ILI) was investigated for one influenza season in health care organizations in Minnesota (Miller et al. 2004). Visual inspection of ILI counts and influenza and pneumonia deaths indicated that ILI counts rose several weeks before the peak in the number of deaths. A CUSUM detection algorithm signaled a confirmed influenza outbreak one day before the first virologically confirmed isolate. When these analyses were repeated with age-stratified data (age >65 years), the algorithm signaled 24 days earlier (Miller et al. 2004).

The CUSUM algorithm was also used to detect trends in fever and respiratory distress indicative of influenza at seven hospitals in Virginia (Yuan, Love, and Wilson 2004). In one of these hospitals, syndromic data revealed an increase in these syndromes 7 days earlier than an increase in sentinel influenza surveillance (Yuan, Love, and Wilson 2004).

A syndromic surveillance system based in Colorado identified unusual clusters of ILI using three statistical models (Ritzwoller et al. 2005). These were the small area method (SMART; small area regression and testing), spatiotemporal method, and a purely temporal method (spatiotemporal scan statistic using 100% of the area). These algorithms were used to compare the timeliness of syndromic chief complaint data with laboratory-confirmed influenza cases. They found that, despite both data sources showing substantial increases during the same calendar week, there was a greater absolute increase in syndromic surveillance episodes (Ritzwoller et al. 2005).

Heffernan and colleagues (2004) applied the temporal scan statistic to emergency department chief complaints. The signal produced from respiratory and fever syndromes provided the earliest indication of community-wide influenza activity in New York City for the 2001–2002 influenza season. The signal occurred 14 days before an increase in the number of positive influenza isolates and 21 days before an increase in the number of sentinel ILI reports (Heffernan et al. 2004). However, the size of these increases and the method for determining the presence of an increase were not described.

Benefits of the aberration detection method:

- The method can be based on simple thresholds or mathematical formulas.
- The method can be used to answer the fundamental question of when an outbreak can be detected.

Limitations of the aberration detection method:

- An increase in a time series could be due to variability within the time series such as seasonality and day-of-week effects.
- Numerous algorithms can be applied to surveillance data, and, for each algorithm, parameter selection affects the time at which the algorithm will alert.
- Algorithms cannot replace the need for local knowledge and experience.

1.4 Correlation

In terms of correlation, timeliness is defined as the time lag at which the correlation between two data sources is significant (Johnson et al. 2004). Specifically, the correlation between two time series is calculated, and then one of the series is moved in time relative to the other, representing different time lags. The correlation is calculated for each time lag, and the timeliness of one data source relative to another is determined by the correlation coefficients that are statistically significant (see Box 1.3).

The cross-correlation function (CCF) calculates a numerical value that describes the similarity of two curves over a defined period with two identical curves having a CCF value of one (Suyama et al. 2003). Prior to computing the CCF, the data have to be normalized to satisfy the assumption of normality. A significant CCF at a specific time lag "x" indicates that the peak in one data source occurs "x" time periods before the peak in another data source. A significant CCF at a lag of zero indicates the peaks occurred at the same time (Suyama et al. 2003). The Spearman rank correlation is another method used to determine correlation, which is based on ranking data, and can be applied when the assumption of normality is violated (Doroshenko et al. 2005).

As shown in Figure 1.3, similar time series have a high correlation (close to 1.0), and dissimilar time series have a low correlation (close to 0). When interpreting correlation values, low correlations may be statistically significant due to the randomness and variability in biosurveillance data sources.

Timeliness has been assessed by correlation methods, including the CCF (Espino, Hogan, and Wagner 2003; Hogan et al. 2003; Ivanov et al. 2003; Johnson et al. 2004; Magruder 2003) and the Spearman rank correlation (Doroshenko et al. 2005).

Espino and colleagues (2003) determined the CCF of regional and state influenza activity to emergency room telephone triage based on 10 hospitals in a large city. They found that emergency room telephone triage was 7 days (correlation 0.25) ahead of state influenza activity and 28 days (correlation

BOX 3: HOW TO CALCULATE TIMELINESS—CORRELATION

1. Construct a time series for each data source
   a. Plot the frequency (number of cases) on the y-axis
   b. Plot time on the x-axis. Time can be recorded by day, date, month, etc.

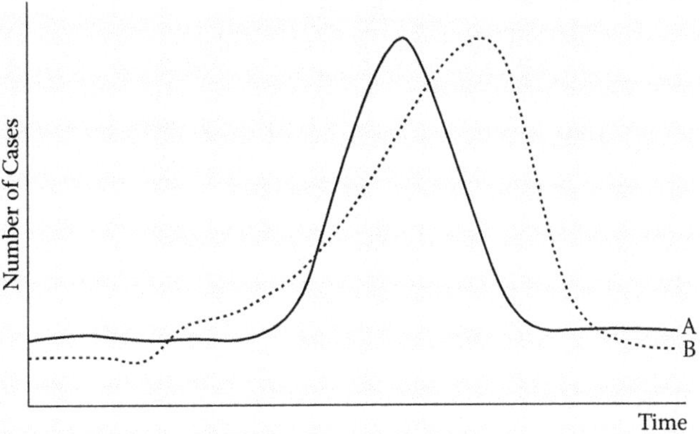

2. Calculate the correlation between the two time series. This will determine the correlation at zero lag.
3. Move one data source along the x-axis for a period of time, for example, 7 days.
4. Calculate the correlation between the two time series. This will determine the correlation at 7 days lag.
5. Repeat the above steps for each time lag to be calculated.
6. Plot time lag (x-axis) against the calculated correlation coefficients (y-axis).
7. Identify on the plot the maximum correlation for the two time series.

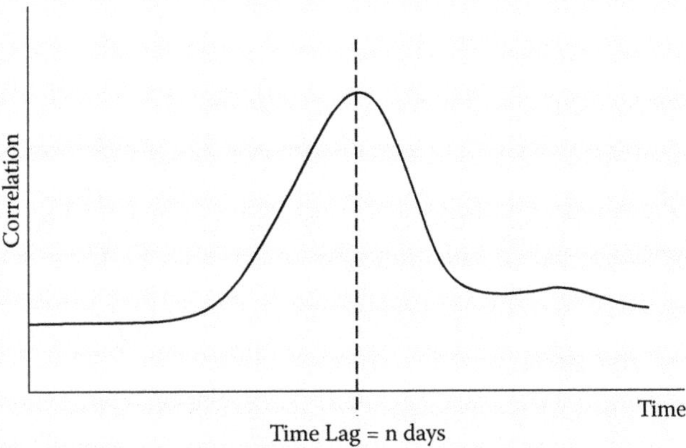

8. The timeliness is quoted as the time lag when the correlation is at a maximum
   a. Timeliness A = Time lag (n)

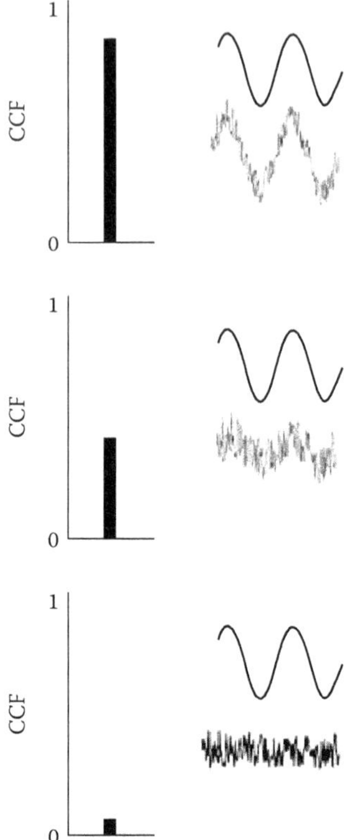

FIGURE 1.3
Demonstration of cross-correlation function (CCF)—decrease in similarity of two curves decreases the overall CCF magnitude. (From Suyama et al. 2003. Surveillance of infectious disease occurrences in the community: an analysis of symptom presentation in the emergency department. *Acad Emerg Med* 10 (7): 753–63.)

0.25) ahead of regional influenza activity. Hence, at this peak correlation, emergency room telephone triage was on average 17.5 days ahead of all influenza activity.

Magruder (2003) found that after controlling for day-of-week and holiday effects, the CCF peaked between 0.86 and 0.93 for OTC sales and physician diagnoses. At this peak correlation, OTC sales were on average, 2.8 days (range 2–7 days) ahead of physician diagnoses based on two influenza seasons (Magruder 2003).

Johnson et al. (2004) investigated the correlation using the CCF between influenza article access on the Internet and CDC surveillance data. Although there was a moderately strong correlation between Web access and influenza reports (range 0.71–0.80), the timeliness of this method was variable, and hence the authors could not draw any strong conclusions (Johnson et al. 2004).

One pediatric study used both the CCF and an exponentially weighted moving average (EWMA) to determine the timeliness of free-text chief complaints in the emergency department to respiratory discharge diagnoses (Ivanov et al. 2003). The mean timeliness calculated across different values of the weighting parameter in the EWMA analysis varied from –11.7 to 32.7 days with an overall mean of 10.3 days (95% CI –15.2:35.5). Cross-correlation analyses of the three outbreaks studied resulted in an average timeliness of 7.4 days (95% CI: −8.3, 43.3) (Ivanov et al. 2003).

This combined aberration detection–correlation method was also used by Hogan and colleagues (2003). The CCF and EWMA algorithm were used to determine the timeliness of sales of OTC electrolyte products for the detection of respiratory and diarrheal outbreaks (Hogan et al. 2003). Over the 3-year study period, the correlation of electrolyte sales to hospital diagnoses based on raw data was 0.9 (95% CI 0.87–0.93) and OTC sales preceded diagnoses by 1.7 weeks (95% CI 0.5–2.9) for respiratory and diarrheal outbreaks.

Doroshenko and colleagues (2005) applied an autoregressive moving average model and Spearman rank correlation to assess the timeliness of calls to a national telephone advice service and ILI sentinel reporting. They found statistically significant but weak correlations up to 21 days lag, suggesting that ILI calls occurred 7–21 days earlier than an increase in consultations recorded by a sentinel surveillance network (Doroshenko et al. 2005).

Lemay and colleagues (2008) applied an autoregressive moving average model and CCF to assess the timeliness of emergency department ILI presentations and laboratory-confirmed influenza by age group. This retrospective study showed a strong correlation between the isolation of influenza viruses and patient consultations to the ED for ILI in four of five seasons. When the ILI consultations were divided by age group, consultations for children less than five years were more likely to be correlated with laboratory-confirmed influenza cases than consultations for other age groups. Statistically significant correlations were found for the fever and respiratory/fever syndromes in four seasons with a lag of 7–28 days (lags of greater than 28 days were not included in the analyses) for children under 5 years.

Suyama and colleagues (2003) determined whether any temporal correlations existed between emergency department (ED) symptom presentations (nausea, vomiting, headache, etc.), and health department (HD) data for infectious disease (e.g., meningitis). Cross-correlation functions were calculated for a 3-day crossover period between ED syndrome presentation and HD disease identification. This was based on the period in which a temporal relationship between ED and HD data may be of clinical significance. Syndrome presentations were based on 73 infectious diseases (class A) reportable to the Ohio Department of Health. CCFs were found to be significant (CCF > 0.074) for all syndromes combined, gastrointestinal syndromes, pulmonary syndromes, and central nervous system syndromes. It was found that for all syndromes combined, ED presentations preceded HD identification by 1 day (CCF = 0.112).

Lazarus et al. (2002) investigated correlation using the Spearman rank correlation between ambulatory-care episodes of lower respiratory syndrome and hospital admissions for lower respiratory syndrome over a 3-year period.

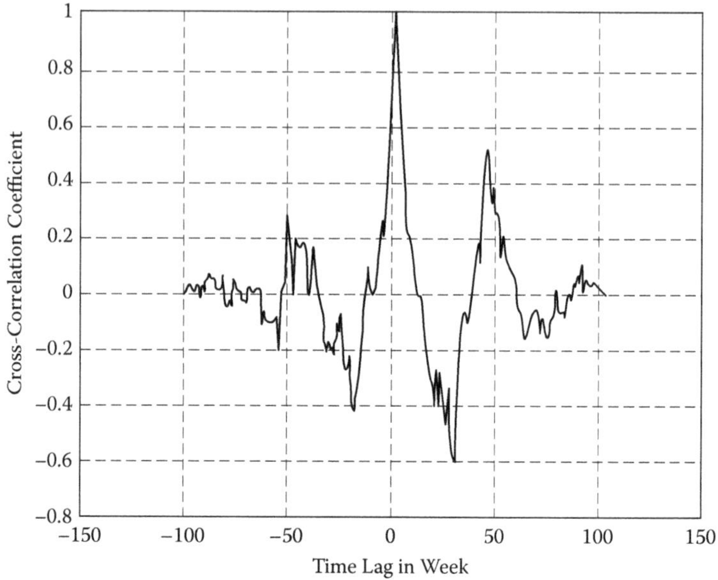

FIGURE 1.4
Cross correlation between "respiratory" (RS) and the "pneumonia and influenza" (P and I) deaths: maximum correlation occurs when RS and "influenza chief complaints" (IS) are 2 weeks earlier than the P and I curve. (From Tsui et al. 2002. Value of ICD-9-coded chief complaints for detection of epidemics. *J Am Med Inform Assoc* 9: S41–S47.)

Overall, ambulatory-care episodes were highly correlated (correlation = 0.92) with hospital admissions, and they preceded them by 2 weeks.

Tsui et al. (2002) measured the value of ICD-9 coded emergency department chief complaints for influenza surveillance. They applied a detection system based on a standard algorithm (the Serfling method) and the cross-correlation function. The timeliness of "respiratory" (RS) and "influenza" (IS) chief complaint ICD-9 codes were compared with national pneumonia and influenza (P and I) deaths. The time to detection for RS and IS data based on the algorithmic method was one week earlier than P and I deaths. In this study, the cross-correlation function demonstrated that the signal provided by ICD-9-coded chief complaints occurred 2 weeks earlier than the signal provided by P and I data (see Figure 1.4) (Tsui et al. 2002).

Benefits of the correlation method:

- This method is useful for showing that variation in one data source can predict changes in another data source (Suyama et al. 2003).

Limitations of the correlation method:

- This method requires data collected over a continuous period of time (i.e., cannot have missing data, e.g., weekend data).

- Correlation coefficients cannot determine the thresholds for triggering an alert.
- Correlation coefficients cannot be used to define a change or level that might be indicative of disease occurrence or an outbreak (Suyama et al. 2003).

1.5 Data Timeliness and Accuracy

As outlined by Buckeridge and colleagues (2002), data sources that are chronologically distant from diagnostic information are timely but not as specific as data sources that are chronologically closer to diagnosis. However, there is a trade-off between data timeliness and specificity/accuracy. For example, OTC sales have the benefit of timeliness, but are not very specific. A rise in sales of antidiarrheal remedies may be associated with an increase in the incidence of diarrheal illness or may be unrelated, such as store specials and sale items. It would be difficult to make a public health decision based solely on increased OTC sales because it does not contain any patient-specific data (Berger, Shiau, and Weintraub 2006). Therefore, the timeliness of a data source is only valuable if the signal is accurate and specific enough to inform public health decision making (Berger, Shiau, and Weintraub 2006).

Timely signals and alerts generated by surveillance activities may not always correspond to an actual increase in disease. A system based on ED chief complaints found that over the course of 277 days, 59 signals were investigated and found not to correspond to an outbreak of communicable disease (Terry, Ostrowsky, and Huang 2004). A system implemented for the 2002 Olympic Games tracked emergency department presentations using real-time surveillance (Gesteland et al. 2003). During the 2-month period of the Olympics, the system's detection algorithms alerted twice, and neither of these alarms corresponded to a real outbreak.

Timeliness provided by a biosurveillance system can only be useful if a process of aberration verification and investigation occurs and is supported by and integrated into the activities of the local health department on a sustained basis (Berger, Shiau, and Weintraub 2006).

1.6 Conclusions

Although in its infancy, the field of biosurveillance has been the subject of multiple studies and scientific debate. The main reason for investigating this surveillance method is the promise of earlier outbreak detection. Timeliness is one metric used to assess the potential of data sources for early outbreak detection.

The methods for determining timeliness include peak comparison, aberration detection comparison, and correlation. The peak comparison method is retrospective and can be used as a preliminary measure to determine the potential timeliness of one data source compared to another. However, comparing the peaks of two time series does not address the question of when an outbreak would be detected, and the peak is not always the feature of interest. The peak comparison method does not account for the size or the width of the peaks in each time series. An earlier peak in one data source does not necessarily translate to a timelier source of data when a detection algorithm is applied in a prospective setting. For example, an algorithm may alert first in one data source yet have a later peak in comparison to another.

The aberration detection method is used to answer the fundamental question of when an outbreak would be detected. However, a weakness of this method to be considered when comparing results based on timeliness is the bias associated with algorithm selection. Numerous algorithms can be applied to surveillance data, and for each algorithm, parameter selection affects the time at which the algorithm will alert. Hence, interpreting the timeliness of one data source in a particular study location can be affected by the appropriateness of the algorithm and the parameters of the model. Therefore, algorithm parameters should be set to detect a defined increase that will satisfy an algorithmic alert in the data and reflect the temporal features (day-of-week, seasonality) for a specific location. A sensitivity analysis should also be conducted to investigate algorithm parameters.

Several studies that used the aberration detection method compared the date of alert in one data source with the date of the peak in the gold standard or reference data source. This introduces bias as prediagnostic data sources would be expected to alert earlier than the peak in the gold standard. This could be further biased by setting a low threshold value, thus resulting in an earlier date of detection relative to the peak and hence increasing the timeliness of the data source (see Figure 1.5). In order to find a better estimate of timeliness between two data sources, the alerts generated by an algorithm on both sources should be compared if a well-established indicator does not exist.

An alert may also result from an increased daily count due to variability within the time series. These may exist in the form of known variability, such as seasonal effects, day-of-week effects, or unknown variability.

As discussed, the basis of outbreak detection by statistical methods is the process of interpreting and responding to alerts. These may be true alerts during an epidemic or false alerts generated by artifacts within the data.

Aberrations in the data are not necessarily caused by an outbreak (Hutwagner et al. 2003). Ultimately, once a statistical aberration is detected, it should be evaluated to determine its epidemiological or clinical significance (Hutwagner et al. 2003). The development of new algorithms for outbreak detection continues and, concurrently, the bias associated with algorithm selection. However, prospectively, alerts should not be dismissed purely on

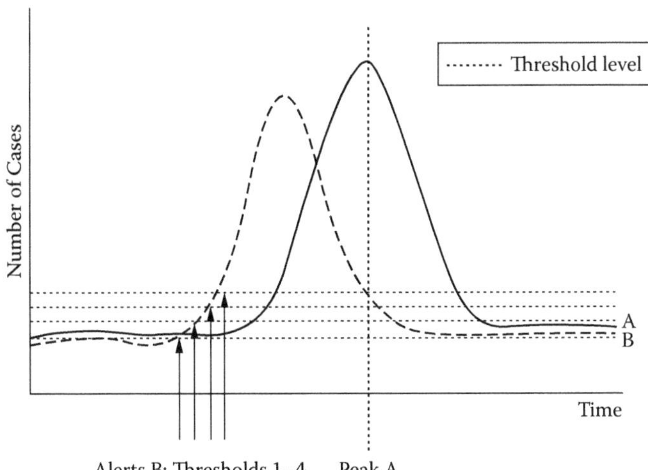

FIGURE 1.5
Peak comparisons to alert with varying thresholds.

the basis of timing alone, as these may identify an unusually early seasonal increases or the emergence of an unknown agent.

Algorithms will not replace the need for local knowledge and experience. The definition of an outbreak requires the description and interpretation of relationships between cases, and algorithms will only alert one to the possibility of such an event based on past experience. O'Brien and Christie (1997) explained that the investigator must decide whether changes might be real or artifactual, and that algorithms may therefore be regarded as an adjunct to other methods of interrogating surveillance data.

As with peak comparison, correlations produce a preliminary measure of potential. In some studies, authors used the cross-correlation function as part of an initial, exploratory analysis (Lazarus et al. 2002; Lewis et al. 2002; Sebastiani et al. 2006) while for others, the result of the correlation analyses was the main outcome (Davies and Finch 2003; Hogan et al. 2003; Najmi and Magruder 2004; Tsui et al. 2002).

Correlation is not biased by algorithm selection and provides a measure of the relationship between two data sources. However, a limitation of this method is that it is sensitive to large variations in the amplitude of the time series (Magruder 2003), such as long and short wavelengths (Bloom, Buckeridge, and Cheng 2007). Bloom and colleagues (2007) suggested that researchers should stipulate the feature scale length of interest and filter the data appropriately prior to the application of the CCF or the results may be ambiguous and misleading. CCFs are useful in showing that one data source is more timely than another; however, they cannot be used to define a change or level that might be indicative of a disease occurrence or outbreak as with aberration detection (Suyama et al. 2003).

1.7 Future Work

Our knowledge of the effectiveness of biosurveillance as a tool to detect disease outbreaks is currently limited (Sosin 2003). There is little consensus as to which data sources, algorithms for detection, and reporting technologies are the most timely (Bravata et al. 2004). Reports of timeliness vary by detection algorithms, locations, populations, and methods.

To date, no strong conclusion regarding the most timely sources have been reached, because of the lack of rigorous methodologies and limited standardization between studies. The simultaneous analyses of several data sources in a single location would improve the validity of comparisons. Evaluations that determine how the integration of several data sources affects timeliness and accuracy are also required (Bravata et al. 2004). However, when assessing the suitability of a data source for early warning, timeliness is only one component to be considered.

Research is required to determine the most appropriate statistical tools for detecting an aberration above the baseline and the clinical or public health significance of these statistical aberrations (Buehler et al. 2003; Mostashari and Hartman 2003; Reingold 2003). Biosurveillance data vary by location and type of outbreak, and hence the performance of aberration detection methods must be evaluated specifically (Zhu et al. 2005).

Given the nonspecific nature of some conditions and events that are the focus of biosurveillance, there are concerns regarding not only the rate of false alerts but also whether the data under surveillance are likely indicators of the disease of interest (Koo 2005). Future work should involve real-time surveillance and monitoring of potential data sources for surveillance. This would give insight into the public health response to alerts and the perceived usefulness in a prospective setting.

Research to identify the timeliness of biosurveillance data sources is essential for guiding surveillance efforts. For future timeliness studies, correlation and peak comparisons can be used to give preliminary results regarding potential; however, aberration detection methods are required for evaluating outbreak detection.

References

Berger, M., R. Shiau, and J.M. Weintraub. 2006. Review of syndromic surveillance: implications for waterborne disease detection. *J Epidemiol Community Health* 60 (6): 543–50.

Bloom, R.M., D.L. Buckeridge, and K.E. Cheng. 2007. Finding leading indicators for disease outbreaks: filtering, cross-correlation, and caveats. *J Am Med Inform Assoc* 14: 76–85.

Bravata, D.M., K.M. McDonald, W.M. Smith, C. Rydzak, H. Szeto, D.L. Buckeridge, C. Haberland, and D.K. Owens. 2004. Systematic review: surveillance systems for early detection of bioterrorism-related diseases. *Ann Intern Med* 140 (11): 910–22.

Buckeridge, D.L, H. Burkom, M. Campbell, W.R. Hogan, and A.W. Moore. 2005. Algorithms for rapid outbreak detection: a research synthesis. *J Biomed Inform* 38 (2): 99–113.

Buckeridge, D.L, J. Graham, M.J. O'Connor, M.K. Choy, S.W. Tu, and M.A. Musen. 2002. Knowledge-based bioterrorism surveillance. *Proc AMIA Symp* :76–80.

Buehler, J., R. Berkelman, D. Hartley, and C. Peters. 2003. Syndromic surveillance and bioterrorism-related epidemics. *Emerg Infect Dis* 9 (10): 1197–204.

Dailey, L., R.E. Watkins, and A.J. Plant. 2007. Timeliness of data sources used for influenza surveillance. *J Am Med Inform Assoc* 14: 626–631.

Davies, G.R., and R.G. Finch. 2003. Sales of over-the-counter remedies as an early warning system for winter bed crises. *Clin Microbiol Infect* 9 (8): 858–63.

Doroshenko, A., D. Cooper, G.E. Smith, E. Gerard, F. Chinemana, N.Q. Verlander, and A. Nicoll. 2005. Evaluation of syndromic surveillance based on national health service direct derived data—England and Wales. *MMWR* 54 (suppl): 117–22.

Espino, J.U., W.R. Hogan, and M.M. Wagner. 2003. Telephone triage: a timely data source for surveillance of influenza-like diseases. *AMIA Annual Symp Proc*: 215–19.

Gesteland, P.H., R.M. Gardner, and F.C. Tsui. 2003. Automated syndromic surveillance for the 2002 Winter Olympics. *J Am Med Inform Assoc* 10: 547–54.

Heffernan, R., F. Mostashari, D. Das, A. Karpati, M. Kulldorff, and D. Weiss. 2004. Syndromic surveillance in public health practice, New York City. *Emerg Infect Dis* 10 (5): 858–64.

Hogan, W.R., F.C. Tsui, O. Ivanov, P.H. Gesteland, S. Grannis, J.M. Overhage, J.M. Robinson, and M.M. Wagner. 2003. Detection of pediatric respiratory and diarrheal outbreaks from sales of over-the-counter electrolyte products. *J Am Med Inform Assoc*, 10 (6): 555–62.

Hopkins, R.S., F. Mostashari, D.M. Sosin, and J.W. Ward. 2003. Syndromic Surveillance: Reports from a national conference, 2003. *MMWR* 53 (suppl): 3.

Hutwagner, L., W. Thompson, G.M. Seeman, and T. Treadwell. 2003. The bioterrorism preparedness and response early aberration reporting system (EARS). *J Urban Health* 80 (2): i89–i96.

Irvin, C.B., P.P. Nouhan, and K. Rice. 2003. Syndromic analysis of computerized emergency department patients' chief complaints: an opportunity for bioterrorism and influenza surveillance. *Ann Emerg Med* 41 (4): 447–52.

Ivanov, O., P.H. Gesteland, W. Hogan, M.B. Mundorff, and M.M. Wagner. 2003. Detection of pediatric respiratory and gastrointestinal outbreaks from free-text chief complaints. *AMIA Annu Symp Proc*: 318–22.

Johnson, H.A., M.M. Wagner, W.R. Hogan, W. Chapman, R.T. Olszewski, J. Dowling, and G. Barnas. 2004. Analysis of web access logs for surveillance of influenza. *Medinfo*: 1202–6.

Koo, D. 2005. Leveraging syndromic surveillance. *J Public Health Manag Pract* 11 (3): 181–83.

Kulldorff, M. 1997. A spatial scan statistic. *Communications in Statistics—Theory and Methods*, 26: 1481–96.

Kulldorff, M., ed. 1999. *Spatial scan statistics: models, calculations, and applications.* Boston: Birkhauser.

Lawson, A., and K. Kleinman, eds. 2005. *Spatial and syndromic surveillance for public health*. 1st edn. West Sussex, England: John Wiley and Sons, Ltd.

Lazarus, R., K.P. Kleinman, I. Dashevsky, C. Adams, P. Kludt, A. DeMaria, and R. Platt. 2002. Use of automated ambulatory-care encounter records for detection of acute illness clusters, including potential bioterrorism events. *Emerg Infect Dis* 8 (8): 753–60.

Lazarus, R., K.P. Kleinman, I. Dashevsky, A. DeMaria, and R. Platt. 2001. Using automated medical records for rapid identification of illness syndromes (syndromic surveillance): the example of lower respiratory infection. *BMC Public Health* 1:9. http://www.biomedcentral.com/1471-2458/1/9 (accessed October 13, 2008).

Lemay, R., A. Mawudeku, Y. Shi, M. Ruben, and C. Achonu. 2008. Syndromic surveillance for influenzalike illness. *Biosecurity and Bioterrorism: Biodefense Strategy, Practice and Science* 6 (2): 161–70.

Lenaway, D.D. and A. Ambler. 1995. Evaluation of a school-based influenza surveillance system. *Public Health Rep* 110 (3): 333–37.

Lewis, M.D., J.A. Pavlin, J.L. Mansfield, et al. 2002. Disease outbreak detection system using syndromic data in the Greater Washington DC area. *Am J Prev Med* 23: 180–86.

Magruder, S. 2003. Evaluation of over-the-counter pharmaceutical sales as a possible early warning indicator of human disease. *Johns Hopkins APL Technical Digest* 24 (4): 349–53.

Mandl, K.D., J.M. Overhage, M.M. Wagner, W.B. Lober, P. Sebastiani, F. Mostashari, J.A. Pavlin, P.H. Gesteland, T. Treadwell, E. Koski, L. Hutwagner, D.L. Buckeridge, R.D. Aller, and S. Grannis. 2004. Implementing syndromic surveillance: a practical guide informed by the early experience. *J Am Med Inform Assoc* 11 (2): 141–50.

Miller, B., H. Kassenborg, W. Dunsmuir, J. Griffith, M. Hadidi, J.D. Nordin, and R. Danila. 2004. Syndromic surveillance for influenza-like-illness in ambulatory care network. *Emerg Infect Dis* 10 (10): 1806–11.

Moore, A., G. Cooper, F. Tsui, and M.M. Wagner. 2002. *Summary of biosurveillance-relevant statistical and data mining technologies*. http://www.autonlab.org/autonweb/showPaper.jsp?ID=moore-biosurv (accessed October 10, 2008).

Mostashari, F., and J. Hartman. 2003. Syndromic surveillance: a local perspective. *J Urban Health* 80 (2): i1–7.

Mostashari, F., A. Fine, D. Das, J. Adams, and M. Layton. 2003. Use of ambulance dispatch data as an early warning system for communitywide influenza-like illness, New York city. *J Urban Health* 80: i43–49.

Najmi, A.H., and S.F. Magruder. 2004. Estimation of hospital emergency room data using OTC pharmaceutical sales and least mean square filters. *BMC Med Inform Dec Mak* 4:5. http://www.pubmedcentral.nih.gov/articlerender.fcgi?artid=419503 (accessed October 13, 2008).

O'Brien, S.J., and P. Christie. 1997. Do CuSums have a role in routine communicable disease surveillance? *Public Health* 111 (4): 255–58.

Proctor, M.E., K.A. Blair, and J.P. Davis. 1998. Surveillance data for waterborne illness detection: an assessment following a massive waterborne outbreak of *Cryptosporidium* infection. *Epidemiol Infect* 120: 43–54.

Quenel, P., W. Dab, C. Hannoun, and J. Cohen. 1994. Sensitivity, specificity and predictive positive values of health service based indicators for the surveillance of influenza A epidemics. *Int J Epidemiol* 23: 849–55.

Reingold, A. 2003. If syndromic surveillance is the answer, what is the question? *Biosecur Bioterror* 1 (2): 77–81.

Ritzwoller, D., K. Kleinman, T. Palen, A. Abrams, J. Kaferly, W. Yih, and R. Platt. 2005. Comparison of syndromic surveillance and a sentinel provider system in detecting an influenza outbreak—Denver, Colorado, 2003. *MMWR* 54 (suppl): 151–56.

Rodman, J.S., F. Frost, and W. Jakubowski. 1998. Using nurse hot line calls for disease surveillance. *Emerg Infect Dis* 2: 329–32.

SAS. 2005. *Statistical Process Control.* http://support.sas.com/rnd/app/qc/qc/qcspc.html (accessed October 10, 2008).

Sebastiani, P., K.D. Mandl, P. Szolovits, I.S. Kohane, and M.F. Ramoni. 2006. A Bayesian dynamic model for influenza surveillance. *Stat Med* 25: 1803–16.

Sosin, D. 2003. Syndromic surveillance: the case for skilful investment. *Biosecur Bioterror* 1 (4): 247–53.

Stoto, M., R. Fricker, A. Jain, J.O. Davies-Cole, C. Glymph, G. Kidane, G. Lum, L.H. Jones, and C.M. Yuan. 2005. Evaluating statistical methods for syndromic surveillance, *ASA-SIAM.*

Suyama, J., M. Sztajnkrycer, C. Lindsell, E.J. Otten, J.M. Daniels, and A.B. Kressel. 2003. Surveillance of infectious disease occurrences in the community: an analysis of symptom presentation in the emergency department. *Acad Emerg Med* 10 (7): 753–63.

Terry, W., B. Ostrowsky, and A. Huang. 2004. Should we be worried? Investigation of signals generated by an electronic surveillance system—Westchester County, New York. Syndromic surveillance: reports from a national conference, 2003. *MMWR* 53 (suppl): 190–95.

Tsui, F.C., M.M. Wagner, V. Dato, and C.C. Ho Chang. 2002. Value of ICD-9-coded chief complaints for detection of epidemics. *J Am Med Inform Assoc* 9: S41–S47.

Wagner, M.M., A.W. Moore, and R. Aryel, eds. 2006. *Handbook of biosurveillance.* Burlington: Academic Press.

Welliver, R.C., J.D. Cherry, K.M. Boyer, J.E. Deseda-Tous, P.J. Krause, J.P. Dudley, R.A. Murray, W. Wingert, J.G. Champion, and G. Freeman. 1979. Sales of non-prescription cold remedies: a unique method of influenza surveillance. *Pediatr Res* 13 (9): 1015–17.

Wong, W.K., and A.W. Moore. 2006. Classical time-series methods for biosurveillance. In *Handbook of biosurveillance,* Ed. M.M. Wagner, A.W. Moore, and R. Aryel, 605. Burlington: Academic Press.

Yuan, C.M., S. Love, and M. Wilson. 2004. Syndromic surveillance at hospital emergency departments—southeastern Virginia. *MMWR* 53(suppl): 56–58.

Zhu, Y., W. Wang, D. Atrubin, and Y. Wu. 2005. Initial evaluation of the early aberration reporting system—Florida. *MMWR* 54 (suppl): 123–30.

2

Simulating and Evaluating Biosurveillance Datasets

Thomas H. Lotze
Applied Mathematics and Scientific Computation Program
University of Maryland
College Park, Maryland

Galit Shmueli
Department of Decision, Operations & Information Technologies and Center for Health and Information Decision Systems
University of Maryland
College Park, Maryland

Inbal Yahav
Robert H.Smith School of Business
University of Maryland
College Park, Maryland

CONTENTS

KEYWORDS Simulation, Time series, Multivariate, Goodness of fit, Disease outbreak

2.1 Motivation

The field of biosurveillance involves the monitoring measures of diagnostic and prediagnostic activity for the purpose of finding early indications of disease outbreaks. By providing early notification of potential outbreaks, the aim is to provide public health officials the opportunity to respond earlier and thus more effectively. Although the field has grown in importance and emphasis in the past several years, the research community involved in designing and evaluating monitoring algorithms has not grown as expected. A major barrier has been data accessibility: typically researchers do not have access to biosurveillance data unless they are part of a biosurveillance group. In fact, after parting from a biosurveillance group, researchers lose their data access. This means that a very limited community of academic researchers works in the field, with a nearly impenetrable barrier to entering it (especially for statisticians or other nonmedical academics). Furthermore, the confinement of each research group to a single source of data and the lack of data sharing across groups "leaves opportunity for scientific confounding" (Rolka, 2006).

While simulated data have their own difficulties, they seem to be a necessity for modern biosurveillance research. Buckeridge et al. (2005) explain:

> [They] are appealing for algorithm evaluation because they allow exact specification of the outbreak signal, perfect knowledge of the outbreak onset, and evaluators can create large amounts of test data ...

The International Society for Disease Surveillance (ISDS) has recognized the paucity of data (both authentic and realistic simulations) as an issue that hinders the field's progression, and is currently working to create a data repository for publicly available datasets. It recently sponsored a contest using simulated data, but required all participants to delete the data after the completion of the contest. There is a serious need for datasets, which simulation holds promise for alleviating.

The first implementation of wholly simulated biosurveillance data in the form of daily counts is the publicly available simulated background and outbreak datasets by Hutwagner et al. (2005). The background series are generated from a negative-binomial distribution with parameters set such that "means and standard deviations were based on observed values from national and local public health systems and biosurveillance surveillance systems. Adjustments were made for days of the week, holidays, postholiday periods, seasonality, and trend." Other research, such as Fricker et al. (2008), has simulated background data using an additive combination of terms representing level, seasonal and day-of-week effects, and random noise. Our approach, as described in Section 2.2, is similar in that we set or estimate levels and temporal patterns from authentic data. However, our approach is more general in that it captures two key dependence structures: autocorrelation and cross-correlation. In particular, we include 1-day autocorrelation, which has been shown to be a major property of biosurveillance daily time series (Burkom et al., 2007) and generate multivariate rather than univariate data: we generate a set of time series rather than a single time series at a time. Thus, there can be a dependence structure between these series (in the form of cross correlations).

More recently, Siddiqi et al. (2007) developed a simulation method based on linear dynamical systems, also known as *Kalman filters*. They model the observed series as a linear transformation from a series of latent variables, find a stable linear transformation for those latent variables, and use this transformation to re-create similar data and to extend it into the future. They modify standard Kalman filter methods, incrementally adding constraints to create a system whose linear transformation remains stable (with eigenvalues less than 1). This method seems very promising, and we recommend using the methods described here to evaluate its effectiveness at mimicking authentic data.

Finally, we note that to evaluate an algorithm's performance on biosurveillance data, one must be able to simulate outbreak signals within the data. It is common practice to evaluate algorithms by seeding real biosurveillance data with simulated outbreak signals (e.g., Burkom et al., 2007; Goldenberg et al., 2002; Reis and Mandl, 2003; Stoto et al., 2006, and many others). However, simulating these outbreak signals accurately is even more difficult than simulating the background biosurveillance data, as known examples of outbreak signatures in health care seeking behavior are even more difficult to obtain. We emphasize that generating a realistic multivariate outbreak signal must be based on epidemiological and other relevant domain knowledge.

2.2 Data Simulation

2.2.1 Overview

As noted in Buckeridge et al. (2005), the main challenge is "complexity of simulating background and outbreak signal," and in particular,

> To allow for meaningful evaluation of diverse algorithms, both normal and outbreak data must be simulated in a manner that ensures sufficient complexity and validity in terms of factors such as spatial patterns, temporal patterns, and joint distributions of variables. As a simulation model grows to meet these requirements, the number of parameters increases, the ability to verify the model becomes difficult, and ultimately it becomes more difficult to ensure the validity of the simulated data.

Our approach is thus to identify those features that seem central in authentic data, estimate the appropriate parameters from authentic data, and use them to stochastically generate new data. In particular, we use the statistical structure of authentic multivariate time series derived from biosurveillance data in order to simulate background data that have the same structure. We can even mimic a particular dataset, thereby generating one or more stochastic duplications of it.

Our method for simulating multivariate time-series data includes several prominent patterns that have been shown by various empirical studies to exist in biosurveillance time series. Day-of-week (DOW) is a common pattern. In emergency department visits in the United States, daily counts are typically lower on weekends and high during the week (Burkom et al., 2007), but can also exhibit other daily patterns (e.g., Brillman et al., 2005; Reis and Mandl 2003), or none (Fricker 2006). Grocery stores tend to have more traffic on weekends, and therefore medication sales appear higher on weekends (e.g., Goldenberg et al., 2002). Another common pattern is abnormal behavior on holidays and postholidays (e.g., Fienberg and Shmueli, 2005; Zhang et al., 2003) due to holiday closings (e.g., schools) or limited operation mode (e.g., pharmacies, hospitals). Another pattern exhibited by some series is seasonal cyclical behavior such as annual or biannual (summer/winter) fluctuations. The daily frequency of collection also leads to nonnegligible short-term autocorrelation (see, e.g., Burkom et al., 2007; Lotze et al., 2008). Finally, there are also dependencies between series that manifest as cross correlations.

Our simulator begins by generating "simple" multivariate time series that include autocorrelation and cross correlation, and then add to them DOW, seasonal, and holiday effects.

2.2.2 Creating Initial Multivariate Data

We generate a set of initial multivariate data from a multivariate normal distribution in the following way: a vector of means, a vector of variances, and a correlation matrix (or equivalently, a vector of means and a covariance matrix) are provided by the researcher. In addition, a few optional parameters can be specified: (1) a vector of autocorrelations to induce autocorrelations into each series; (2) a random seed for ensuring repeatability of generation; and (3) the length of the series to be generated.

A covariance matrix is created from the variance vector and the correlation matrix. If there is no autocorrelation, the covariance matrix is used to generate a series of independent multivariate normal random data. In the presence of non-zero autocorrelation, the covariance matrix is used to generate the first day of data, and each subsequent day of data are then generated from the conditional multivariate normal distribution given counts on the previous day. This maintains the same covariance overall but also includes autocorrelation. Specifically, we represent the vector of values on k series at day t as $\tilde{X}_t = \begin{pmatrix} X_{1,t} \\ \vdots \\ X_{k,t} \end{pmatrix}$, with mean $\tilde{\mu} = \begin{pmatrix} \mu_1 \\ \vdots \\ \mu_k \end{pmatrix}$ and covariance matrix Σ. The bivariate distribution of $\tilde{X}_{t+1}$ and $\tilde{X}_t$ is

$$\begin{pmatrix} \tilde{X}_t \\ \tilde{X}_{t+1} \end{pmatrix} = \begin{pmatrix} X_{1,t} \\ \vdots \\ X_{k,t} \\ X_{1,t+1} \\ \vdots \\ X_{k,t+1} \end{pmatrix} : N\left(\begin{pmatrix} \tilde{\mu} \\ \tilde{\mu} \end{pmatrix}, \begin{pmatrix} \Sigma & C \\ C & \Sigma \end{pmatrix} \right), \tag{2.1}$$

where C is a diagonal matrix with elements ci (i = 1, … ,k) on the diagonal, where $ci = Cov(Xi,t, Xi,t_+1)$ is the lag-1 autocovariance of series i. Then, given the values on day t, the conditional distribution of the next day (with the given covariance Σ and autocovariance C) is

$$\tilde{X}_{t+1} \mid \tilde{X}_t : N(\tilde{\mu}^*, \Sigma^*), \tag{2.2}$$

where $\tilde{\mu}^* = \tilde{\mu} + C\Sigma^{-1}(\tilde{X}_t - \tilde{\mu})$ and $\Sigma^* = \Sigma - C\Sigma^{-1}CT$.

Data generated from this conditional distribution provide a multivariate dataset with the given means, covariance, and autocorrelation structure.

The next step is to add effects such as DOW and seasonality to the initial data. To do that, we first "label" the initial data by creating indicators for DOW, day, month, and year. Now each day of data has a calendar date attached to it.

2.2.3 Adding Effects of Holidays, Seasonality, and DOW

The inclusion of the three types of patterns to the initial data is done sequentially. We describe a certain order, but if all components are entered either multiplicatively or additively (rather than a mix), then the order of pattern inclusion does not matter.

2.2.3.1 Holidays

Holiday effects are added either in multiplicative form (the new point is a fraction of the original) or in additive form (the new point is the original, with some amount subtracted). Holidays can be specified at any point in the series; the default is to use multiplicative holiday effects on all federal holidays (derived from the office of personnel management site, www.opm.gov/fedhol: New Year's Day, birthday of Martin Luther King, Jr., Washington's Birthday, Memorial Day, Independence Day, Labor Day, Columbus Day, Veterans Day, Thanksgiving Day, and Christmas Day).

2.2.3.2 Seasonality

Seasonality is added in either additive or multiplicative form. It can be a scalar (in which case, it modifies a shifted sine wave function with a period of 365.25 days, $f = sin(2\pi * x/(365.25) + 2)$) or a fully specified vector. The default is to add no seasonality; a multiplicative one-half-scale sine wave appears to be a good approximation for respiratory seasonality.

2.2.3.3 Day-of-Week (DOW)

The DOW pattern can be multiplicative or additive, and must be fully specified as a vector containing an index for each day. By default, it is set to multiplicative, with weekends set to one-third of weekday values.

In each of these steps, the dataset is normalized to maintain the same means (by dividing by or adding the appropriate amount to the series overall). However, the covariance does increase as the effects are applied uniformly to each series.

Finally, after all patterns of interest are added, the series are rounded to integers and bounded to be nonnegative in order to yield valid count data.

2.3 Mimicking Existing Dataset Qualities

In addition to generating a general type of multivariate time series with specific temporal and dependence patterns, our data simulator can also be used to mimic a multivariate authentic dataset, thereby producing a new semiauthentic dataset. The authentic dataset and its semiauthentic mimic have the same statistical structure, yet they differ in their actual daily counts. This combination means that the resulting semiauthentic datasets are useful for purposes of research (e.g., algorithm development and evaluation), yet avoid data disclosure concerns such as privacy and confidentiality.

Another important use of simulated datasets that are "copies" of the same authentic dataset is for purposes of randomization and Monte Carlo testing. The ability to test an algorithm on multiple versions of the same data structure helps avoid overfitting and gives more accurate estimates of model performance.

In the following, we describe how the different statistical components of the authentic data are estimated. These are then used to create the mimicked dataset.

Estimating DOW patterns. Given a dataset, the method of ratio to moving averages (RMA) is used to estimate DOW indices. A vector of seven indices is created separately for each series, in order to capture the weekly pattern for that series.

Estimating seasonality. The data are smoothed using a 7-day moving average. A smoothing spline is fit to the smoothed data, and this spline is then evaluated at each daily point. These daily points are then used as the seasonality components. For more details on the smoothing spline, see Chambers and Hastie (1992).

Estimating holiday effects. Holiday dates are copied from the original dataset, if any are present. This vector is used to identify that days should have holiday effects in the mimicked dataset.

Estimating series means. The mean for each simulated series is determined from the mean of the corresponding original series, excluding holidays (if any).

Estimating series variances and autocorrelations. To determine the variance and autocorrelation of the authentic series devoid of seasonal patterns, we use a Holt–Winters exponential smoother on each series separately and obtain a series of residuals (actual daily counts minus predicted daily counts). This residual series should not contain trends, DOW, or seasonal effects. We then compute the autocorrelation, variance, and correlation matrix of the residual series, which is later used as input for the simulator.

Some or all of the previous estimated parameters are then fed into the data simulator, thereby yielding a simulated mimicked version of the authentic multivariate data. The original dataset and its mimic contain the same statistical characteristics but are different stochastic realizations (i.e., the counts are not identical).

2.4 Evaluating Simulation Effectiveness

A crucial component of using simulation to mimic authentic data is verifying that the simulated data retain the key characteristics of the original data. This is done by testing whether the simulated data come from the same distribution as the original authentic data. If they come from the same distribution, then the simulation method should be trustworthy and provide valid results; if not, then the differences between the original and simulated data can provide distorted and unrealistic results.

Of course, given a finite amount of original data, there exist an infinite number of distributions that could generate that data. The distribution tests used here merely attempt to confirm that the simulation method is within that space of possible models, specifically those that have a reasonable chance of generating the data. We must use domain knowledge (such as our awareness of which characteristics are relevant) to further constrain the possible simulation models. Goodness-of-fit tests of the simulated data should be considered as relative measures of consistency; it is known that distributional tests become extremely sensitive with large amounts of data, and so may reject even the most useful simulations.

In addition, it should be considered that a mimic method will only be useful if it accurately captures the randomness of the underlying distribution. If a mimic is simply a duplicate of the original data, it is clearly not a good additional test, nor does it avoid any privacy concerns. Similarly, a mimic that merely adds random noise to the original is not providing a new authentic set of possible data; it is simply providing the original data with extra variation.

2.4.1 Univariate χ^2 Tests

The first method for evaluating the closeness between distribution of authentic and mimic data is a series of simple χ^2 tests. To test a mimic against its original dataset, we take each univariate data series and split it by day of week. The values for a single day of week are then formed into bins; an example of the binning process is given in Figure 2.1. The width of the bin varies by density, determined such that there are at least 10 observations in each bin. The original data are split and binned in the same fashion, and these two sets of counts (mimicked and original) are tested for distributional equality using a χ^2 test (with degrees of freedom equal to $k - 1$, where k = the number of bins). An FDR (Benjamini and Hochberg 1995) significance correction is used to account for multiple testing across multiple series. The χ^2 tests can also be repeated for each DOW separately with FDR correction, not only to inform us whether there are issues with our simulation but also to point us toward the reasons for those issues.

2.4.2 Multivariate Tests

The preceding χ^2 tests can only uncover univariate disparities between the original and mimicked data. To also consider the covariance between the series, we consider multivariate goodness-of-fit tests. While it is not obvious that such a test can be performed in a distribution-free manner, several methods have been developed to do so (notably, Bickel 1969; Friedman and Raisky 1979; Schilling 1986; Kim and Foutz 1987; Henze 1988; Hall and Tajvidi 2002).

In this chapter, we use the nearest-neighbors test described in Schilling (1986), because of its asymptotic normality and computational tractability. Under this test, the nearest k neighbors are computed for the combined sample. Each of the nearest neighbors is then used to determine an indicator variable, whether or not it shares the same class as the neighboring point. The statistic T, the proportion of k-nearest neighbors sharing the same class, is used to test equality of distributions. If both samples have the same size and come from the same distribution, T will approach 0.5 as the sample size increases. If the two samples differ in distribution, then T will tend to be larger than 0.5. With an appropriate correction, T has an approximate standard normal distribution. For an example, see Figure 2.2.

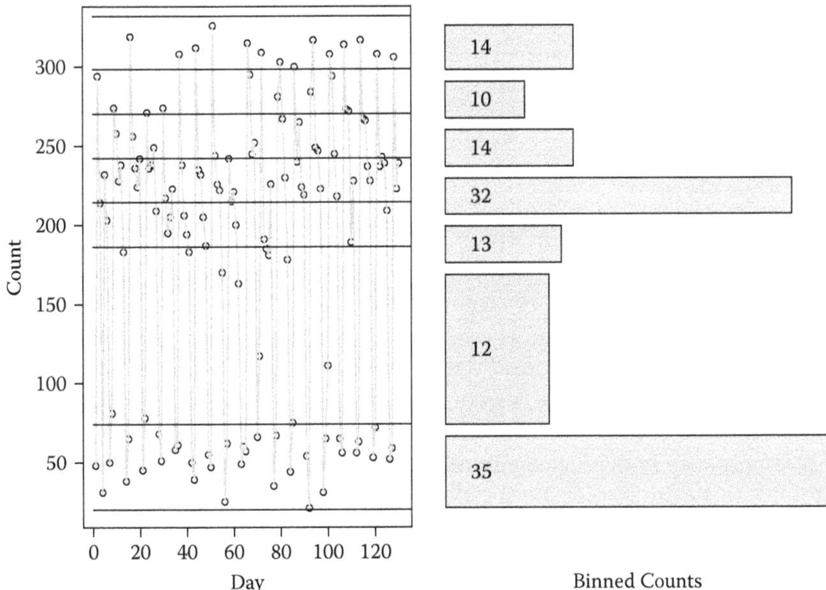

FIGURE 2.1
A portion of a single time series being binned.

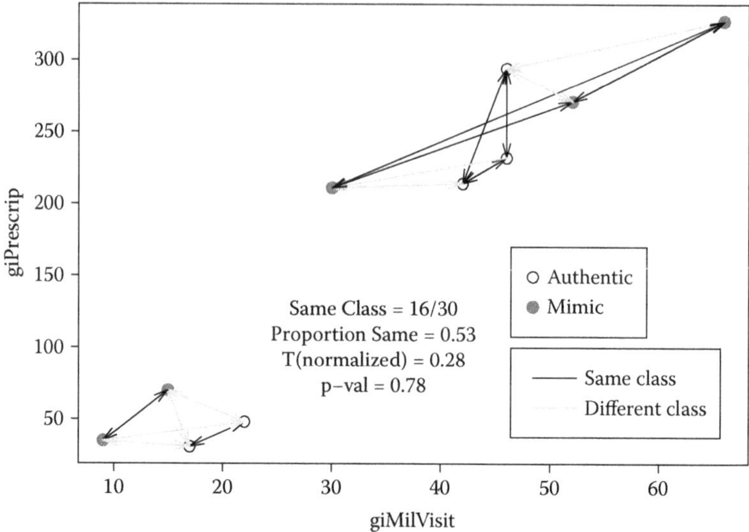

FIGURE 2.2
A simple example of the knn test for multivariate distribution equality, using only two series and 5 points from authentic and mimic. Each point is labeled as whether it is authentic or mimic; the three nearest neighbors are computed, and an arrow is drawn connecting each point to its three neighbors. The line is black if they are both the same type of point; gray if different. The number of neighbor links that are the same is summed, then normalized, and finally tested. Here, there is not enough evidence to reject the null hypothesis, so we conclude that the authentic and mimic distributions may be the same.

2.5 Outbreak Signature Simulation

2.5.1 Overview

We also consider the simulation of outbreak signatures to be added to the background data. In order to compare the performance of biosurveillance algorithms in terms of true and false alert rates and timeliness, we simulate not only background data but also outbreaks signatures that can be injected into the background data. Because in biosurveillance, the nature of the outbreak signatures is generally unspecified, algorithms are tested across different types and sizes of outbreak signatures.

Most researchers evaluating algorithm performance have added simulated outbreak signatures to authentic data. Many studies add a fixed number of additional cases, a linearly growing number of cases, or an exponentially growing number of cases to the authentic data (Goldenberg et al., 2002; Reis et al., 2003; Reis and Mandl 2003; Mandl et al., 2004; Stoto et al., 2006) in order to provide a variety of different possible outbreak signal shapes. Single-day "spike" signals and multiday lognormal curves are also popular (Burkom 2003b; Burkom et al., 2007), as they have some epidemiological basis. Spike outbreak signals occur when the disease onset and spread is faster than the rate of reporting for the health sources, or when the disease effect is rapid and tightly peaked. Lognormal outbreak signals are more common: many diseases are seen to have a lognormal distribution after time of infection to when symptoms develop and are reported (incubation time).

Buckeridge et al. (2004) has proposed a realistic model that includes modeling of anthrax patterns using a plume model for dispersion as well as modeling incubation period and behavior of the infected population. Wallstrom et al. (2005) present a software tool (HiFide) for modeling cryptosporidium outbreak signals and influenza in univariate health series. Both of these models are based on real outbreaks. STEM (Ford et al., 2006) is a software plug-in that can be used to quickly generate outbreak signals with a variety of infection parameters, over real geographic transportation networks. Other methods, which simulate individual cases (Wong et al., 2002) or spatiotemporal data (Cassa et al., 2005; Watkins et al., 2007), can be adapted to generate daily counts.

However, we again caution that such outbreak signal simulations can currently only be judged via domain knowledge; there is not enough data to compare their accuracy using statistical tests. For this reason, our outbreak simulator extends outbreak simulation to the multivariate case. Because an outbreak will likely manifest in multiple related series, we must be able to simulate an outbreak signal which occurs in each. The simulator can generate both spike and lognormal shapes, in a variety of sizes (increased number of affected cases, possibly different for different series) and shapes; it allows flexibility to tailor the outbreak generation as appropriate for the comparison.

In addition, we provide a novel labeling system that takes the multivariate nature of the data into account. There is still debate as to what time period of an outbreak it is valuable to detect. For example, if a detected alert occurs after the peak of the disease effect, it is not very useful to the public health practitioners. In general, for univariate series, the debate is between counting any alert during an outbreak versus counting only alerts that occur before the peak of the disease outbreak signal. For the multivariate case, this is even more complicated, as the peaks may occur at different times in different series. For this reason, instead of only two labels (normal/outbreak), we use four labels as follows:

0—no outbreak signal on that day

a—outbreak before any series have peaked

b—outbreak between the first and the last series' peak

c—outbreak after all series have peaked

Note that labels are applied to days, not to single series. An example is shown in Figure 2.3, where a single lognormal outbreak signal was placed on day 10 and injected into both series. Until day 9, the label is 0. On day 10, an

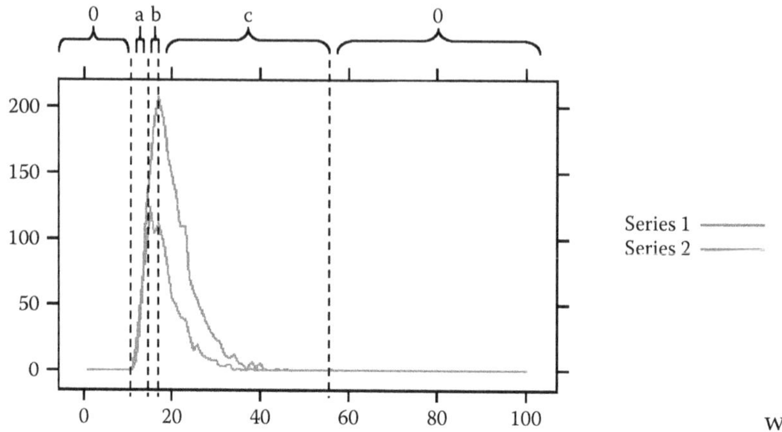

FIGURE 2.3
Data labeling.

outbreak signal starts, and hence the label is *a*. The outbreak signal reaches its peak in series 2 on day 12 and in series 1 on day 14. The outbreak label for days 12–14 is therefore *b*. Finally, on day 15, the number of cases decreases, and the corresponding outbreak label is *c*.

Finally, we also allow for an outbreak to be generated and then modified according to the same effects (DOW, holiday, seasonal, etc.) as the simulated background data. Such a modification is possible with simulated background health data, as the parameters are unknown in actual data. Although it is unknown whether outbreak signals are subject to the same effects as the background health data, a reasonable assumption is that the same reasons that keep people from showing up in no-outbreak scenarios (weekend, weather, etc.) will affect them equally when they are sick due to a "normal" cause or a "disease outbreak" cause.

2.5.2 Outbreak Signature Types

The outbreak signature simulation enables the user to generate two types of signatures: a single-day (multivariate) spike and a multiple-day (multivariate) log-normal progression. As in the data simulator, we start with an "initial" outbreak signature, and then add to it patterns such as seasonality, DOW, and holidays.

To create the initial outbreak signature, one must set for each series *noutbreak*, the increase in the total number of cases throughout the outbreak manifestation period (which can be thought of as the total number of cases added due to the outbreak). Users can either manually define a vector of additional cases for each series, or they can specify the increase in the series mean in terms of a multiple of the standard deviation.

Algorithm 1 Create log-normal outbreak
Input: {μ, σ, *numCases*}
samples = Generate *numCases* samples from a log-normal distribution with mean = μ and sd = σ
outbreak = histogram(sample)
trim t% last cases from outbreak

2.5.2.1 Single-Day Spike

Generating a single-day spike outbreak requires either specifying *noutbreak* directly for each series, or it can be set as a multiple of the standard deviation of the initial series:

$$n_{outbreak} = const \times std$$

We anticipate that some users will be more comfortable with specifying the total count increase directly, while others will prefer to determine the increase in terms of standard deviations (as is customary in statistical process control). In general, we consider small-to-medium spike sizes, because biosurveillance systems are designed to detect early and more subtle indications of a disease outbreak.

2.5.2.2 Lognormal Outbreak Signature

A lognormal progression is a reasonable epicurve model, because as Burkom (2003a) describes, the incubation period distribution of many infectious diseases tends to be lognormal, with distribution parameters dependent on the disease agent and route of infection. Generating a lognormal signature such as the spike requires specifying the size of the outbreak $n_{outbreak}$. The main difference is that this quantity now spans over more than a single day such that $n_{outbreak}$ is in fact the area under the lognormal curve. Similar to the spike, $n_{outbreak}$ can either be set directly or as a multiple of the standard deviation of the series (excluding DOW, seasonal, and holiday effects).

In addition to the signature size, the user must specify its shape, determined by the lognormal distribution parameters μ and σ. The peak of the outbreak signature (which corresponds to the mode of a lognormal distribution) is approximately on day $\exp \mu - \sigma^2$. We then trim the latest t% of the cases to avoid long tails. This process is summarized by algorithm 1, and an example of a simulated lognormal outbreak is given in Figure 2.4.

2.5.2.3 Adding Effects to Initial Outbreak Signatures

To this "initial" outbreak, effects such as DOW, seasonal patterns, and holidays can be added in the same way that they are added to the initial simulated data (see Section 2.3).

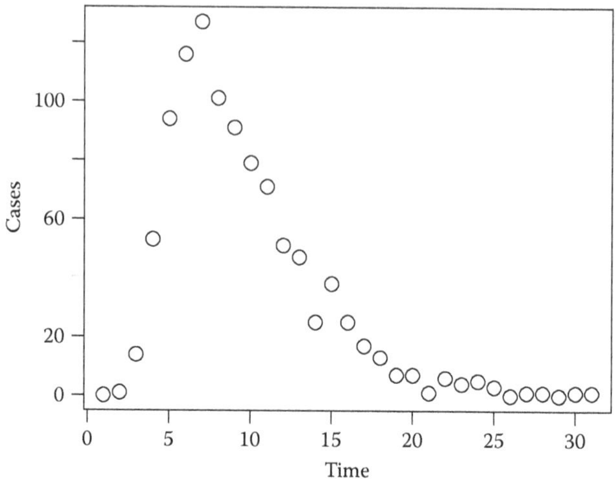

FIGURE 2.4
Log-normal outbreak with 1000 cases. Outbreak shape: $\mu - 2\ \sigma - 0.5$.

2.6 Example: Mimicking a BioALIRT Dataset

2.6.1 Mimicking Background Health Data

To illustrate the product of the data simulator, we mimic a set of authentic multivariate daily counts taken from the BioALIRT program conducted by the U.S. Defense Advanced Research Projects Agency (DARPA) (Siegrist and Pavlin 2004). We use a dataset of six series from a single city, where three of the series are indicators of respiratory symptoms and the other three of gastrointestinal symptoms. The series come from three different data sources: military clinic visit diagnoses, filled military prescriptions, and civilian physician office visits, all within a particular U.S. city. Figure 2.5 displays the six series of daily counts over a period of nearly 2 years.

To mimic this six series dataset, we estimate the different explainable patterns using the mimicker, and then generate a mimicked copy of the original dataset. Figure 2.6 displays the six mimicked series. This dataset is clearly very similar to the authentic dataset in its overall appearance in terms of count levels and patterns. To better see the similarity in structure with respect to the cyclic behavior (seasonality in Resp and DOW in both Resp and GI),

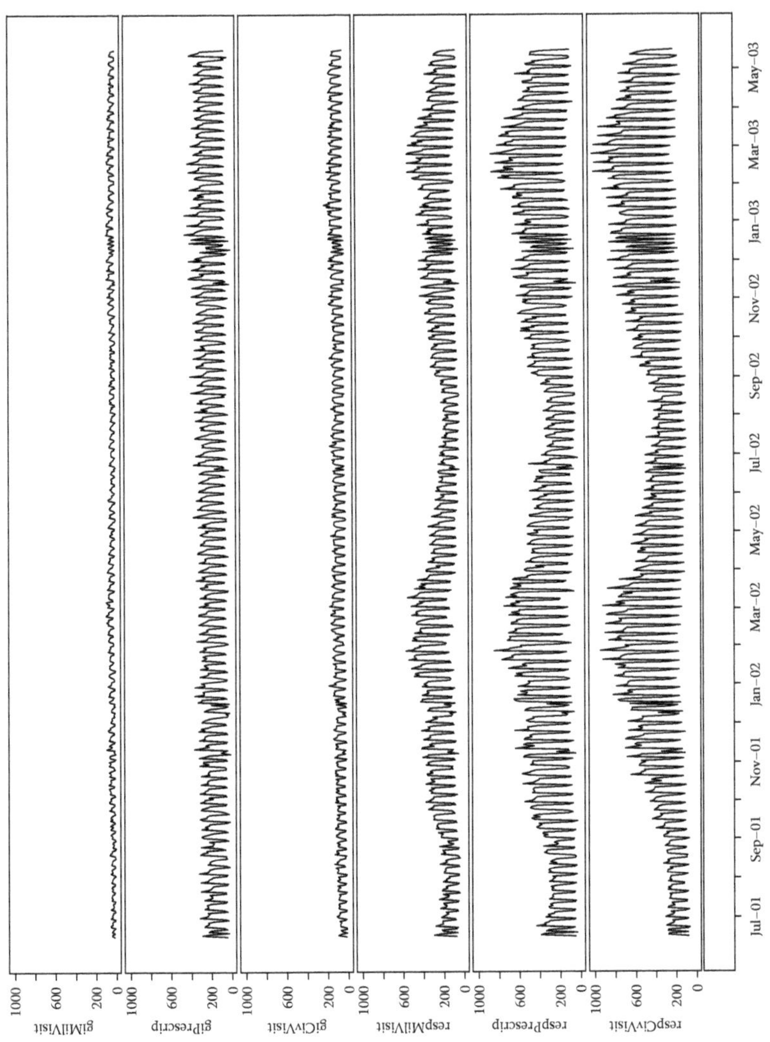

FIGURE 2.5
Authentic data: Daily counts of respiratory- and gastrointestinal-related doctors' visits (military and prescription) and filled prescriptions for a particular given U S city.

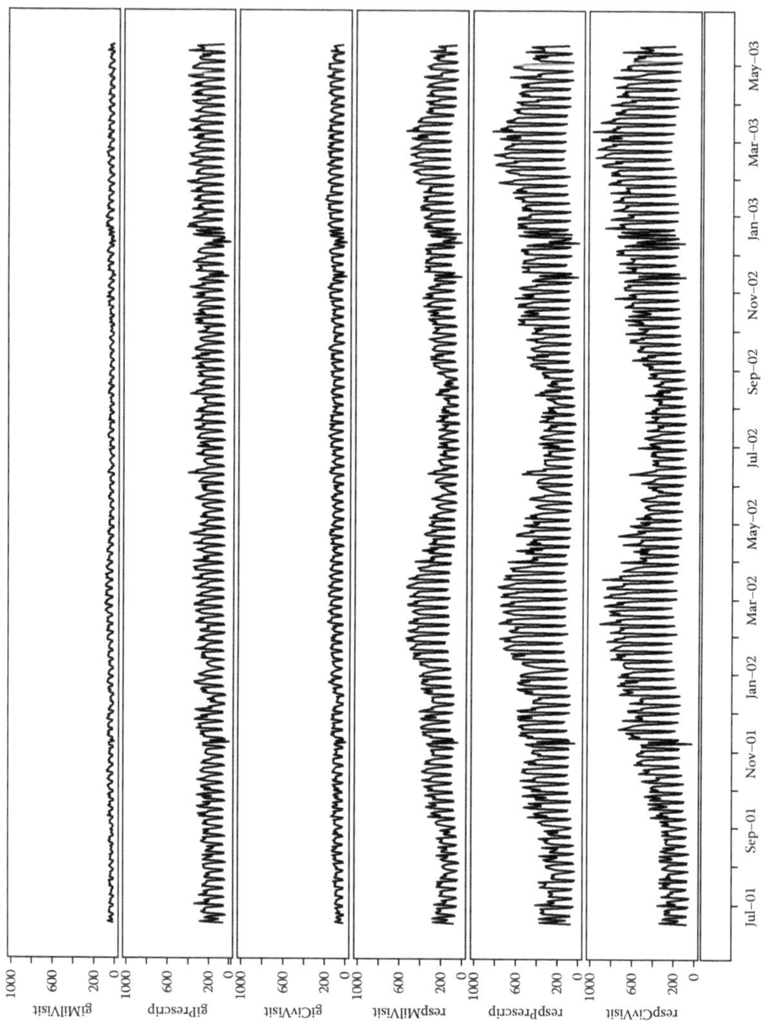

FIGURE 2.6
Mimicked daily counts of the authentic data in Figure 2.5.

Figures 2.7, 2.8, and 2.9 show the pairs of authentic (black) and mimicked (gray) series on different temporal scales: daily, weekly, and monthly.

Although the authentic dataset and mimicked dataset appear very similar, they are far from identical. By generating the mimicked dataset stochastically, we obtain a different realization from the same process. To see how the daily counts differ between the authentic and mimicked data, see Figure 2.10, which displays the differences between the daily counts of each authentic series and its mimicked counterpart. We see that the differences are in the order of magnitude of tens of counts. There are also several days with extreme deviations between the authentic and mimicked series. These are mostly on days that are either non-federal holidays (e.g., Christmas Eve and New Year's Eve) or federal holidays on which "business is as usual" in many areas (e.g., Columbus Day). This emphasizes the importance of specifying all *relevant* holidays in the particular area where the data are collected or simulated.

2.6.2 Distribution Testing

We now consider the tests of distributional equivalence. The multivariate nearest-neighbor test gives a raw statistic of 0.536, which after standardization provides a *Z*-score of 3.62, with a p-value of 0.000293. These p-values should be viewed cautiously, because due to the sample size of $n = 1400$, it will be very sensitive to any differences in distribution. Comparing it to another earlier simulation method using different DOW variances shows improvement, compared to the alternative method's standardized Z-score of 33.3. Still, the value is quite low, leading us to consider the univariate $\chi 2$ tests.

When the individual DOW scores are considered for each series, we find significant deviations in four categories: giMilVisit on Sun (p-val = 0.000915); giMilVisit on Sat (p-val = 0.000225); giPrescrip on Sun (p-val = 0.000045); and giCivVisit on Sun (p-val = 0.000060).

Examining individual bin comparisons, we see that the mimics have less variance on weekends than the original, suggesting that a negative binomial with increased variance might improve the simulation method. Figure 2.11 shows differences in Sundays for GI Civilian visits.

Outbreaks can then be inserted into this simulated dataset, to provide labeled semiauthentic health data. Such data are necessary in order to apply many detection or classification algorithms.

2.6.3 Outbreak Insertion

In the next step, we simulate an outbreak signature and then insert it into the mimicked data. For illustration, we simulated a lognormal outbreak signature with parameters $\mu = 0, \sigma = 1$, and *noutbreak* $\sim N(2\sigma, 2)$. Figure 2.12 displays

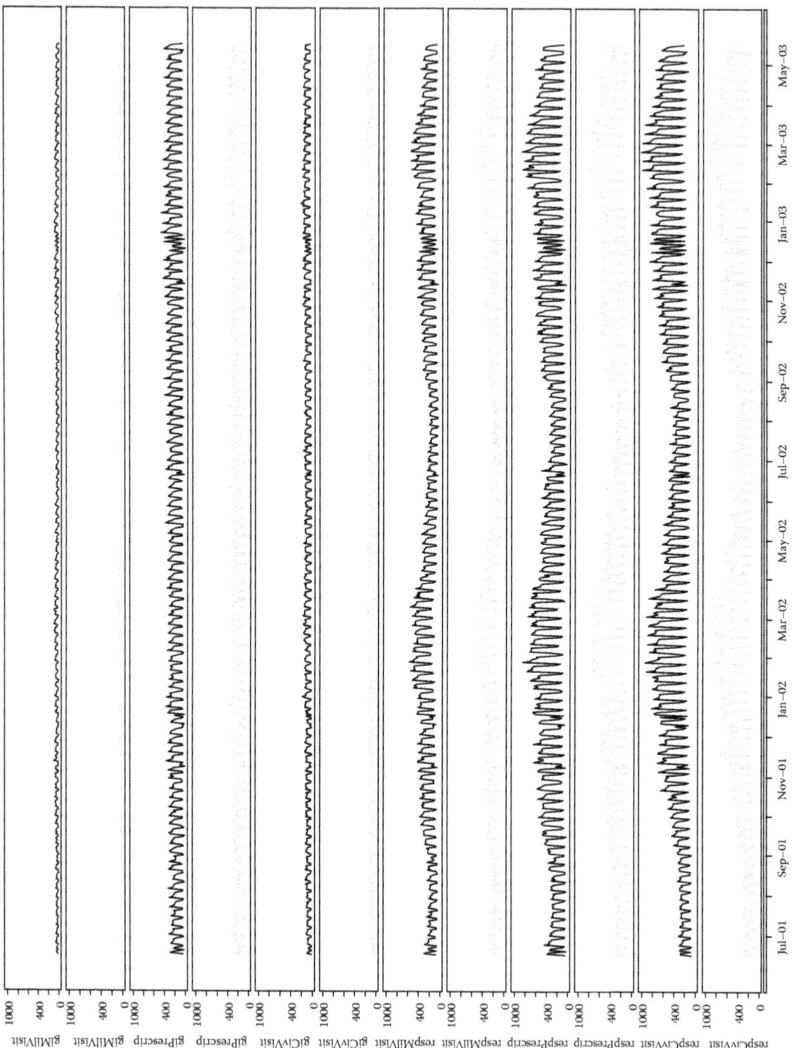

FIGURE 2.7
Authentic (black) and mimicked (gray) series, displayed at daily frequency. Series are in the same order as in Figures 2.5 and 2.6.

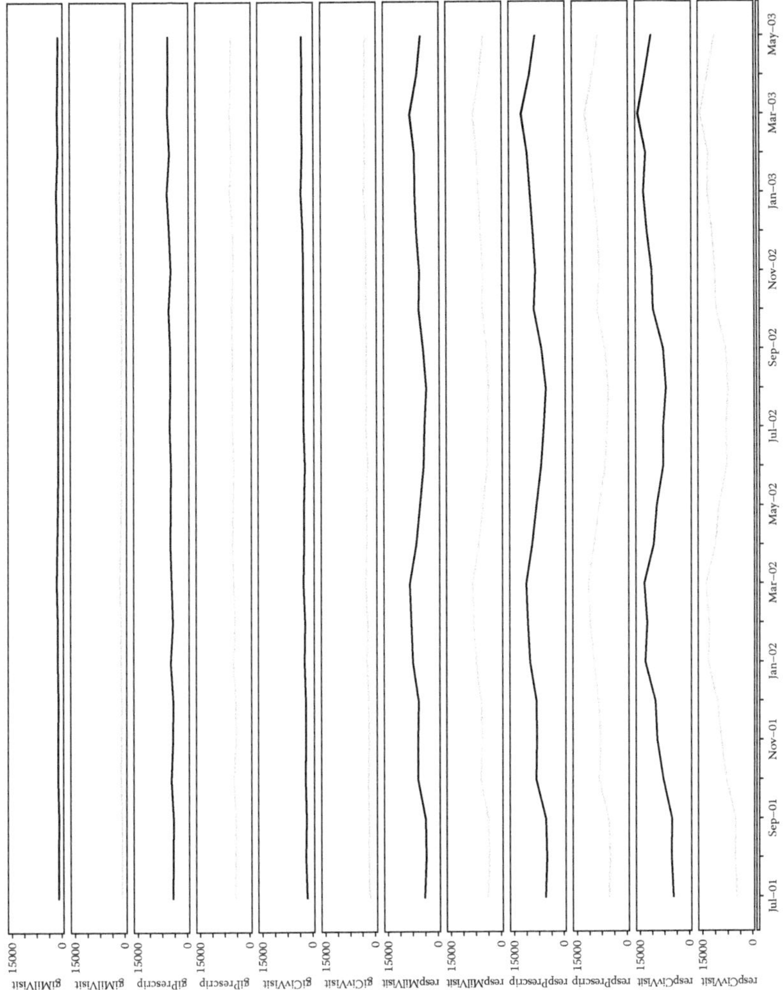

FIGURE 2.8
Authentic (black) and mimicked (grey) series, displayed at weekly frequency. Series are in the same order as in Figures 5 and 6.

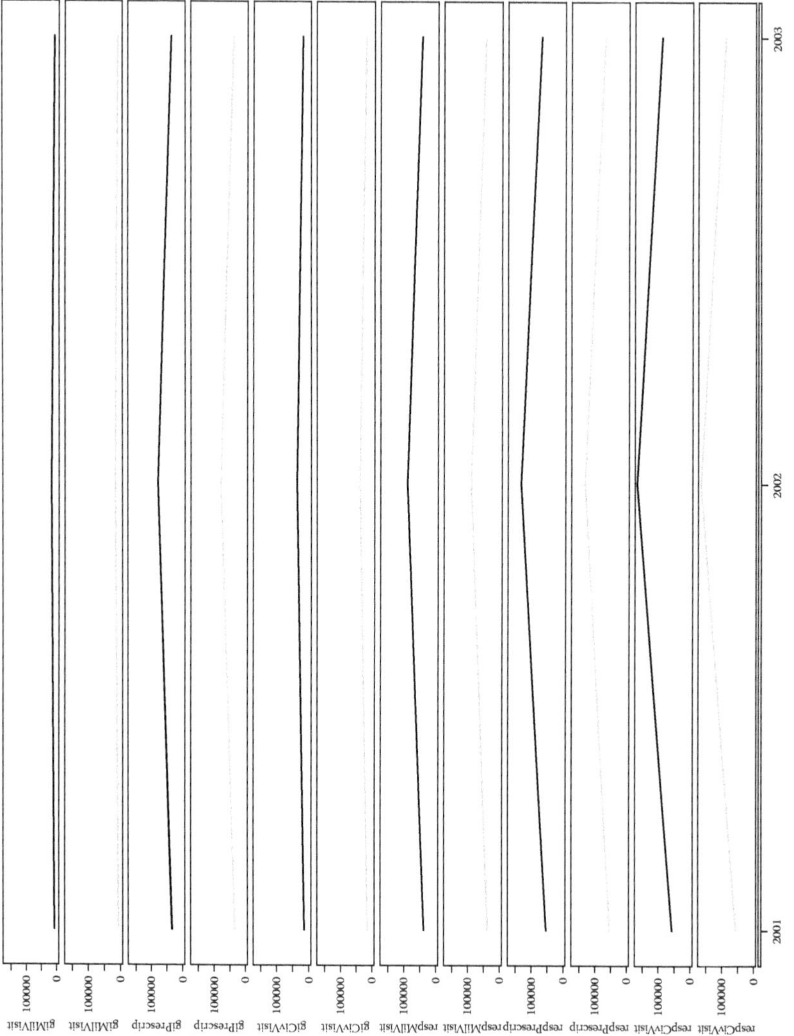

FIGURE 2.9
Authentic (black) and mimicked (grey) series, displayed at monthly frequency. Series are in the same order as in Figures 5 and 6.

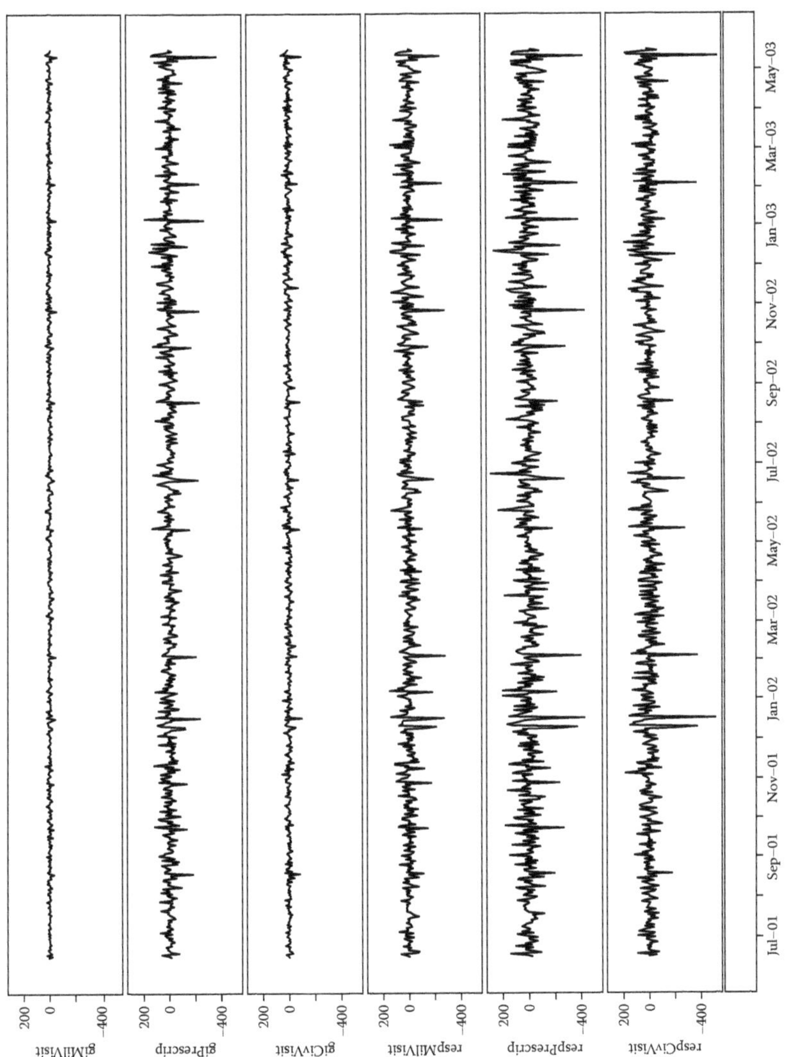

FIGURE 2.10
Daily count deviations between each of the six authentic series and their mimics.

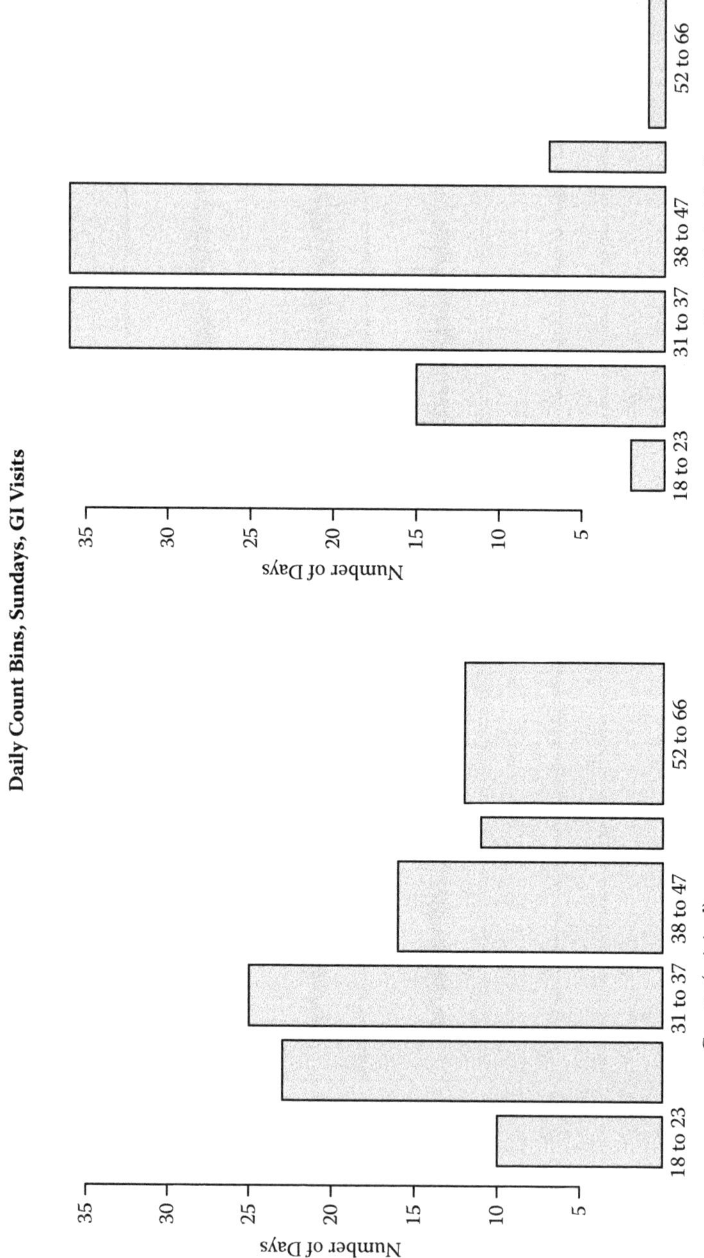

FIGURE 2.11
An indication of a difference between authentic and mimicked data: the mimicked series tend to have lower variance than the authentic data.

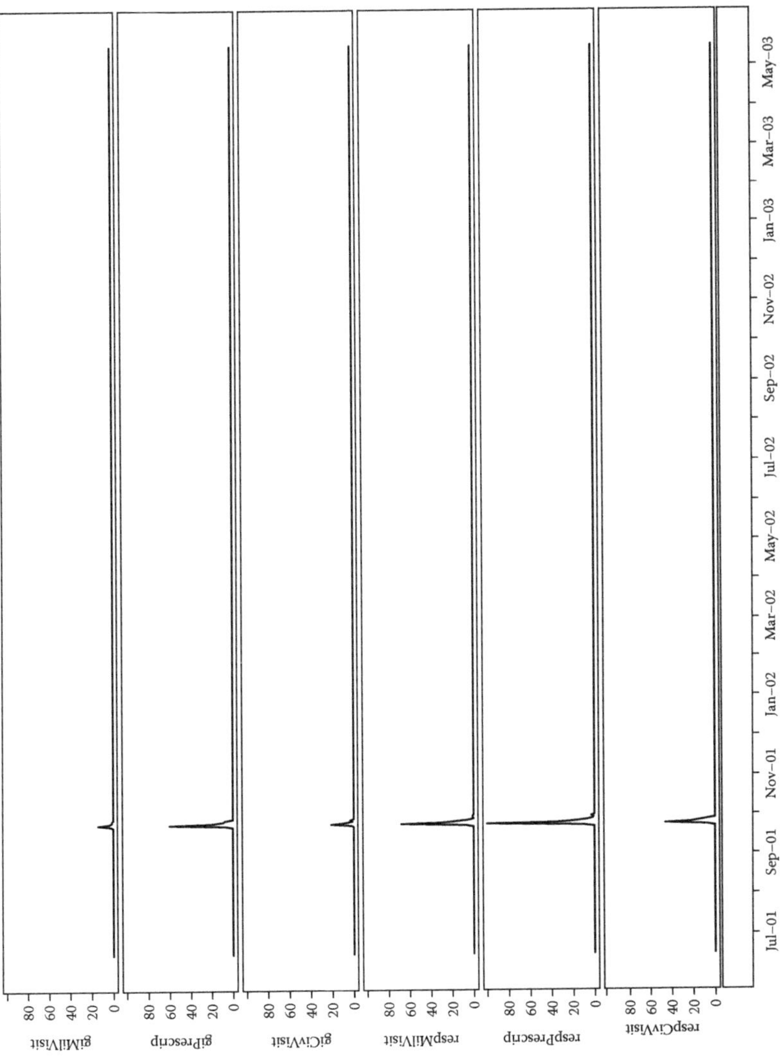

FIGURE 2.12
Simulated lognormal signature of an outbreak that starts on October 8, 2001 (Monday), after incorporating the explainable patterns.

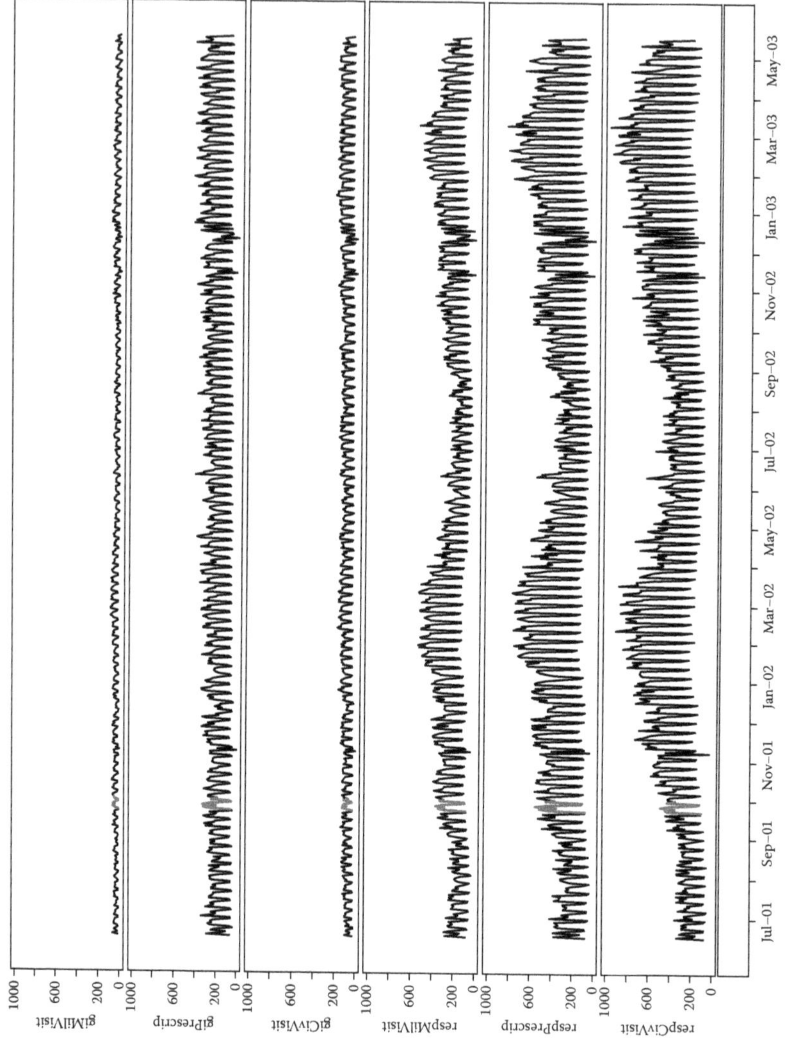

FIGURE 2.13
Final labeled data: mimicked data with inserted outbreak. During the outbreak, the line is bold and colored.

the simulated outbreak signature. Before inserting it into the mimicked dataset, we first add the explainable effects to the outbreak data.

Now the simulated outbreak signature (that includes the explainable patterns) is inserted into the mimicked data, and labels are applied to each day according to the labeling scheme described in the previous section. The end result can be seen in Figure 2.13.

This entire process can then be repeated, inserting outbreaks on different days, to create multiple datasets with different outbreak locations. This provides a large number of example datasets with similar background data and outbreak type, but which are stochastically different. Thus, it allows a researcher to run an algorithm many times and summarize the results, estimating an algorithm's average performance in terms of false alerts and outbreaks detected.

2.7 Summary and Future Work

2.7.1 Future Work

There are several potential improvements that could be made to the mimic methodology. We anticipate that adding more lags to the mimic will increase the accuracy of patterns captured. While most of the autocorrelation is captured by a single day lag, additional lags still hold higher-level information about the series. In addition, a more elaborate spline fitting to estimate seasonal components would be valuable and could potentially allow for extension of mimics to longer series.

An alternative method for simulating health data is to simulate individual-level activities within a city (such as visiting an ED or purchasing medication). This was proposed and implemented in WSARE 3.0 (Wong et al., 2003). These simulated individual-level events could then be aggregated to the level of biosurveillance health series of the type examined here. Alternatively, one could also modify WSARE's Bayesian method, using the conditional probabilities of case given combinations of characteristics as sufficient statistics from original health data, as another testable way to generate simulated series.

The evaluation tests considered here are unable to detect certain types of deviations between the authentic and mimicked datasets. For example, since the temporal factor is not considered, they will be unable to find differences in autocorrelation and other time-related deviations. For example, if all Saturday values were randomly reordered, the test results would be identical. Similarly, if the daily observations were reordered to have the same marginal distribution, but a different autocorrelation, this ordering would not cause a change in the test results. In addition, these tests will not find cases where the simulated data is too *close* to the original, such as when there is simple random variation around the original data points. As described earlier, however, this is an undesirable property of a mimic simulation. Tests for such scenarios should also be considered.

Ultimately, the best test of the mimicked data will be whether algorithms perform equally well on the mimicked data and on authentic data. If detection algorithms perform on authentic data as well as on mimicked data, we can be confident that our mimicked series are useful for testing and comparing algorithms. We can test this by simulating and injecting outbreak signatures, then testing the performance of various algorithms on authentic versus simulated data.

2.7.2 Summary

An R package for the mimic and outbreak functions is freely available at projectmimic.com, along with 10 simulated datasets mimicked from an authentic biosurveillance dataset. The R package is easily installed and contains extensive help for all functions, with example code. The datasets contain 2 years of data, with six health indicators from a single region. We encourage researchers to freely use the code or datasets provided.

By making the code and algorithms public and freely available, we hope to lower the barriers to entry and allow more researchers to become involved in biosurveillance. By providing a mechanism for generating mimics, we hope to encourage data holders to make mimics freely available. By providing a mechanism for testing mimics, we hope to evaluate methods for mimicking time-series data and to improve such methods.

In conclusion, we believe that simulation can be an effective way of generating new, semiauthentic datasets for public research, free from privacy, confidentiality, and proprietary constraints. The tests presented here provide checks on the validity of the simulation, and allow us to consider further improvements in simulation of health data. By doing this, we hope to enable many more researchers to consider the many challenges, in particular statistical, in biosurveillance (see Shmueli and Burkom 2010 for a survey of such challenges) and to provide an opportunity for rapid advancement of both research and practical solutions.

Acknowledgments

We thank Dr. Howard Burkom and Sean Murphy from the Johns Hopkins Applied Physics Laboratory for useful discussion and suggestions. The research was partially funded by NIH grant RFA-PH-05-126. Permission to use the data was obtained through data use agreement #189 from TRICARE Management Activity. For the first author, this research was performed under an appointment to the U.S. Department of Homeland Security (DHS)

Scholarship and Fellowship Program, administered by the Oak Ridge Institute for Science and Education (ORISE) through an interagency agreement between the U.S. Department of Energy (DOE) and DHS. ORISE is managed by Oak Ridge Associated Universities (ORAU) under DOE contract number DE-AC05-06OR23100. All opinions expressed in this paper are the author's and do not necessarily reflect the policies and views of DHS, DOE, or ORAU/ORISE.

References

Benjamini, Y. and Y. Hochberg (1995). Controlling the false discovery rate: A practical and powerful approach to multiple testing. *Journal of the Royal Statistical Society B 57*, 289–300.

Bickel, P. (1969). A distribution free version of the Smirnov two sample test in the *p*-variate case. *The Annals of Mathematical Statistics 40 (1)*, 1–23.

Brillman, J. C., T. Burr, D. Forslund, E. Joyce, R. Picard, and E. Umland (2005). Modeling emergency department visit patterns for infectious disease complaints: Results and application to disease surveillance. *BMC Medical Informatics and Decision Making 5:4*, 1–14.

Buckeridge, D. L., H. Burkom, M. Campbell, W. R. Hogan, and A. W. Moore (2005). Algorithms for rapid outbreak detection: A research synthesis. *Journal of Biomedical Informatics 38*, 99–113.

Buckeridge, D. L., H. Burkom, A. Moore, J. Pavlin, P. Cutchis, and W. Hogan (2004). Evaluation of syndromic surveillance systems—design of an epidemic simulation model. *MMWR Morb Mortal Wkly Rep. 53 Suppl.*, 137–143.

Burkom, H. S. (2003a). Biosurveillance applying scan statistics with multiple, disparate data sources. *Journal of Urban Health 80*, 57–65.

Burkom, H. S. (2003b). Development, adaptation and assessment of alerting algorithms for biosurveillance. *Johns Hopkins APL Technical Digest 24* (4), 335–342.

Burkom, H. S., S. P. Murphy, and G. Shmueli (2007). Automated time series forecasting for biosurveillance. *Statistics in Medicine 26*, 4202–4218.

Cassa, C. A., K. Iancu, K. L. Olson, and K. D. Mandl (2005). A software tool for creating simulated outbreaks to benchmark surveillance systems. *BMC Medical Informatics and Decision Making 5:22*.

Fienberg, S. E. and G. Shmueli (2005). Statistical issues and challenges associated with rapid detection of bio-terrorist attacks. *Statistics in Medicine 24 (4)*, 513–529.

Ford, D. A., J. H. Kaufman, and I. Eiron (2006). An extensible spatial and temporal epidemiological modelling system. *International Journal of Health Geographics 5:4*.

Fricker, R. D., Jr. (2006). Directionally sensitive multivariate statistical process control methods with application to syndromic surveillance. *Advances in Disease Surveillance 3:1*.

Fricker, R. D., Jr., B. L. Hegler, and D. A. Dunfee (2008). Comparing syndromic surveillance detection methods: Ears versus a cusum-based methodology. *Statistics in Medicine 27 (17)*, 3407–29.

Friedman, J. H. and L. C. Rafsky (1979). Multivariate generalizations of the Wald-Wolfowitz and Smirnov two-sample tests. *The Annals of Statistics 7(4)*, 697–717.

Goldenberg, A., G. Shmueli, R. A. Caruana, and S. E. Fienberg (2002). Early statistical detection of anthrax outbreaks by tracking over-the-counter medication sales. *Proceeding of the National Academy of Sciences 99*, 5237–5240.

Hall, P. and N. Tajvidi (2002). Permutation tests for equality of distributions in high-dimensional settings. *Biometrika 89(2)*, 359–374.

Henze, N. (1988). A multivariate two-sample test based on the number of nearest neighbor type coincidences. *The Annals of Statistics 16(2)*, 772–783.

Hutwagner, L., T. Browne, G. M. Seeman, and A. T. Fleischauer (2005). Comparing aberration detection methods with simulated data. *Emerging Infectious Diseases Feb.*

Kim, K.-K. and R. V. Foutz (1987). Tests for the multivariate two-sample problem based on empirical probability measures. *The Canadian Journal of Statistics / La Revue Canadienne de Statistique 15(1)*, 41–51.

Lotze, T., S. P. Murphy, and G. Shmueli (2008). Preparing biosurveillance data for classic monitoring. *Advances in Disease Surveillance.*

Mandl, K., B. Reis, and C. Cassa (2004). Measuring outbreak-detection performance by using controlled feature set simulations. *Morbidity and Mortality Weekly Report 53 Suppl*, 130–136.

Reis, B. and K. Mandl (2003). Time series modeling for syndromic surveillance. *BMC Medical Informatics and Decision Making* 3(2).

Reis, B. Y., M. Pagano, and K. D. Mandl (2003). Using temporal context to improve biosurveillance. *Proceedings of the National Academy of Sciences 100(4)*, 1961–1965.

Rolka, H. (2006). *Statistical Methods in Counter-Terrorism: Game Theory, Modeling, Syndromic Surveillance and Biometric Authentication*, Chapter Emerging Public Health Biosurveillance Directions, pp. 101–107. Springer.

Schilling, M. F. (1986). Multivariate two-sample tests based on nearest neighbors. *Journal of the American Statistical Association 81(395)*, 799–806.

Shmueli, G., and Burkom, H. S. (2010). Statistical Challenges Facing Early Outbreak Detection in Biosureveillance. *Technometrics* Vol 52 (1), pp. 39–51.

Siddiqi, S. M., B. Boots, G. J. Gordon, and A. W. Dubrawski (2007). Learning stable multivariate baseline models for outbreak detection. *Advances in Disease Surveillance 4*, 266.

Siegrist, D. and J. Pavlin (2004). Bio-ALIRT biosurveillance detection algorithm evaluation. *Morbidity and Mortality Weekly Reports (MMWR) 53 (suppl)*, 152–158.

Stoto, M., R. D. Fricker, A. Jain, J. O. Davies-Cole, C. Glymph, G. Kidane, G. Lum, L. Jones, K. Dehan, and C. Yuan (2006). Evaluating statistical methods for syndromic surveillance. In A. Wilson, G. Wilson, and D. H. Olwell (Eds.), *Statistical Methods in Counter-Terrorism: Game Theory, Modeling, Syndromic Surveillance and Biometric Authentication*, pp. 141–172. ASA-SIAM.

Wallstrom, G. L., M. Wagner, and W. Hogan (2005). High-fidelity injection detectability experiments: A tool for evaluating syndromic surveillance systems. *Morbidity and Mortality Weekly Report 54 Suppl*, 85–91.

Watkins, R. E., S. Eagleson, S. Beckett, G. Garner, B. Veenendaal, G. Wright, and A. J. Plant (2007). Using gis to create synthetic disease outbreaks. *BMC Medical Informatics and Decision Making 7:4.*

Wong, W.-K., A. Moore, G. Cooper, and M. Wagner (2002). Rule-based anomaly pattern detection for detecting disease outbreaks. In *Proceedings of the 18th National Conference on Artificial Intelligence.* MIT Press.

Wong, W.-K., A. Moore, G. Cooper, and M. Wagner (2003). Bayesian network anomaly pattern detection for disease outbreaks. In *Proceedings of the Twentieth International Conference on Machine Learning*, pp. 808–815. Menlo Park, California: AAAI Press.

Zhang, J., F. Tsui, M. Wagner, and W. Hogan (2003). Detection of outbreaks from time series data using wavelet transform. In *AMIA Annual Symposium Proceedings*, pp. 748–752.

3

Remote Sensing-Based Modeling of Infectious Disease Transmission

Richard K. Kiang
NASA Goddard Space Flight Center
Greenbelt, Maryland

Farida Adimi
NASA Goddard Space Flight Center
Greenbelt, Maryland
and
Wyle International
McLean, Virginia

Radina P. Soebiyanto
NASA Goddard Space Flight Center
Greenbelt, Maryland
and
University of Maryland at Baltimore County
Baltimore, Maryland

CONTENTS

3.1 Introduction

In recent years, using remote sensing for modeling infectious disease transmission has become an increasingly popular and important technique. A significant amount of research has been conducted on how remote sensing can be used for assessing disease risks and enhancing public health organizations' abilities for decision making. The most well-known examples are the early warning techniques for malaria developed by various research groups for different regions of the world (e.g., Thomson et al. 1996; Hay et al. 1998; Rogers et al. 2002; Abeku et al. 2004; Teklehaimanot et al. 2004; Omumbo et al. 2004; Thomson et al. 2006). Early warnings of more intense malaria transmissions or possible outbreaks allow public health organizations to implement countermeasures, such as larval and vector controls, distribution or retreatment of bed nets, and public awareness campaigns, so as to strengthen public health support and readiness. While there are usually no estimates done on how many lives are saved through these initiatives, such techniques can clearly help reduce human suffering and avert tragedies.

Similar approaches have been applied for the control of other infectious diseases, including a number of the World Health Organization (WHO)-designated neglected tropical diseases (NTD). As many of the victims of NTDs are among the world's poorest, it is a very promising prospect that remote sensing can be a cost-effective approach to help control these diseases in developing countries.

In this chapter, we will describe the environmental and contextual determinants of a number of the more important infectious diseases, ranging from those that are more familiar and have afflicted humans since the ancient times to the more recent ones such as H5N1 avian influenza, which is still actively present in certain parts of the world. Remote sensing data can provide information on necessary geophysical parameters. Techniques for ground cover classification, which can be necessary for identifying ground cover types and extracting certain environmental and contextual information, will be explained. A number of statistical and biological modeling techniques that can utilize remotely sensed geophysical parameters to model disease risks will also be discussed.

3.2 Environmental Determinants for the Transmission of Infectious Diseases

Infectious diseases are caused by pathogenic microbial agents such as viruses, bacteria, protozoa, parasites, and fungi. Diseases are contagious or communicable if they can be transmitted among humans or transmitted within or across species. Agents of infection include contaminated objects or media, as well as vectors that carry pathogens from one host to another. Vectors are considered to be either mechanical or biological. Mechanical vectors are those that are not infected by pathogens themselves. Biological vectors are those that do become infected and also play an integral role in a pathogen's life cycle. The vectors for common infectious diseases are often arthropods (such as mosquitoes, sand flies, and ticks) or mammals (such as mice, birds, and bats). Environmental conditions have a definitive influence on the propagation of vectors and, to a lesser extent, on the development of pathogens. Although not a topic of this chapter, environmental conditions may also influence disease transmission between humans by modulating the contact rates among humans.

In this section, we will discuss the environmental determinants for some of the more well-known infectious diseases, as well as those for the more recent H5N1 avian influenza, which has affected a significant part of the world and caused human deaths in at least 12 countries.

3.2.1 Malaria

Malaria is a parasitic disease caused by a number of *Plasmodium* species. It is transmitted by infected female *Anopheles* mosquitoes. Malaria is endemic in a significant part of the world's tropical regions, including sub-Saharan Africa, South and Southeast Asia, and Latin America. The WHO estimates more than 500 million cases (and 1 million deaths) of malaria occur every year worldwide. Climate and environmental conditions play an important role in the spread and transmission of malaria (Kiang et al. 2006). For example, rainfall provides mosquitoes breeding sites. It also increases humidity, which prolongs their life span. However, that the lack of rainfall has also been shown to create new breeding sites, such as pools and puddles in some regions; as such, little rainfall can increase vector population as well. Alternatively, intense and prolonged rainfall may flush away larval habitats and reduce malaria transmission (Kovats 2003). Natural bodies of water such as ponds and streams serve as breeding sites as well. Temperature is another factor that can influence the transmission of malaria. Warmer temperature accelerates larval and vector development (Craig 1999) and shortens the sporogonic cycle; this prolongs the time a mosquito can transmit malaria. Warmer air holds more moisture. Suitable or relative humidity is needed for the survival of *Anopheles* mosquitoes. Studies have shown that optimal relative humidity is between 55% and 80% for active malaria transmission to occur in India (Bhattacharya 2006). Vegetation, which is associated with mosquito breeding, feeding, and resting sites, is another important factor for malaria transmission.

3.2.2 Dengue Fever

Dengue fever or dengue is a viral disease transmitted by infected *Aedes aegypti* and *A. albopictus* mosquitoes. Similar to malaria, dengue fever is most prevalent in the Tropics. Four related serotypes are involved in the diseases. However, there is no cross-protection among serotypes. A severe form of the disease is dengue hemorrhagic fever, which can be fatal. According to the WHO, about 2.5 billion people, or 40% of the world's population, are currently at risk for this disease. Dengue is considered an urban disease as it is predominately found in urban areas. For example, *A. aegypti* breeds in stagnant water such as flower vases, uncovered barrels, buckets, and discarded tires. A dengue vector study done near Bangkok, Thailand (Strickman and Kittayapong 2002), demonstrated that mosquito larvae responsible for dengue fever were spatially correlated and predominately concentrated in specific regions of the study area. In addition, this study showed that the abundance of larvae prevails in wet seasons compared to hot and cool seasons. A longitudinal study conducted in an endemic area of northern Thailand (Vanwambeke et al. 2006) showed that the outbreak of dengue in 2002 was correlated with the location of the individuals and the type of land cover around the houses, such as irrigated fields and orchards. On the other hand, this study discovered that, unlike malaria, temperature and precipitation do not seem to correlate with the occurrence of dengue fever in Northern Thailand.

3.2.3 West Nile Virus

West Nile virus (WNV) is an infectious disease transmitted by a few species of mosquitoes, and can infect birds, horses, humans, and other animals. In humans, WNV can cause inflammation of the brain or its lining, which can lead to encephalitis or meningitis. In the United States, WNV is transmitted by certain types of *Culex* and *Aedes* mosquitoes. Human cases of WNV in Iowa (USA) between 2002 and 2006 were investigated by De Groote et al. (2008). They found that human WNV incidents were associated with unique landscape, and, to some extent, average precipitation, minimum temperature, and dew points. In a study examining the WNV incidents in California during the summer of 2003, it was concluded that above average temperature and rainfall were probably the important causes for WNV outbreaks (Reisen 2004). A landscape-based model was developed to derive avian WNV risk maps for Mississippi (Cooke 2006)—road density, stream density, slope, and normalized difference vegetation index (NDVI) were all demonstrated to be significant factors in the WNV occurrences.

3.2.4 Rift Valley Fever

Rift Valley fever (RVF) is a viral infectious disease transmitted by some species of *Aedes* mosquitoes. It primarily affects livestock but can also be transmitted to humans. RVF leads to abortion in pregnant, infected domestic livestock. As such, it has devastating economic implications and can lead to meat shortages and scarcities. RVF largely affects some regions in Africa and, recently, certain parts of the Middle East, including Saudi Arabia and Yemen. Outbreaks of RVF in Africa are associated with heavy rainfall and flooding (Davies et al. 1985). Studies have also shown associations between deviations in vegetation growth and RVF outbreaks in Saudi Arabia and Yemen in 2000; such anomalies in the NDVI measurements were used as an early warning for possible RVF outbreaks there (Anyamba et al. 2006).

In addition, Linthicum et al. (1999) examined RVF outbreaks in East Africa from 1950 to 1998 and observed that RVF outbreaks to be closely related to anomalies in the Pacific and Indian Oceans' sea surface temperatures and vegetation index data.

3.2.5 Filariasis

Lymphatic filariasis is a parasitic disease caused by three nematode species: *Wuchereria bancrofti, Brugia malayi, and Brugia timori. Wuchereria bancrofti* is the most common species, estimated to cause approximately 100 million infections annually. Lymphatic filariasis is one of the neglected tropical diseases designated by the WHO.

If not properly treated, filariasis infection may lead to elephantitis. Although the case mortality is low, the social stigma carried by the disease is significant. Fortunately, antihelminthic treatments for filariasis are effective and cost-effective. Mass treatment with just one dose each of two drugs may stop the transmission (The Carter Center 2009). Hence, the WHO considers lymphatic filariasis to be an eradicable disease.

Humans are the definitive hosts for the parasites responsible for lymphatic filariasis. Quite a few mosquito species, including those belonging to *Aedes, Anopheles, Culex, Mansonia,* and *Ochlerotatus,* may serve as the intermediate hosts. The broad spectrum of mosquito species involved in filariasis transmission makes targeted larval control challenging. On the other hand, malaria bed nets can provide general protection for filariasis if the particular filariasis vector species are among those that feed during the night.

The same remote sensing parameters—precipitation, temperature, vegetation, humidity, and elevation—as in malaria can be used for assessment of filariasis risks (Sabesab et al. 2006).

3.2.6 Leishmaniasis

Leishmaniasis is a disease caused by the *Leishmania* parasites and transmitted by phlebotomine sand flies. Leishmaniasis has two forms: cutaneous and visceral. The latter is more serious, with a nearly 100% rate of mortality if left untreated. Most leishmaniases are zoonotic, and natural reservoirs of the disease include domestic or wild animals, such as dogs and rodents. After being bitten by infected female sand flies, humans may not necessarily become infected except for those who are immunodepressed. Today, coinfection of leishmaniasis and HIV has emerged as a significant problem. AIDS greatly increases the risk of visceral leishmaniasis infection, and visceral leishmaniasis infection accelerates the onset of AIDS. Among intravenous drug users, sharing needles can also lead to direct human-to-human transmission of leishmaniasis. Plowing and compacting soil to destroy rodent habitats or removing the vegetation on which vector rodents feed can help reduce the rodent reservoir and number of associated cases of cutaneous leishmaniasis.

Additionally, controlling stray dogs and providing insecticide-treated collars can help reduce the dog reservoir and associated cases of visceral leishmaniasis. However, observing or inferring animal reservoirs and habitats from satellites is difficult. Instead, disease prevalence has been found to be statistically related to precipitation, temperature, vegetation, and elevation. These remotely sensed parameters have been used to estimate climate-based risks for visceral leishmaniasis transmission (Nieto et al. 2006).

3.2.7 Cholera

Cholera is caused by the bacteria *Vibrio cholerae*. The disease was believed endemic to the Indian subcontinent as early as 500 B.C. before it spread to other parts of the world. Through proper filtering and chlorination of water supplies, cholera largely has disappeared in developed countries, but it is still a significant problem in the developing world. The disease may spread quickly if it is not managed properly through sterilization and decontamination. Oral rehydration is the predominant and most effective treatment. Without it, an infected person may die in just a few hours after symptoms appear.

Cholera-causing bacteria have been shown to be naturally attached to planktonic copepods (Hug et al. 1983). Planktonic copepods are groups of small crustaceans, which are food but also parasitic to many kinds of marine mammals and invertebrates. In some coastal areas, during a planktonic bloom, a glass of untreated or unfiltered water may contain several copepods. Because planktonic copepods graze on phytoplankton and transport carbon to ocean depths, planktonic copepods play a necessary role in the ocean's carbon cycle and are an integral component of the Earth's ecosystem. As a result, it will not be possible to eradicate cholera by eliminating copepods. Instead, the only ways to protect against this disease may be improved living standards and sanitation practices, proper treatment of drinking water, improved public health surveillance and response, and early warning and vaccination.

The environmental determinants associated with cholera are those that promote the growth of planktonic copepods, including sea surface temperature, ocean height, and plankton blooms (Colewell 2004). All these parameters, along with coastal brackish and estuarine ecosystems where the bacteria may be present, can be remotely sensed. In addition, remote sensing can also monitor El Niño events, which affect weather patterns and ocean temperature for a significant portion of the world. The prediction of El Niño is a topic actively studied by climate researchers.

3.2.8 Schistosomiasis

Schistosomiasis is a parasitic disease transmitted by five species of *Schistosoma*; one species causes urinary schistosomiasis, and the other four cause intestinal schistosomiasis. Schistosomiasis is one of the 14 neglected tropical diseases, tends to affect the poorest communities of the world, and is the second most devastating disease after malaria globally. The distribution of Schistosomiasis species is geographically dependent. With approximately 90% of all the cases in the world, Africa bears the majority of the burden of this disease.

Human transmission of schistosomiasis is through the intermediate hosts of certain species of freshwater snails. Larvae can be released daily from snails, depending on ambient temperature and light; these then can attach to and penetrate human skin. Farm animals may be infected by some species of *Schistosoma* as well. Swimming, playing, or working in infected water bodies can lead to infection. Eggs of schistosomes may also be present in an infected person's stool or urine. In the poorest communities where there is inadequate hygiene and waste management, eggs may recontaminate or cross-contaminate bodies and/or sources of water, completing the transmission cycle.

The ecology of the snail (as the intermediate host) provides insight on how remote sensing can be used for the detection, control, and prevention of schistosomiasis (Yang et al. 2005). Temperature, type of vegetation/ground cover, bodies of water, precipitation, flood, irrigation, and water transport projects and farms have all been related to the presence and movement of these snails. Because remote sensing is a practical tool for monitoring and measuring these environmental and socioeconomic factors, it is possible to use this method as a tool for risk assessment and control.

3.2.9 Avian Influenza (AI)

Since 1996, when the highly pathogenic avian influenza (HPAI) H5N1 virus was isolated in China, the disease has spread across Asia to Europe and Africa. As of June 2009, there have been 432 human cases worldwide with 262 deaths. Indonesia has been the country hardest hit with 141 human cases and 115 deaths.

AI, which is caused by influenza Type A viruses, is a common infectious disease among many species of wild birds. The Type A viruses are normally of low pathogenicity to wild birds as well as to domestic poultry (when initially infected). In a dense poultry population, however, the virus can mutate very efficiently and may become highly pathogenic in the course of several months (Kida and Sakoda 2006). Infection in poultry with an HPAI virus such as H5N1 results in severe mortality. Globally, approximately 250 million poultry have been lost in recent years due to H5N1 and massive culling.

Fortunately, the H5N1 virus has not yet mutated into a form that is easily transmittable to humans. So far, human-to-human transmission is limited to prolonged, close contact with infected humans. However, coinfection of HPAI and human influenza viruses in humans or pigs may produce, through genetic reassortment or adaptation, deadly strains of an influenza virus that could be H5N1 or another highly pathogenic subtype. The worry among the world's nations is that such an event could lead to a worldwide pandemic reminiscent of the 1918 pandemic.

Excluding the possible transmission to humans and other mammals, as currently understood, the AI transmission loop involves migratory, sedentary, and backyard birds and poultry. Migratory and sedentary birds first transmit, or spill over, low pathogenic AI (LPAI) virus to poultry either directly or through backyard birds. Domestic poultry then transmit, or spill back, HPAI virus to other birds—including migratory birds—directly or indirectly. The infected migratory birds, if still fit to fly, can then spread the virus to other regions. A confounding factor to this cycle is that the avian influenza virus is apathogenic to some species of ducks. Though they may appear unaffected and healthy, ducks which are really infected but asymptomatic may transmit the virus to other poultry and birds. Aside from migration, other means through which HPAI H5N1 can spread includes transboundary and in-country movement of poultry products and by-products, as well as legal and illegal wild bird trades.

Avian influenza viruses survive well in water, especially at low temperatures. In some areas, the virus may survive in water through the entire winter. Therefore, water bodies and wetlands where wild birds and domestic birds may mingle are a risk. Moreover, because the AI virus transmits through fomites, areas near the transportation routes to where poultry farms dominate are also considered at-risk. Other meteorological and environmental parameters may have direct or indirect roles in promoting avian influenza transmission. These parameters may influence, for example, the survival of H5N1 virus, the availability of grazing fields for free range poultry, the selection of refueling and molting areas, and the seasonal migration and weather-induced movements for certain species. These meteorological and environmental parameters can be conveniently derived from satellite data.

3.3 Remote Sensing as a Means of Acquiring Environmental Information

Satellites offer continuous temporal and spatial observations of the Earth, and provide an uninterrupted data flow pertaining to its climate and the environmental conditions. Therefore, remote sensing is a vital technology for studying the relationship between these conditions and infectious diseases. In addition, anomalies and deviation from normal environmental and climatic conditions that are observed in remote sensing data are useful for assessing risks of infectious disease outbreaks. Several of the current Earth observation satellite missions provide data products pertaining to the environmental and contextual determinants of infectious diseases. Some of these missions are summarized in the next sections.

3.3.1 Satellites, Sensors, Measurements, and Data Products

There are two types of remote sensing instruments: passive and active sensors. Passive sensors measure the radiance reflected by or emitted from the Earth's surface at different wavelength bands, depending on the nature of the geophysical parameters to be measured. Active sensors, on the other hand, measure ground reflected radiation originally emitted from the sensors. Radar and LIDAR are two common types of active sensors. In the following sections, we describe a few of the passive sensors currently being flown that can measure some of the climatic and environmental factors pertaining to the diseases described earlier in this chapter.

3.3.1.1 Landsat

The Landsat series (USGS 2009a) began in 1972 with the first Landsat 1 mission, followed by several others: Landsat 2, Landsat 3, Landsat 4, Landsat 5, and the most recent Landsat 7, which was launched in April 1999. Both Landsat 5 and Landsat 7 are still collecting data. Landsat 5 was launched in 1994 and carries the multispectral scanner (MSS) with four spectral bands ranging from visible to near infrared with a ground resolution of 57 m × 79 m. Landsat 5 also carries a Thematic Mapper (TM), which consists of an array of seven spectral bands from the visible to mid-infrared (30 m) and a thermal band (120 m). Landsat 7 carries an Enhanced Thematic Mapper Plus (ETM+) with eight spectral bands, including the visible to the mid-infrared with a spatial resolution of 30 m, a thermal band with 60 m spatial resolution, and a panchromatic band with a spatial resolution of 15 m. Landsat missions provide several land products, including radiometrically and geometrically corrected, and terrain-corrected data. Through ground cover classification techniques, Landsat data can be used for identifying potential larval habitats of large dimension and certain contextual determinants.

3.3.1.2 Advanced Very High Resolution Radiometer (AVHRR)

The Advanced Very High Resolution Radiometer (AVHRR) (Applied Physics Laboratory 2009) is carried onboard the National Oceanic and Atmospheric Administration (NOAA) Polar Orbiting Satellites (POES). It collects global daily information about the land, ocean, and the atmosphere. The first AVHRR sensor was launched in October 1978 onboard the TIROS-N satellite, and the two sensors onboard the most recent NOAA-12 and NOAA-14 missions are still collecting data. A typical AVHRR sensor has five bands ranging from visible and mid-infrared to thermal bands. Among AVHRR data products are vegetation indices and logs of sea surface temperature.

3.3.1.3 Tropical Rainfall Measuring Mission (TRMM)

The Tropical Rainfall Measuring Mission (TRMM) (Goddard Space Flight Center 2009a) includes five sensors: the Precipitation Radar (PR), TRMM Microwave Imager (TMI), the Visible and Infrared Scanner (VIRS), the Cloud and Earth Radiant Energy Sensor (CERES), and the Lightning Imaging Sensor (LIS). TMI is the sensor responsible for providing rainfall information by measuring the intensity of microwave radiation at five distinct frequencies ranging between 10.7 and 85.5 GHz. TRMM is a collaborative mission between the United States and Japan. As precipitation is the most important environmental determinants for most infectious diseases, TRMM has made a definitive contribution to reducing morbidity and mortality due to infectious disease in humans.

3.3.1.4 Global Precipitation Measurement (GPM)

The next generation satellite to measure global precipitation is the Global Precipitation Measurement (GPM) mission (Goddard Space Flight Center 2009b). The GPM will consist of a core satellite and up to eight satellites to form a constellation. It will extend precipitation measurements to higher latitudes and implement more frequent sampling. It is expected to be launched around 2013 or 2014. GPM will provide high temporal resolution precipitation data with greater accuracy and more complete coverage.

3.3.1.5 Terra and Aqua

The Terra and Aqua missions are part of the Earth Observing System (EOS), which gathers information about the Earth's ecosystem, including its land, ocean, and atmosphere. Terra was launched in late 1999 and started providing data in early 2000. Nearly 2 years later, Aqua was launched and began providing complementary data. The Moderate-resolution Imaging Spectroradiometer (MODIS) (Goddard Space Flight Center 2009c), a key instrument onboard Terra and Aqua, has 36 bands spanning from the visible to the long-wave infrared. Two of these bands have a 250 m resolution and are dedicated for the study of land, cloud, and aerosol boundaries. Land, cloud, and aerosol properties are collected by five other bands with 500 m resolution. The remaining 1-km bands are devoted to observations pertaining to the atmosphere, surface parameters, and water vapor. Kiang et al. (2006) has used several MODIS products, including surface reflectance, the Land Surface Temperature (LST), the Normalized Difference Vegetation Index (NDVI), and water vapor, to estimate and predict malaria prevalence.

The Advanced Spaceborne Thermal Emission and Reflection Radiometer (ASTER) (Jet Propulsion Laboratory 2009a) is also onboard the EOS Terra spacecraft. ASTER operates from the visible to the thermal infrared spectrum with a spatial resolution of 15 m, 30 m, and 90 m for the thermal bands. ASTER provides data for a variety of research applications, such as monitoring of surface climatology, vegetation, volcanoes, flooding, coastal erosion, and soil mapping. ASTER data is useful for ground cover classification.

3.3.1.6 EO-1

As part of the NASA New Millennium Program, EO-1 (USGS 2009b) is the first mission that was developed with advanced technologies to build smaller and less costly spacecraft. EO-1 was launched in November 2000. Three instruments are being flown on board the EO-1 spacecraft. The Advanced Land Imager (ALI) has ten bands: one panchromatic, six visible/near infrared, and three shortwave infrared bands. The panchromatic band has a spatial resolution of 10 m, the rest of the bands have a resolution of 30 m. Hyperion is another instrument on board EO-1; it is a hyperspectral imager covering the wavelength range from 0.4 to 2.5 μm in 220 bands with a 30 m resolution. Data from the Hyperion observations can be used for applications concerning agriculture, environmental management, and detailed land classification. Terrain and geometrically corrected radiometric products are generated from ALI's and Hyperion's observations. The third instrument is an atmospheric corrector capable of providing more accurate reflectance measurements for other land imagers through its atmospheric correction algorithms.

3.3.1.7 RADARSAT

RADARSAT (Canadian Space Agency 2009) is an environmental monitoring satellite for the land and ocean. The first RADARSAT-1 with a finest resolution of 8 m was launched in November 1995. The second RADARSAT-2 with a finest resolution of 3 m was successfully launched in late 2007. RADARSAT data uses include land cover classification and identification of potential larval habitats.

3.3.1.8 Commercial Satellites

Among the high-resolution commercial sensors are Ikonos and QuickBird; data from these sensors are provided through commercial vendors, and they typically include corrected radiometric products. Ikonos, with 1 m resolution, was launched in September 1999, and Quickbird, with an even higher resolution of 60 cm, was launched in October 2001. Because of their high resolution, both Quickbird and Ikonos data can be used for land cover classification that involves small-surface objects, such as ponds or ditches.

3.3.2 Space Shuttles—Shuttle Radar Topography Mission (SRTM)

The Shuttle Radar Topography Mission (SRTM) (Jet Propulsion Laboratory 2009b) was conducted from the Space Shuttle *Endeavour* in February 2000.

The goal of the mission was to collect global high-resolution digital topography data. Digital elevation models (DEM) constructed from the SRTM data are useful for modeling infectious diseases where transmission depends on terrain elevation.

3.3.3 Google Earth and Virtual Earth

Google Earth (Google 2009) offers maps, terrain, and satellite images of the Earth. Although, in general, Google Earth does not provide raw remote sensing data or environmental parameters, its visual images could be used in identifying land cover features and navigation. Virtual Earth, which has been renamed as "Bing Maps for Enterprise" (Microsoft 2009), is another tool that could be used to navigate to specific locations and integrate the remote sensing data or other images for further analysis. While using Google Earth or Bing Maps data for quantitative analyses such as classifications can be straightforward, the images these programs offer are ideal for qualitative analyses. In fact, a growing number of studies have relied on the imagery ability of these tools for selecting test sites and generally characterizing ground cover.

3.4 Ground Cover Classification Methods

Ground cover can be inferred from remote sensing imagery data using classification methods. Some typical ground cover types or classes important in infectious disease transmission include bodies of water, rice fields, pastures, forests, wetlands, orchards, roads, urban and suburban areas, dwellings, buildings, etc. Contextual determinants for disease transmission, such as deforestation, road building, and other anthropogenic modification of ecosystems, can be inferred from ground cover or changes in ground cover over time. Some typical classification techniques for ground cover are discussed in the following sections.

3.4.1 The Parallelpiped Method

The parallelpiped method is one of the simplest classification methods. It uses the lower and upper values in each spectral dimension to construct a multidimensional parallelpiped for each class. Pixels falling within the parallelpiped of the class are classified with that class. The lower and upper limits can be estimated using class mean and standard deviation. Because of its simplicity, this method requires a short computing time. However, it is also less accurate because of the difficulty of considering spectral correlation between bands. Parallelpipeds constructed after principal component analysis or with eigenvalue decomposition may avoid some problems (Strang 2006).

3.4.2 The Maximum Likelihood Estimator (MLE) Method

The maximum likelihood estimator (MLE) method, one of the most common classification methods, is a procedure based on finding the values of the model parameters that maximizes the likelihood function or distribution. The likelihood function is calculated based on statistics, and data can take the form of a normal, Poisson, Bayesian, or Bernoulli distribution, among others. In remote sensing applications, normal distributions are often assumed. After establishing class type from training sites, a pixel/entity from application sites is assigned to the classification that has the highest likelihood value (Duda et al. 2000).

3.4.3 The Neural Network Method

Unlike the maximum likelihood estimator and parallelpiped methods, the neural network (NN) method does not require the knowledge of the model's distribution function and, therefore, belongs to the nonparametric class of statistical methods. The NN method is a powerful universal approximator. Quite a few types of neural networks can be used for the unsupervised and supervised classification of remote sensing data (Principe et al. 2000). Some examples where neural networks have been used in ground cover, vegetation, and land use classification can be found in the literature (Bocco et al. 2007; Debeir et al. 2001).

3.4.4 Spatial Techniques

In most ground cover classifications, only spectral information associated with a pixel is used. That is, a pixel is assumed an isolated entity unaware and independent of all the neighboring pixels. This assumption may be sufficiently valid when the size of a pixel is large. However, for remote sensing data with high spatial resolution or when pixel size is on the order of 1 m, per-pixel spectral classification is no longer adequate and may result in low classification accuracy. The information of the neighboring pixels or neighborhood can be included in the classification by using textural or contextual information of the neighborhood (Petrou and Sevilla 2006). Only by including spatial information can accuracy in classification be restored.

3.5 Modeling Techniques with Utilization of Remote Sensing Data

Quantitative study of infectious disease transmission dates back as early as 1760, when Daniel Bernoulli investigated the effect of inoculation on the spread of smallpox (Blower and Bernoulli 2006). Since then, a broad spectrum of modeling frameworks has been developed, with statistical to mechanistic approaches and aims and different purposes for each method. A mathematical model is most commonly used for predicting disease risk (incidence) given previous data on the disease cases. As we have previously discussed in this chapter, infectious disease transmissions are influenced by environmental and ecological factors, which can be characterized by remote sensing data. One can use remote sensing data in a mathematical model as the predictors for disease risk. For indirectly transmitted diseases such as vectorborne ones, remote sensing data can be used in a model to predict the geographic distribution and abundance of the vector and disease prevalence.

Often, direct relationships between disease transmission and environmental and ecological factors are not clearly understood. Typically, this calls for a statistical modeling to predict disease risk. The widely used statistical model is generally a correlation-based approach that does not require extensive knowledge on the biology of the disease. On the other hand, when sufficient detail on the biology of the disease is known, one may use biological-based modeling, such as the compartmental Susceptible Exposed Infected Recovered (SEIR) Model. Such models as the SEIR model often not only offer information for risk prediction but also provide an understanding of the quantitative nature of disease transmission. We will discuss both statistical and biological models that are commonly used in the following sections.

3.5.1 Statistical Modeling

Statistical-based modeling generally uses a correlative approach to infer the empirical relationship between the independent and the dependent variables. Since we are dealing here with modeling techniques using remote sensing data, the independent variables, or predictors, in this chapter typically refer to environmental factors. The dependent variables, or outcome, can be the disease incidence or the presence (or absence) of disease.

Again, statistically based models are popular due to their ease of use as they do not require detailed knowledge about disease transmission mechanisms. Although models of this type have good predictive power, it should be noted that statistical models are based on correlation from past data. This means that the model assumes no evolution in the transmission dynamics. Hence, any nonlinearity in the transmission process, which may be embedded in the data, cannot be captured in the model.

3.5.1.1 Logistic Regression

Logistic regression falls under the category of generalized linear models, and it is the most common statistical technique for predicting the probability of disease occurrence using environmental variables. The method does not need to assume any underlying distribution of the independent variables, which is, again, convenient as detailed mechanisms regarding disease transmission is often unknown.

Logistic regression models the independent variables to be linear with respect to the logarithm of the odds of the outcome (*logit*). If p denotes the probability of a disease occurrence, and xi is the environmental variable i, then

$$\log\left(\frac{p}{1-p}\right) = \beta_0 + \beta_1 x_1 + \beta_2 x_2 + \ldots + \beta_i x_i + \ldots + \beta_N x_N \tag{3.1}$$

and

$$p = \frac{1}{1 + e^{-(\beta_0 + \beta_1 x_1 + \beta_2 x_2 + \ldots + \beta_i x_i + \ldots + \beta_N x_N)}} \tag{3.2}$$

The methods in logistic regression will estimate the parameters βi while minimizing the error between data and predicted value. One can then take the exponent of the parameter ($e^{\beta i}$) to determine the amount of change in the outcome for a unit increase in the environmental variable i. The predictive accuracy of the model can be evaluated using receiver–operator characteristic (ROC) curve analysis (Brooker et al. 2002). Briefly, predictions on disease risk are calculated based on the probability threshold, and, as ROC varies across this threshold, the specificity and sensitivity of the model can be obtained. The Akaike Information Criterion (AIC) is often used to eliminate variables that do not contribute significantly to the model (Miller 2002).

3.5.1.2 Regression Trees

Another statistical tool for modeling infectious diseases with remote sensing data is called Classification and Regression Trees (CART) (Breiman et al. 1984). CART is a nonparametric, decision tree-based method that is widely applicable given that it does not assume any underlying distribution for both the predictor and response variables. Typically, a regression tree is generated when the outcome variable is continuous, whereas a classification tree is used for categorical outcome variable. Since our interest is in predicting disease occurrence rates, we will briefly discuss regression tree method in the following text.

CART uses binary recursive partitioning in building the tree. Starting with a root of the tree, the method splits the data into two child nodes that maximizes the homogeneity within these nodes. The partitioning continues iteratively with each of the resulting child nodes. For each iteration, CART will find the most suitable (optimized) partitioning given previous actions (partitioning in the parent node). When further partitioning is no longer possible, the node becomes the terminal node.

This method is attractive since it is easy to interpret the branching decisions. In addition, the CART method supports wide ranges of data formats that can be sparse in nature. It is best used as an exploratory tool, for example, to determine important independent variables, but it does not have good predictive power (Gaudart et al. 2005).

3.5.1.3 ***Neural Network***

The neural network (NN) method is an information processing method analogous to the functioning of the brain. It has remarkable capabilities in many applications, including pattern recognitions. As described earlier in this chapter (Section 3.4.3), the NN method is a powerful tool for ground cover classifications. This method is suitable when little is known about the underlying process of the disease transmission. Generally, NN have a good predictive power. Assessing exactly how prediction is made using the predictors, however, may be less obvious.

Typical NNs consist of interconnected nodes arranged in layers, with the independent variables acting as input and the dependent variables as output. Each node carries a threshold function, while each connection carries weight. For the nodes in the first layer, they will take the NN inputs through its weighted connections and evaluate them using the threshold functions. The outputs from these nodes, in turn, will be fed to the nodes in the next layer—as determined by the topology—for further evaluation, and so forth. The weights that connect the nodes are determined during the training phase by minimizing the error between the predicted output and the outcome data.

We have applied NN to model malaria transmission in Thailand using precipitation, temperature, relative humidity, and vegetation index data as the independent variables (Kiang et al. 2006). Our study shows a distinct dependency of malaria incidences with meteorological and environmental variables. Using various NN approaches, we also showed the trade-off between training and testing accuracy as the architecture complexity increases.

3.5.1.4 ***Genetic Algorithms***

Genetic algorithm (GA) is a search technique inspired by Darwin's evolution theory commonly used in optimization problems. For a given problem, GAs search for a solution in each iteration by evolving the current solution. The search typically begins with a set of candidate solutions called *populations*, which are subject to further evaluation on their "fitness." The objective function typically serves as the fitness function. Based on this fitness function, the current population is chosen randomly and subsequently modified (mutated or crossed over) to form a child generation of the population. The algorithm now enters the next iteration, and, again, it will evaluate the fitness of the new population and so forth until it reaches stop criteria—that is, either a new population does not have better fitness than the previous one, the objective function is satisfied, or it has reached the maximum number of population generated. In general, GA performs well especially in a complex search spaces, although the solution may only be local optima.

The most common application of GAs in epidemic modeling is through the use of the Genetic Algorithm for Rule Prediction (GARP) (Stockwell and Peters 1999). This is a method widely used in the biodiversity discipline, and it projects the potential distribution of animals and plants in unknown areas based on a set of if–then rules relating point-occurrence data and associated geographical and environmental variables. The GA is used to develop or search the rules that ultimately give the best description of the species distribution based on ecological and environmental factors. Consequently, with the if–then constraints, one can determine the species distribution in an unknown area and possibly at different times, given particular ecological and environmental information. In infectious disease transmission studies, GARP can be used to predict the geographical distribution of disease vectors in indirectly transmitted diseases (this approach is also known as Ecological Niche Modeling [ENM]). Levine et al. (2004), for example, has successfully used GARP to predict the geographical location of *Anopheles gambiae* complexes in Africa using 12 environmental layers of the available 14. Beard et al. (2003) used GARP to predict the distribution of the vector for Chagas disease, *Triatoma gerstaeckeri*, in southern Texas. In addition to predicting vector distribution, GARP can also be employed to project disease incidence as demonstrated by Peterson et al. (2004) in their filovirus disease study. In that case, GARP was appropriate to use since neither the filovirus reservoir nor the transmission mechanism was known.

3.5.1.5 Ecological Niche Modeling (ENM)

Ecological Niche Modeling (ENM) relates ecological niche with a species' geographical distribution. Ecological niche describes a set of conditions needed by a species to maintain its population without any immigration (Peterson 2006). In ENM, recorded existence of a species in any area is characterized by its environmental factors. Based on this collective information, ENM predicts the spatial distribution of the said species in an unsampled area or landscape. In terms of infectious disease modeling, ENM is suitable for predicting the geographical distribution of the vector. However, it should be noted that this is not exactly equivalent to predicting the risk and prevalence of a disease. Occurrence of vector does not directly relate to the probability of disease transmission, and, therefore, further modeling is needed to relate a vector's distribution with transmission probability. Refer to Soberon and Peterson (2005) for further details on ENM.

3.5.2 Biological Modeling

The most classical approach for modeling epidemiological phenomena is biology-based modeling. Formulation is typically derived from the principles of disease transmission and based on the current knowledge of biological mechanisms. However, it is more often the case that not much disease biology is known and replacements with assumptions are necessary. As such, an advantage of this method is that one can test the current understanding of disease transmission using the model; a discrepancy between the model outcome and data would indicate a missing process. In the following, we will discuss three biological-based modeling methods: the compartmental SEIR model, agent-based simulation, and Markov chain Monte Carlo (MCMC).

3.5.2.1 SEIR

One of the most widely used biological modeling frameworks is the compartmental, deterministic, ordinary differential equation (ODE)-based model describing the dynamics of the host population. Hosts are divided into categories such as susceptible, exposed, infected, and recovered (SEIR), as represented by the state variables. The "exposed" compartment is for those who are in the latent period, when one is infected but not yet infectious; "recovered" is for those who have gained immunity. Immunity can either be permanent or temporary, depending on the disease control. In the case of temporary immunity, the recovered individual may go back into the "susceptible" class. There are various ways to divide the host population, and this section only describes the method that is most commonly used along with the general formulation. Readers, who are interested in the detailed treatment of the SEIR model, are referred to Anderson and May (1991).

For a directly transmitted disease (Figure 3.1), any susceptible individual moves to the exposed class when contact with the infectious class results in disease transmission. This transmission is conventionally formulated using

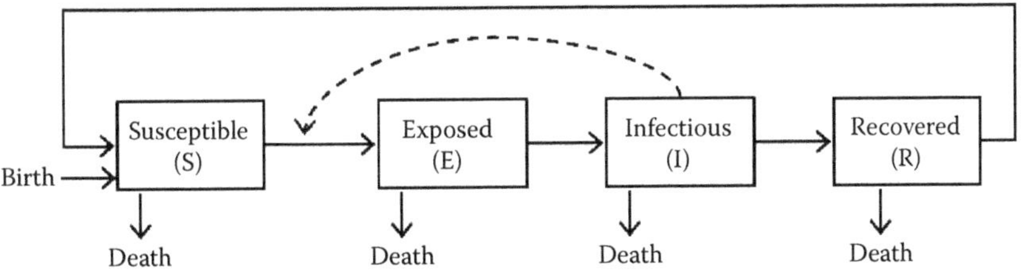

FIGURE 3.1
Diagram representing a simple SEIR model for a directly transmitted disease in a closed population. The model assumes the disease is not inheritable, and therefore, all births go into susceptible class. Transition from susceptible to exposed is due to contact with the infectious, as indicated by the dashed line.

the mass action principle, where the net rate of new infection is proportional to the product of the *densities* of the susceptible and infectious populations, and a homogenous mixing between the two populations is assumed. If we let S and I to be the density of the susceptible and infectious populations, respectively, and β be the probability that a contact results in a successful transmission, then the infection rate is βSI. The transmission parameter, β, depends on a vast range of social, environmental, and epidemiological factors (Anderson and May 1991), and may be derived from epidemiological data. Various alternatives for formulating disease transmission exist as well (McCallum et al. 2001), with the most popular being: $\beta S\ (I/N)$, where N indicates the total population density. With this formulation, the transmission rate now takes into account the abundance of the infected per individual in the total population. Naturally, the choice of transmission formula depends on the characteristics of the disease under study.

With the state variables denoting density of the said population, the SEIR model illustrated in Figure 3.1 can be written using mass-balance as

$$\frac{dS}{dt} = \alpha N - \beta SI + \phi R - \mu S \tag{3.3}$$

$$\frac{dE}{dt} = \beta SI - \sigma E - \mu E \tag{3.4}$$

$$\frac{dI}{dt} = \sigma E - \gamma I - \mu I \tag{3.5}$$

$$\frac{dR}{dt} = \gamma I - \phi R - \mu R \tag{3.6}$$

Here, α and μ are birth and death rates, respectively. σ is the rate of exposed individual moving into the infectious category, typically calculated as the inverse of the latent period. γ is the recovery rate, while φ is the rate for the immunity to disappear.

When the disease transmission is indirect, another species serves as an intermediary host for the pathogen. In this case, the model will include the dynamics of the intermediate host population as shown in Figure 3.2. Transmission occurs when the susceptible primary host comes in contact with infected intermediary host (vector).

As we have previously mentioned, the transmission rates β depends on many things, including environmental factors. One of the environmental factors that have long been recognized to characterize infectious disease pattern is seasonality (Fisman 2007). When the new infection case pattern

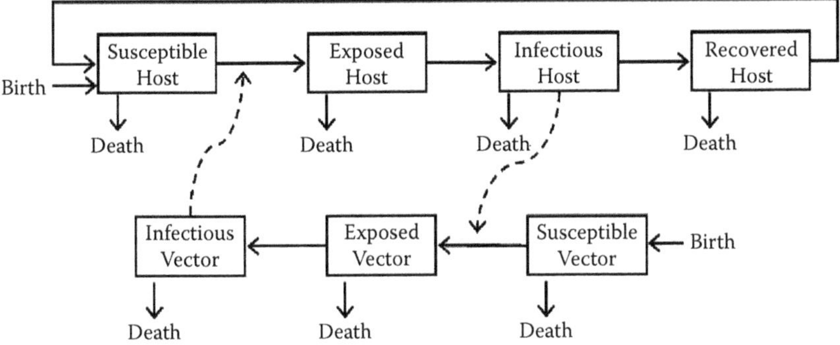

FIGURE 3.2
SEIR model for vectorborne disease. Transmission occurs in two ways: from vector to the primary host and conversely.

follows seasonal trends, such as influenza, one of the common approaches to modeling such conditions is the use of a forcing function in the transmission parameter, β. Dusthov et al. (2007) demonstrated this for influenza where he produced a persistent oscillation in the number of the infected individuals.

By using the compartmental division, the SEIR method model assumes that every individual in each category is homogenous. For example, all susceptible individuals are equally prone to the disease, regardless of their genetic composition or comorbidity. Furthermore, this deterministic model describes average or typical behavior of the population in each category.

3.5.2.2 Agent-Based Simulation

The Agent-Based Model (ABM) or individual-based model is a computing-intensive model that concurrently simulates a set of interacting individuals and is widely used to represent social networks. The individual can represent the host, vector, or a collection of hosts such as a farm. Unlike SEIR, ABM is capable of capturing the heterogenic properties of individuals and their associated spatial landscapes. In addition, ABM can take into account movements between individuals and represent transmission as being dependent on distance. Overall, ABM provides great flexibility in terms of representing a biologically realistic system. However, the more details included in the model, the greater the increase in both the number of parameters in the model as well as in the efforts needed to estimate these parameters.

Keeling et al. (2001) demonstrate the use of ABM for the spread of foot-and-mouth disease in the United Kingdom. Here, the individuals represent farms, which are categorized as susceptible, exposed, infectious, or recovered. With the model considering the dynamics of the disease spread between farms, Keeling et al. demonstrated the benefit of several control strategies. A major effort in the development of large-scale ABM in epidemics is led by a collaborative group called MIDAS (Models of Infectious Disease Agent Study).

3.5.2.3 Markov Chain Monte Carlo

An alternative to the deterministic SEIR model is a stochastic model using a Markov chain Monte Carlo (MCMC) approach, which also incorporates the biology of a disease. MCMC is a well-established method with a vast range of applications; hence, there is immense literature available on this method. (Readers are referred to Gilks et al. [2005] for thorough discussion on MCMC.) Briefly, however, MCMC refers to a suite of methods that, in general, draws samples from a target probability distribution. The states in an MCMC model typically represent the disease stages, similar to the SEIR, and possess Markov property wherein the condition of one's state is independent of previous states and depends only on the current time. These states are governed by transition probability.

MCMC is an attractive method for many reasons. It permits the flexible modeling of variations in the infectious period over time (O'Neill 2002), which cannot be modeled using SEIR framework. MCMC also allows the model to reflect the stochastic nature of some disease transmission. Finally, it avoids identification problems that are a large obstacle in applying the more deterministic SEIR model. Morton and Finckenstadt (2005) describe an example of how MCMC methods can be used in modeling infectious diseases, such as measles incidence.

3.5.3 Additional Methods

We have not yet exhausted all of the existing modeling frameworks, which may be equally important, due to the scope of this book. For example, geostatistical techniques that concern clustering, cluster detection, interpolation, and disease mapping can certainly be used in conjunction with remote sensing data and are very important to disease risk prediction. Readers are referred to other publications for more information on such techniques (i.e., Elliott et al. 2000).

3.6 Conclusions

Remote sensing is an effective way to measure geophysical parameters important to the transmission of infectious diseases. Risk assessments derived from statistical or biological models using these parameters can reduce the morbidity and mortality due to these diseases. Properly implemented countermeasures based on the risk assessments may also reduce the possibility for insecticide resistance and damage to the environment.

As new satellites with advanced sensors are continued to be developed and launched, there will be more satellite data that will be more suitable for disease modeling, risk assessments, and surveillance. As Earth and climate science advance, climate prediction models that rely on satellite measurements as input will also be able to better predict future precipitation, surface temperature, and other parameters that influence disease transmission. Consequently, we anticipate that using remote sensing will have an increasingly important role for public health in the future.

One must still bear in mind, however, that certain contextual determinants important to disease transmission cannot be captured or measured by remote sensing. Such contextual determinants may include the strengthening or deterioration of public health infrastructure at a location, availability of new treatments, reduced sensitivity of drugs, emergence of drug-resistant pathogens, military conflicts or warlike conditions, and significant population movements. When all of these and other contextual determinants do not exist or are more or less unchanged, however, environmental determinants are indeed the more important factors to be used for modeling disease risk.

References

Abeku T.A., S.J. De Vlas, G.J.J.M. Borsboom, et al. 2004. Effects of meteorological factors on epidemic malaria in Ethiopia: a statistical modelling approach based on theoretical reasoning. *Parasitology* 128:585–93.

Anderson, R.M., and R.M May. 1991. *Infectious Diseases of Human: Dynamics and Control*. Oxford University Press.

Anyamba A., J.P. Chretien, P.B.H. Formenty, et al. 2006a. Rift Valley Fever potential, Arabian Peninsula. *Emerging Infectious Diseases* 12:518–20.

Anyamba A., J.P. Chretien, J. Small, C.J. Tucker, and K.J. Linthicum. 2006b. Developing global climate anomalies suggest potential disease risks for 2006–2007. *International Journal of Health Geographics* 5:60 (December). http://www.ij-healthgeographics.com/content/5/1/60.

Applied Physics Laboratory. 2009. AVHRR Imagery. http://fermi.jhuapl.edu/avhrr/index.html (accessed August 24, 2009).

Beard, C.B., G. Pye, F.J. Steurer, et al. 2003. Chagas disease in a domestic transmission cycle, Southern Texas, USA. *Emerging Infectious Diseases* 9:103–5.

Blower, S., and D. Bernoulli. 2008. An attempt at a new analysis of the mortality caused by smallpox and of the advantages of inoculation to prevent it. *Rev. Med. Virol.* 14:275–88.

Bocco M., G. Ovando, S. Sayago, and E.Willington. 2007. Neural network models for land cover classification from satellite images, *Agricultura Tecnica* 67:414–421.

Breiman, L, J.H. Friedman, R.A. Olshen, and C.J. Stone. 1984. *Classification and Regression Trees*. Wadsworth International Group, Bemont, California.

Brooker, S., S.I. Hay, and D.A.P. Bundy. 2002. Tools from ecology: useful for evaluating infection risk models? *Trends in Parasitology* 18:70–74.

Canadian Space Agency. 2009. RADARSAT-1. http://www.asc-csa.gc.ca/eng/satellites/radarsat1/default.asp (accessed August 24, 2009).

The Carter Center 2009. The Carter Center lymphatic filariasis elimination program. http://www.cartercenter.org/health/lf/index.html (accessed August 24, 2009).

Colwell, R.R. 2004. Infectious diseases and environment: cholera as a paradigm for waterborne disease. *International Microbiology* 7:285–89.

Cooke, W.H., K. Grala, and R.C. Wallis. 2006. Avian GIS models signal human risk for West Nile virus in Mississippi. *International Journals of Health Geographics* 5:36 (August). http://www.ij-healthgeographics.com/content/5/1/36.

Craig M.H., R.W. Snow, and D. le Sueur. 1999. A climate-based distribution model of malaria transmission in sub-Saharan Africa. *Parasitol Today* 15:105–11.

Davies F.G., K.J. Linthicum, and A.D. James. 1985. Rainfall and epizootic Rift Valley fever. *Bull. World Heath Organization* 63:941–43.

Debeir O., P. Latinne, and I. Van Den Steen. 2001. Remote sensing classification of spectral, spatial, and contextual data using multiple classifier systems. *Image Anal Stereol* 20 (Suppl 1): 584–89.

DeGroote J.P., R. Sugumaran, S. Brend, B.J. Tucker., and L.C. Bartholomay. 2008. Landscape, demographic, entomological, and climate associations with human disease incidence of West Nile virus in the state of Iowa, USA. *International Journal of Health Geographics* 7:19 (May). http://www.ij-healthgeographics.com/content/7/1/19.

Duda R.O., P.E. Hart, and D.G. Stork. 2000. *Pattern Classification* (Second Edition). John Wiley & Sons. 650 pp.

Elliott P.J. Wakefield, N. Best, and D. Briggs. 2000. *Spatial Epidemiology – Methods and Applications.* Oxford University Press. 475 pp.

Fisman, D.N. 2007. Seasonality of Infectious Disease. *Annu. Rev. Public Health* 28: 127–43.

Gaudart, J., B. Poudiougou, S. Ranque, and O. Doumbo. 2005. Oblique decision trees for spatial pattern detection: optimal algorithm and application to malaria risk. *BMC Medical Research Methodology* 5:22 (July). http://www.biomedcentral.com/1471–2288/5/22.

Gilks, W.R., S. Richardson, and D. J. Spiegelhalter, Editors. 1995. *Markov Chain Monte Carlo in Practice.* London: Chapman and Hall.

Goddard Space Flight Center. 2009a. Tropical Rainfall Measuring Mission. http://trmm.gsfc.nasa.gov (accessed August 24, 2009).

Goddard Space Flight Center. 2009b. Global Precipitation Measurement. http://gpm.gsfc.nasa.gov (accessed August 24, 2009).

Goddard Space Flight Center. 2009c. MODIS Web. http://modis.gsfc.nasa.gov (accessed August 24, 2009).

Google. 2009. Google Earth. http://earth.google.com (accessed August 24, 2009).

Hay, S.I., R.W. Snow, and D.J. Rogers. 1998. From predicting mosquito habitat to malaria seasons using remotely sensed data: practice, problems and perspectives. *Parasitology Today* 14:306–13.

Hug, A., E.B. Small, P.A. West, M.I. Hug, R. Rahman, and R.R. Colwell. 1983. Ecological relationships between *Vibrio cholerae* and planktonic crustacean copepods. *Appl Environ Microbiol* 45:275–83.

Jet Propulsion Laboratory. 2009a. Advanced Spaceborne Thermal Emission and Reflection Radiometer. http://asterweb.jpl.nasa.gov (accessed August 24, 2009).

Jet Propulsion Laboratory. 2009b. Shuttle Radar Topography Mission. http://www2.jpl.nasa.gov/srtm/mission.htm (accessed August 24, 2009).

Keeling, M.J., M.E.J. Woolhouse, D.J. Shaw, et al. 2001. Dynamics of the 2001 UK foot and mouth epidemic: stochastic dispersal in heterogeneous landscape. *Science* 294:813–17.

Kiang R., F. Adimi, V. Soika, et al. 2006. Meteorological, environmental remote sensing and neural network analysis of the epidemiology of malaria transmission in Thailand. *Geospatial Health* 1:71–84.

Kida H, and Y. Sakoda. 2006. The importance of surveillance of avian and swine influenza, in *International Scientific Conference on Avian Influenza and Wildbirds Proceedings*, Rome, May 30–31, 2006.

Kleinschmidt, I., M. Bagayoko, G.P.Y. Clarke, M. Craig, and D. Le Sueur. 2000. A spatial statistical approach to malaria mapping. *International Journal of Epidemiology* 29:335–361.

Kovats R.S., M.J. Bouma, S. Hajat, E. Worrall, and A. Haines. 2003. El Niño and health. *Lancet* 362:1481–89.

Levine, R.S., A.T. Peterson, and M.Q. Benedict. 2004. Geographic and ecologic distributions of the *Anopheles gamibiae* complex predicted using a genetic algorithm. *American Journal of Tropical and Medicine and Hygiene* 70:105–9.

Linthicum, K.J., A. Anyamba, C.J. Tucker, P.W. Kelley, M.F. Myers, and C.J. Peters. 1999. Climate and satellite indicators to forecast Rift Valley Fever epidemics in Kenya. *Science* 285:397–400.

McCallum, H., N. Barlow, and J. Hone. 2001. How should pathogen transmission be modeled? *Trends in Ecology and Evolution.* 16:295–300.

Microsoft. 2009. Bing Maps. http://www.microsoft.com/maps (accessed August 24, 2009).

Miller, A.J. 2002. *Subset Selection in Regression* (2nd Edition). Chapman and Hall. 238 pp.

Morton, A., and B.F. Finkenstadt. 2005. Discrete time modeling of disease incidence time series by using Markov chain Monte Carlo methods. *Applied Statistical* 54:575–94.

Nieto P., J.B. Malone, and M.E. Bavia. 2006. Ecological niche modeling for visceral leishmaniasis in the state of Bahia, Brazil, using genetic algorithm for rule-set prediction and growing degree day-water budget analysis. *Geospatial Health* 1:115–26.

Omumbo J.A., S.I. Hay, C.A. Guerra, and R.W. Snow. 2004. The relationship between the *Plasmodium falciparum* parasite ratio in childhood and climate estimates of malaria transmission in Kenya. *Malaria Journal* 3 (June). http://www.malariajournal.com/content/3/1/17.

O'Neill, P. D. 2002. A tutorial introduction to Bayesian inference for stochastic epidemic models using Markov Chain Monte Carlo methods. *Mathematical Biosciences* 180:103–14.

Peterson, A.T., J.T. Bauer, and J.N. Mills. 2004. Ecologic and geographic distribution of filovirus disease. *Emerging Infectious Diseases* 10:40–47.

Peterson, A.T. 2006. Ecologic niche modeling and spatial patterns of disease transmission. *Emerging Infectious Diseases* 12:1822–26.

Peterson, A.T. 2007. Ecologic niche modelling and understanding the geography of disease transmission. *Veterinaria Italiana* 43:393–400.

Petrou, M., and P.G. Sevilla. 2006. *Image Processing: Dealing with Texture.* Wiley InterScience. 634 pp.

Principe, J.C., N.R. Euliano, and W.C. Lefebvre. 2000. *Neural and Adaptive Systems—Fundamentals through Simulations.* John Wiley & Sons. 656 pp.

Reisen, W.K., Y. Fang, and V.M. Martinez. 2006. Effect of temperature on the transmission of West Nile virus by *Cules tarsalis. Journal of Medical Entomology* 43:309–17.

Rogers, D.J., S.E. Randolph, R.W. Snow, and S.I. Hay. 2002. Satellite imagery in the study and forecast of malaria. *Nature* 415:710–15.

Sabesan, S., H.K.K. Raju, A. Srividya, and P.K. Das. 2006. Delimitation of lymphatic filariasis transmission risk areas: a geo-environmental approach. *Filaria Journal* 5 (November):12. www.filariajournal.com/content/5/1/12.

Soberon, J., and A.T. Peterson. 2005. Interpretations of models of fundamental ecological niches and species' distributional areas. *Biodiversity Informatics* 2:1–20.

Stockwell, D., and D. Peters. 1999. The GARP modeling systems: problems and solutions to automated spatial prediction. *International Journal of Geographical Information Science* 13:143–58.

Strang, G. 2006. *Linear Algebra and Its Applications. Fourth Edition.* Brooks/Cole. 544pp.

Strickman, D., and P. Kittayapong. 2002. Dengue and its vectors in Thailand: introduction to the study and seasonal distribution of *Aedes* larvae. *American Journal of Tropical Medicine and Hygiene* 67:247–259.

Teklehaimanot, H.D., M. Lipsitch, A. Teklehaimanot, and J. Schwartz. 2004. Weather-based prediction of *Plasmodium falciparum* malaria in epidemic-prone regions of Ethiopia I. Patterns of lagged weather effects reflect biological mechanisms. *Malaria Journal* 3 (November). http://www.malariajournal.com/content/3/1/41.

Thomson, M.C., S.J. Connor, P.J. Milligan, and S.P. Flasse. 1996. The ecology of malaria—as seen from Earth-observation satellites. *Annals of Tropical Medicine and Parasitology* 90:243–64.

Thomson, M.C., F.J. Doblas-Reyes, S.J. Mason, et al. 2006. Malaria early warnings based on seasonal climate forecasts from multi-model ensembles. *Nature* 439:576–79.

USGS. 2009a. Landsat missions. http://landsat.usgs.gov/index.php (accessed August 24, 2009).

USGS. 2009b. Earth Observing 1. http://eo1.usgs.gov (accessed August 24, 2009).

Vanwambeke, S.O., B.HB. van Benthem, N. Khantikul, et al. 2006. Multi-level analyses of spatial and temporal determinants for dengue infection. *International Journal of Health Geographics* 5 (January). http://www.ij-healthgeographics.com/content/5/1/5.

Yang, G-J., P. Vounastsou, X-N. Xhou, J. Utizinger, and M. Tanner. 2005. A review of geographic information system and remote sensing with applications to the epidemiology and control of schistosomiasis in China. *Acta Tropica* 96:117–29.

4

Integrating Human Capabilities into Biosurveillance Systems: A Study of Biosurveillance and Situation Awareness

Cheryl A. Bolstad
SA Technologies
Forest Hill, Maryland

Haydee M. Cuevas
SA Technologies
Forest Hill, Maryland

Jingjing Wang-Costello
SA Technologies
Forest Hill, Maryland

Mica R. Endsley
SA Technologies
Forest Hill, Maryland

Walton John Page
Agilex
Chantilly, VA

Taha Kass-Hout
Atlanta, GA

CONTENTS

4.1 Introduction

Between November 2002 and March 2003, hundreds of people in Guangdong Province of China were hospitalized with a mysterious respiratory illness. On February 15, 2003, one of these individuals traveled to Hong Kong to visit his family. Six days later, he checked into a hotel where he infected 12 other people. Public health investigators later said these 12 individuals spread the illness to many others in Hong Kong, Vietnam, Singapore, Ireland, Germany, and Canada (CDC 2003; National Public Radio 2008). This pattern of infection continued and, by October of that year, severe acute respiratory syndrome (SARS) was reported in nearly 30 different countries, affecting more than 8000 individuals, and causing 774 deaths worldwide (Marley et al. 2004). Six years later, in April 2009, the World Health Organization (WHO) announced the emergence of a novel influenza A (H1N1) virus (also referred to as *swine flu*), which had not previously circulated in humans. This new virus was first reported in early April in Mexico and in the United States and quickly spread via human-to-human contact (CDC 2009). By June 2009, nearly 30,000 confirmed cases had been reported in 74 countries, including 141 deaths (WHO 2009). The rapid global spread of the virus prompted WHO to raise the level of influenza pandemic alert from Phase 5 to Phase 6 (the highest level on WHO's six-point scale) on June 11, 2009, making this outbreak the first influenza pandemic in more than 40 years (WHO 2009).

As these two examples illustrate, the growth of international travel and trade has dramatically accelerated the spread of infectious diseases. As a result, diseases such as SARS and swine flu are able to quickly spread across many countries around the world. Beyond the understandable concerns regarding public health, disease outbreaks can also lead to significant economic consequences by affecting world trade and tourism. For example, in an effort to stop the spread of the swine flu, several countries strongly discouraged or altogether imposed bans on travel to Mexico, and some to the United States and Canada as well. The economic impact of such restrictions can be considerable, and particularly costly for countries already experiencing financial hardship. In Mexico City alone, losses of approximately $88 million a day occurred due to various restrictions on commerce and tourism (Gibbs 2009). Potential losses in tourism revenues presented a challenge to the United States as well as the nation continues to deal with the financial strains of a recession.

In light of these consequences, controlling a disease outbreak in its early stages is absolutely essential to ensure both global public health as well as economic stability. However, early and accurate detection of outbreaks is not easy, as illustrated by the outbreak of cryptosporidosis in Milwaukee, Wisconsin, in early 1993. This outbreak was caused by a breakdown of a water filtration process at a water supplier. Approximately 403,000 individuals in the greater Milwaukee area were infected. On April 7, laboratory tests confirmed that the outbreak was caused by the parasite *Cryptosporidum* oocyst (Mac Kenzie et al.

1994). Upon further review of this event, researchers noted that early indicators regarding this outbreak included increased demands in antidiarrheal medications noticed by a pharmacist on April 1 and increased diarrhea-related calls to local nurse hotlines on April 2 (Rodman, Frost, and Jakubowski 1998). An important lesson learned from the Milwaukee cryptosporidiosis outbreak is that the most crucial sources of data may not always be anticipated or obvious.

To improve international response to disease outbreaks, the WHO established the Global Outbreak Alert and Response Network (GOARN). The GOARN interlinks with a large number of existing networks worldwide to collect disease information and provide alertness and readiness to the global health community in the case of any disease outbreak (Heymann and Rodier 2001). The procedure for outbreak alert and response has the following four phases: (1) collection of reports or rumors of new outbreaks, (2) verification of the collected data, (3) communication of the confirmed facts with national-level partners, and (4) coordination of international assistance when required (Heymann and Rodier 2001). Although the GOARN system represents an important first step toward effective disease control and management, public health professionals and organizations still need useful surveillance tools and systems that can help them access and interpret this information in an accurate and timely manner.

Biosurveillance involves the process of detecting and categorizing diseases and disease outbreaks in people, animals, or plants by monitoring elements in the environment that may cause these diseases. In turn, *biosurveillance systems* are designed to collect existing health-related data and analyze this information for the purpose of detecting disease cases, disease outbreaks, and environmental conditions (e.g., contaminated drinking water in the local area) that increase susceptibility to diseases (Fricker, Hegler, and Dunfee 2008). For example, *Biosense* is an initiative of the United States Centers for Disease Control and Prevention (CDC) intended to "improve the nation's capabilities for conducting real-time biosurveillance and enable health situation awareness through access to existing data from healthcare organizations across the country" (CDC 2007). Another biosurveillance system called *ESSENCE* (Electronic Surveillance System for the Early Notification of Community-Based Epidemics) was developed by the U.S. Department of Defense to detect both naturally occurring outbreaks of disease and potential bioterrorism attacks (Gilmore 2002).

Biosurveillance systems that can support early detection and real-time interpretation of information represent a critical front line of defense for modern epidemic and disease control. However, the effectiveness of biosurveillance systems such as Biosense and ESSENCE will greatly depend upon how well their design supports their user's situation awareness (SA). In this chapter, we argue that enhancing the user's SA is an important design consideration for systems targeted at improving detection and response to disease outbreaks. We first discuss the important role that SA plays in biosurveillance. We then present guidance for developing SA-oriented solutions for optimizing the utility of biosurveillance systems. Our approach will be discussed within the context of a theoretical model of SA, citing the value of conducting an SA requirement analysis and designing SA-oriented systems.

4.2 Theoretical Model of Situation Awareness

According to the theoretical model of SA proposed by Endsley (1995), SA can be defined as "the perception of elements in the environment within a volume of time and space, the comprehension of their meaning, and the projection of their status in the near future." This definition highlights three levels or stages of SA formation: perception, comprehension, and projection (see Figure 4.1). Level 1 SA (perception) involves the sensory detection of significant environmental cues. Perception is an active process whereby individuals extract salient cues from their environment. Level 2 SA (comprehension) involves integrating this information in working memory to understand how the information will impact the individual's goals and objectives (Salas et al. 1995). Level 3 SA (projection) involves extrapolating this information forward in time to determine how it will affect future states

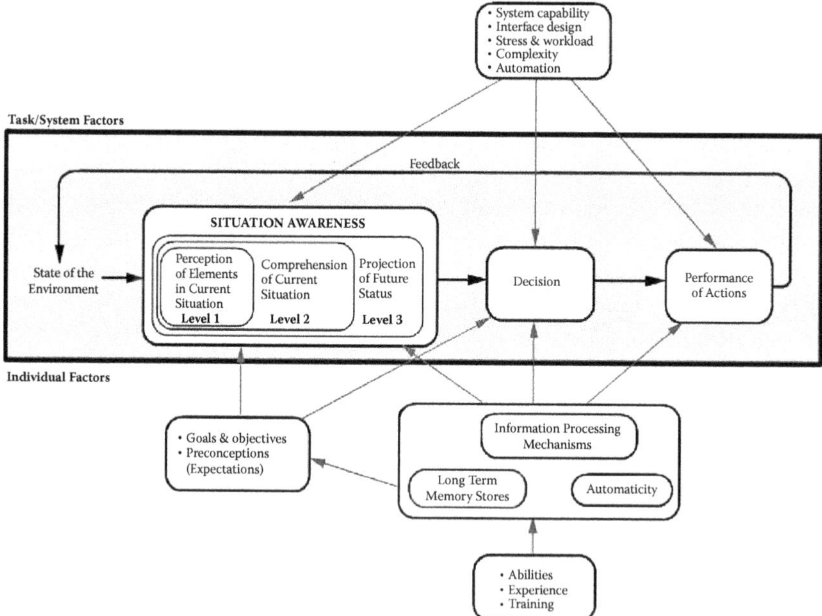

FIGURE 4.1
Theoretical model of situation awareness. (Adapted from Endsley 1995, Toward a theory of situation awareness in dynamic systems, *Human Factors* 37[1]: 32–64.)

of the operational environment (Endsley 1993). Level 3 SA combines what the individual knows about the current situation with his or her mental model or schemata of similar events to predict what might happen next.

4.2.1 Situation Awareness in Biosurveillance

As depicted in Figure 4.1, SA provides the foundation for subsequent decision making and performance in the operation of complex and dynamic systems (Endsley 1995). SA encompasses not only the perception of critical information within the environment but also an increased understanding of the state such that future events can be predicted and proper action can be taken. As such, SA is important throughout the entire process of outbreak detection and management in biosurveillance. When an alert is triggered, the first step for health professionals is to identify whether a real biological event is present (Level 1 SA—perception). Here, what matters most is that health professionals are provided with and are able to attend to the correct data and information. However, performance at this stage can be influenced by individual differences in training and experience (e.g., novice–expert differences) as well as by the design of the systems available to support the detection of potential threats; these factors can both directly and indirectly influence what information is perceived. For example, experts, as compared to novices, are likely to have developed a greater sensitivity for detecting or recognizing patterns in specific types of data through training, extensive experience in conducting biosurveillance, better-focused attention, or more effective use of data representations (Garrett and Caldwell 2009). In turn, this greater sensitivity may enable them to detect events with more accuracy and speed.

The second step in this process requires understanding patterns or trends in the data as well as evaluating the availability of resources to meet the challenge (Level 2 SA—comprehension). For instance, health professionals need to be able to determine whether a series of events, such as a rise in hospital admissions, is due to the normal flu season or an indication of something potentially more serious. Finally, the third step involves predicting the future trends and distribution of the outbreak and the ability to meet the demands of outbreak to decide how best to respond to the alert (Level 3 SA—projection). This includes conducting "what-if" analyses involving social, organizational, economical, environmental, and political trends. For example, if the outbreak involves a highly infectious virus, health professionals will need to notify other state, national, and possibly international agencies to help contain the outbreak and prevent a large scale epidemic. These last two stages (comprehension and projection) are absolutely essential for effective outbreak management and response. As illustrated in Figure 4.2, consideration of the three levels of SA is useful for understanding the types of difficulties biosurveillance professionals face while performing their tasks and also for determining how best to mitigate these challenges.

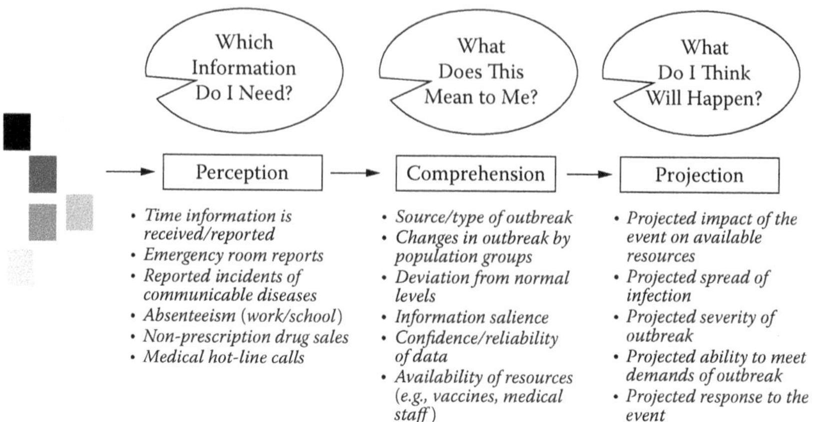

FIGURE 4.2
Illustration of the three levels of situation awareness in biosurveillance.

As noted in the preceding discussion, Endsley's theoretical model of SA illustrates several variables that can influence the development and maintenance of SA within the biosurveillance domain. SA may be affected by the inherent complexity of the tasks involved in monitoring and responding to potential disease outbreaks as well as the design of systems available for monitoring these public health threats. Biosurveillance personnel are often bombarded with too much data, but not enough reliable and interpretable information that they can use to guide their decision making. Adding to this complexity is that sources of information are not always obvious (as learned in the Milwaukee cryptosporidosis outbreak) and biosurveillance systems do not capture "soft" data such as expert opinions. In addition, as evident in the SARS outbreak, threats of epidemics and bioterrorism are constantly evolving, and threat profiles keep changing. As such, early detection has been one of the greatest challenges facing current biosurveillance systems.

As mentioned, individual factors that may affect SA in biosurveillance include the diverse background, training, and experience of biosurveillance personnel and other health professionals. Thus, a major drawback of overlooking user requirements in their original design and creation is that biosurveillance systems may fail to optimally keep the human in the loop. At the organizational level, SA may be negatively influenced by the existence of multiple (and sometimes competing) goals of the various agencies involved. For example, political and organizational boundaries may hinder the sharing of information (e.g., GOARN was not able to perfectly communicate the first indications of the SARS outbreak in China). Yet, as will be discussed in the next section, possessing a similar understanding of the current information (team and shared SA) is absolutely critical in biosurveillance.

4.2.2 Team and Shared Situation Awareness in Biosurveillance

Team SA can be defined as "the degree to which every team member possesses the SA required for his or her responsibilities" (Endsley 1995). By this definition, each team member needs to have a high level of SA on those factors that are relevant for his or her job. Thus, the success or failure of a team depends on the success or failure of each of its team members. In contrast, *shared SA* can be defined as "the degree to which team members possess the same SA on shared SA requirements" (Endsley and Jones 2001). As implied by this definition, certain SA information requirements may be relevant to multiple team members. A major part of teamwork involves the area where these requirements overlap. Therefore, to ensure successful performance, it is important that team members share a common understanding of what is happening on these shared SA elements. However, this does not imply that all information needs to be shared, which would create more workload for the health professionals as they would be forced to sort through a great deal of noise to find the information they need. Instead, what matters most is that team members are able to access and similarly interpret important information on the shared SA requirements that are relevant across their different positions and specializations. For example, when a disease outbreak occurs in multiple countries, physicians within each country need to know the disease symptoms, possible spreading mechanisms, and treatments that have been helpful; this necessitates shared SA across the different doctors regarding the disease. In contrast, government health officials have to know the number of cases within each country and possible links between these cases to determine possible trends; this requires team SA among different government personnel to gather the needed information.

In addition, the detection and control of disease outbreaks often require the creation of ad hoc teams interacting across space and time to coordinate their efforts to achieve a common goal. These teams are composed of individuals with a broad range of specializations within distinct domains (e.g., epidemiologists, physicians, nurses, veterinarians, computer scientists, statisticians, water quality specialists, biologists, and microbiologists) and are drawn from different local, state, and federal health agencies as well as international organizations (Wagner, Moore, and Aryel 2006). The dynamic, fluid, and multidisciplinary nature of these ad-hoc teams may influence their shared SA. For example, ad-hoc teams may have unique shared SA requirements, which differ from those of intact groups that are accustomed to working together, such as specific information regarding their team members' knowledge, skills, and abilities needed to guide assignment of roles and responsibilities (Strater et al. 2009).

Because biosurveillance involves many people from different disciplines and agencies working together to monitor and respond to potential threats to public health, both nationally and internationally, systems need to go beyond keeping one human in the loop, but, more important, support collaboration and sharing of information across these multiple stakeholders and communities of interest. In other words, biosurveillance systems must support not only individual SA but also team SA and shared SA among these geographically distributed entities. Unfortunately, limited research exists that investigates how biosurveillance systems can be effectively used to support their users' SA. To address this issue, we next describe a set of SA-oriented guidelines that specifically target the SA needs of health professionals working in biosurveillance.

4.3 SA-Oriented Guidelines

Ideally, biosurveillance systems should be designed to automatically process large amounts of information in order to rapidly provide public health professionals with the SA they need for early detection and management of potential outbreaks (Mnatsakanyan et al. 2007). Creating system designs that enhance health professionals' awareness of what is happening in a particular situation can dramatically improve their detection and decision-making performance. Yet current biosurveillance systems are data driven in design such that health professionals are "awash with competing bits of data" (Endsley, Bolte, and Jones 2003), that is, systems often provide users with large amounts of data irrespective of the task or goal they are trying to accomplish at that moment. Instead, a well-designed system should simultaneously focus on providing critical data that is structured to support the active goals of the end user while at the same time promoting team and shared SA.

Traditional human factors design methods and principles are insufficient for achieving these requirements in that these primarily address the physical and perceptual characteristics of system components, rather than the way that the integrated system needs to function from a cognitive standpoint. To address this issue, we propose that the design of biosurveillance systems needs to be guided by the Situation Awareness-Oriented Design (SAOD) process. Developed by Endsley and colleagues (see Endsley, Bolte, and Jones 2003) as a means to improve human decision-making and performance through optimizing SA, the SAOD process is user centered and derived from a detailed analysis of the goals, decisions, and SA requirements of the operator. This process has been successfully applied as a design philosophy for systems involving remote maintenance operations, medical systems, flexible manufacturing cells, and military command and control. Two main components of the SAOD process that are particularly relevant in biosurveillance are SA Requirements Analysis and SA-Oriented Design Principles. In our previous work, we have successfully applied these components of the SAOD process to develop information systems that provide SA to public health professionals working in the biosurveillance domain. We next describe these two components in more detail and illustrate how they would be implemented.

4.3.1 SA Requirements Analysis

SA requirements are defined as those dynamic information needs associated with the major goals or subgoals of the operator in performing his or her job. These critical SA requirements can be identified utilizing a Goal-Directed Task Analysis (GDTA), a unique form of cognitive task analysis that involves conducting extensive knowledge elicitation sessions with domain subject matter experts (for a detailed description of this methodology, see Endsley, Bolte, and Jones 2003). The objective of the GDTA is to identify the major goals and decisions that drive performance in a particular job or position as well as to delineate the critical, dynamic information requirements associated with each goal and decision. Figures 4.3 and 4.4 illustrate a hypothetical example of what a portion of a GDTA for health professionals working in the biosurveillance domain might look like. Figure 4.3 shows examples of important top-level goals, and Figure 4.4 illustrates some of the information requirements at each of the three levels of SA for Goal 1.0 "Ensure earliest possible detection of bio events." A complete GDTA is much more comprehensive and detailed.

To support these goals, an effective biosurveillance system needs to synthesize the information available to provide an accurate common picture of the situation for all health professionals who will access and use such a system, thereby ensuring shared SA across all individuals involved. However, one

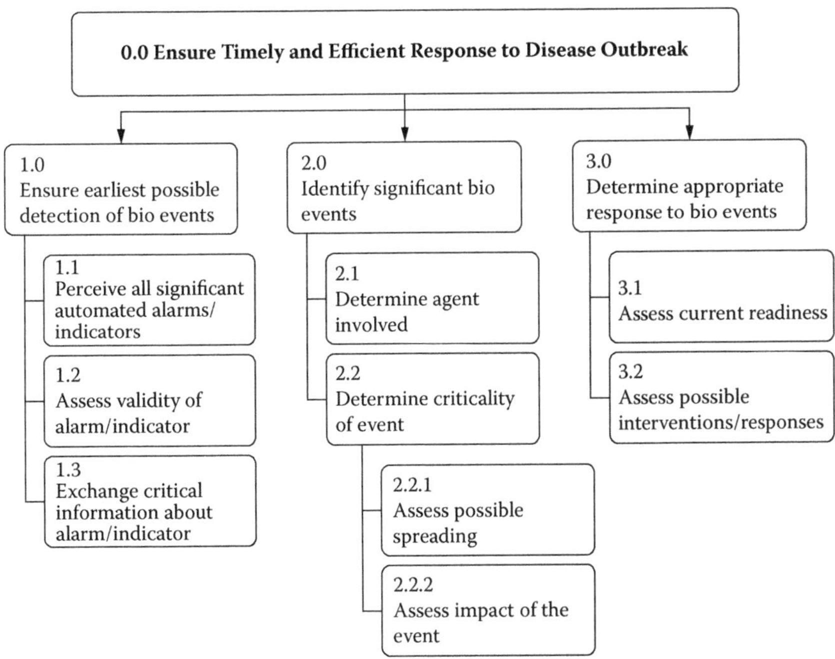

FIGURE 4.3
Hypothetical example of portion of a GDTA for the biosurveillance domain.

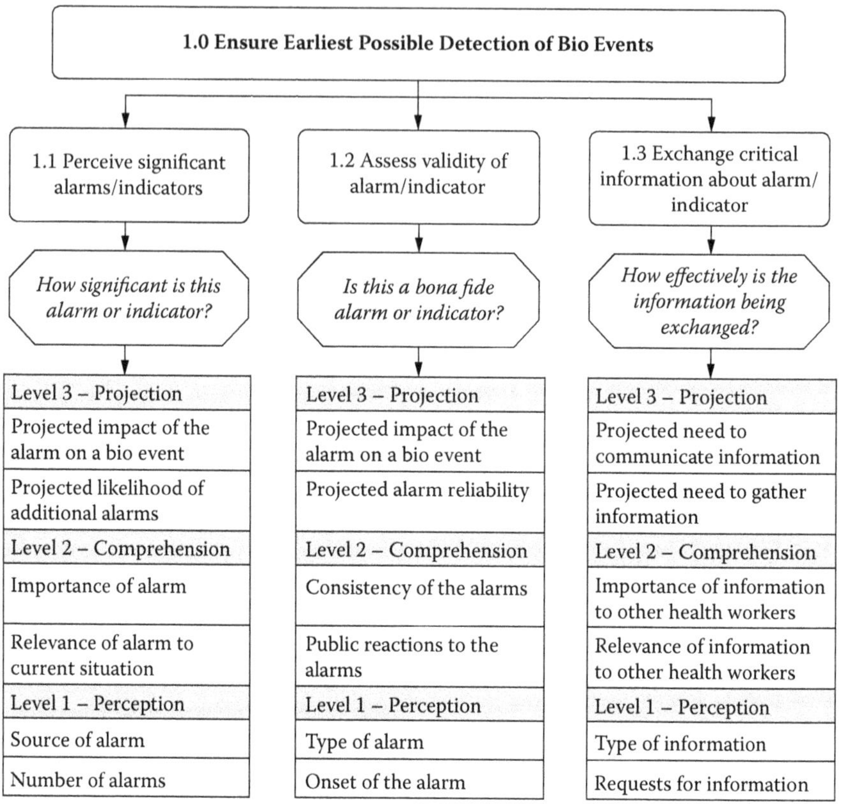

FIGURE 4.4
Hypothetical example of information requirements for a portion of a GDTA for the biosurveillance domain.

of the major challenges in biosurveillance is that the sources of data are infinite. As illustrated in the Milwaukee cryptosporidosis outbreak, both critical sources (e.g., emergency room reports) as well as noncritical sources (e.g., drug store sales on nonprescription drugs) of information are important. As such, biosurveillance systems need to include a broad range of information sources. Yet, the key to maximizing operational efficiency is to determine what information is significant and to validate this information, thus, avoiding collecting data that is not useful. The GDTA methodology can be used to isolate this essential data. In turn, applying SAOD principles (discussed next) will help ensure that biosurveillance systems are designed to optimally present this information to its users.

4.3.2 SA-Oriented Design Principles

The SAOD principles include a set of 50 design principles based on a theoretical model of the mechanisms and processes involved in acquiring and maintaining SA in dynamic complex systems (Endsley, Bolte, and Jones 2003). Supporting the SA of health professionals may be achieved by applying these principles to the design of biosurveillance systems. Because of the limited length of this chapter, we will not present all 50 design principles but will instead provide a few general guidelines based on a hypothetical biosurveillance system.

Organize information around goals. SAOD proposes that effective systems provide information organized around the major goals and subgoals, as identified in the GDTA. For our hypothetical system, three main goals and nine subgoals were identified (refer to Figure 4.3). One possible way to design a system is to create an interface with three separate modules based on the main goals. However, this would not lead to a very usable interface as some functions would be buried under several menu layers. A better approach would be to design a system focusing on the hypothetical subgoals that must be performed to support the top-level goals. Based on these subgoals, five general work areas can be identified: alerts, alert details, assets, readiness, and trends (see Figure 4.5).

The top-level screen lists all current country alerts that are clustered based on some user-defined parameters (e.g., location, type). The second tab decomposes the clustered alerts and provides detailed information on each individual alert, which is needed to determine validity and criticality. The third

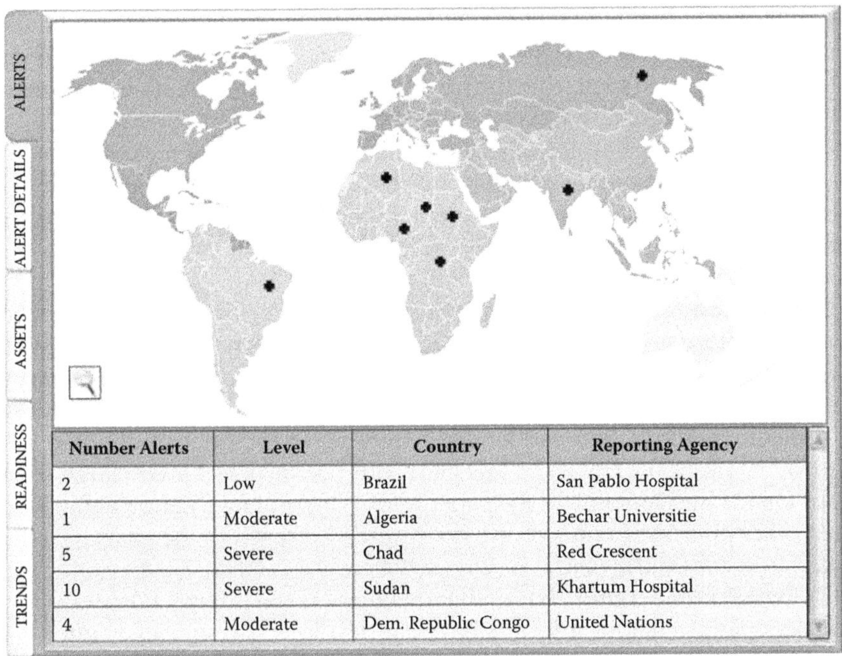

Number Alerts	Level	Country	Reporting Agency
2	Low	Brazil	San Pablo Hospital
1	Moderate	Algeria	Bechar Universitie
5	Severe	Chad	Red Crescent
10	Severe	Sudan	Khartum Hospital
4	Moderate	Dem. Republic Congo	United Nations

FIGURE 4.5
Interface example showing organization around goals.

and fourth tabs provide information on organization readiness and available assets needed to support Goal 3.0 "Determine appropriate response to bio events." The fifth tab provides trending information needed to support Level 3 SA. Additionally, the simplicity of the interface design helps promote team and shared SA as health professional can readily access the same information with ease and communicate this information in a similar fashion.

Present Level 2 SA information directly to support comprehension. System design needs to support interpreting and comprehending all incoming data. This includes mapping and interpretation of alerts, trend data, and environmental and organizational factors as well as being able to distinguish between false alarms and undiagnosed or unconfirmed events. The latter is particularly difficult as many biological events may be unfamiliar to users, and thus may not trigger a disease alert. Instead, each reported case must be interpreted with other information such as similarity to other cases, location of similar cases, and response of the nearby public and government organizations. For example, for common diseases, such as influenza, health professionals look for alarming trends in terms of outbreak rate and mortality. They expect some cases, but need to respond quickly if reports exceed a given threshold. Novel diseases, such as novel influenza A (H1N1), are much more difficult to detect. It took months, several thousand reported flu cases, and over 150 deaths before Mexican health officials realized that the flu symptoms, which villagers in La Gloria, Mexico, were displaying, were actually swine flu (CNNHealth 2009).

Provide assistance for Level 3 SA projections. Many systems do not provide the information needed to predict future states. This is a very demanding part of SA formation and one that novices and even some experts find difficult. As such, biosurveillance systems need to not only present data to support lower levels of SA (detection of a possible outbreak and understanding patterns or trends in the data), but, more important, higher levels of SA to determine the future impact of the information (predicting the future trends and distribution of the outbreak).

Explicitly identify missing information. One of the critical issues in system design is letting end users know both what information is missing and what information is being used in the analysis. For example, a biosurveillance system may provide an alert indicating a possible outbreak of cryptosporidosis in a major city based on a sudden large increase in pharmacy sales of antidiarrheal medications. However, this alert could be incorrect if two large pharmacy chains had coupons in the paper for this type of medication and if sales from other pharmacy chains were not recorded or used in the analysis.

Represent information timeliness. One of the problems facing health professionals is information recency, that is, the timeliness of the information presented. For example, latency of information from developing countries is often not optimal. Thus, health professionals need support for recalculating the current picture once they have received late data. They also need to be able to distinguish between new and past information and be alerted to the data's age as certain diseases can spread so rapidly that even a few hours can significantly reduce the data's usefulness and relevance for predicting trends.

Support assessment of confidence in composite data. Providing health professionals with confidence ratings for the accuracy of the information displayed will support their decision-making as well as alert them to when confirmation of the information is needed (e.g., a coding error for Crimean hemorrhagic fever instead of congestive heart failure). In addition, oftentimes, unreliable system performance (e.g., high false alarms) and lack of human interactions when using a system may be due to design issues that are caused by insufficient information standardization and management. System designs that focus on improving system reliability may mitigate such issues.

Use information filtering carefully. As more sources of data are brought into biosurveillance systems, more new sources are identified. Recently, more attention has been brought to loosely structured sources of data (such as news feeds, Internet search queries), which may offer much earlier detection than structured sources. However, an inherent problem with such sources is that users must sort through a great deal of noise to isolate the information that is most useful and relevant for their tasks. Nevertheless, the complexity of sorting through multiple data sources can be mitigated by designing the tool to carefully filter incoming information based on the goals and SA information requirements of users as identified using the GDTA methodology.

Build a common operating picture to support team operations. This can be accomplished by providing shared information displays and virtual collaborative spaces. Such tools are especially critical for health professionals in the field (e.g., local area doctors) to help establish a shared understanding of the situation. One current program, called Mesh4X by InSTEDD has been designed to support cross-organizational information sharing between different databases, desktop applications, Web sites, and devices (http://code.google.com/p/mesh4x). The system provides synchronization between different software and data types so that researchers can easily share and transfer data that is needed to build a common picture. Even providing a standard mapping tool such as Google Maps will help to build shared SA.

Avoid display overload in shared displays. Data overload is a common problem in many complex interface designs, including biosurveillance systems. The sheer amount and varying types of data that must be considered and analyzed by a biosurveillance system could easily cause the tool to be very cumbersome, complex, and difficult for the end user to utilize and develop good SA. Biosurveillance systems address this by the development of automated detection algorithms, which help focus the user's attention on potential threats, and visualization applications that seek to make patterns in the input data seem more obvious. Yet, the amount of data produced can still be quite difficult to manage. Thus, as noted earlier, to be maximally effective, biosurveillance system interfaces should organize this information around users' goals and critical SA information requirements.

Support transmission of different comprehensions and projections across teams. Tools need to allow sharing of intuitive assessments between biosurveillance personnel and other health professionals. Currently, data analysis and detection tools are not integrated with Listservs and other collaboration tools. Yet, understanding individual interpretations and team consensus is paramount to effective SA and decision-making performance.

4.4 Conclusions

The outcome of the Milwaukee cryptosporidosis outbreak in 1993 may have turned out differently if a syndromic system had been in place at that time that would have detected the outbreak from noncritical sources (e.g., unusually high sales of over-the-counter medications) (Cooper et al. 2006). From a global perspective, the growth of international travel and trade presents a real and significant challenge to effective management of disease outbreaks. Consider, for example, that after about a year following its initial outbreak in November 2002, SARS had spread to about 30 different countries, affecting approximately 8000 individuals. Yet, within just 2 months following its initial outbreak in April 2009, the novel influenza A (H1N1) virus had spread to 74 countries, with nearly 30,000 confirmed cases reported. Without question, timely and accurate detection and response to a potential disease outbreak in its early stages is absolutely essential to ensure both global public health as well as economic stability.

Yet, the development of biosurveillance systems is still in its infancy. To date, the majority of biosurveillance system design, analysis, and evaluation has been geared toward specific data sources and detection algorithms, but less effort has been put into how these systems will interact with their human operators. Yet, overlooking user requirements in the design process can lead to suboptimal human-system performance. Furthermore, not enough attention has been directed toward addressing how biosurveillance systems will support the information needs of dynamic ad-hoc teams composed of individuals working for different organizations, or how these systems will perform in an environment with numerous biosurveillance algorithms, which may provide contradictory interpretations of ongoing events. Companies such as InSTEDD are striving to develop more comprehensive integrated tools that can be effectively used across the broad spectrum of biosurveillance to enable health professionals to adapt to rapidly changing data (Kass-Hout 2008). However, progress toward realizing the full potential of biosurveillance systems is still limited.

To address these challenges, in this chapter, we argued that consideration of the role of SA in biosurveillance is an important design objective. Biosurveillance systems should be designed to support users' SA across all stages of a potential disease outbreak, from initial detection to response to control and management. In addition, systems must support not only the individual user's SA but also provide information to meet the shared SA requirements of the multiple stakeholders and communities of interest involved. We demonstrated how these objectives can be accomplished by applying the GDTA methodology to conduct an SA Requirements Analysis for end users and utilizing SA-Oriented Design Principles to create useful system interfaces. Although not discussed in this chapter, biosurveillance personnel and other health professionals would also benefit from training programs aimed at developing the skills that support their SA. Findings from GDTAs conducted with biosurveillance personnel would guide the specification of important training objectives for how best to support the SA needed to achieve their goals. In addition, training on the roles, methods, and concepts used by other members of the multidisciplinary ad-hoc teams inherent in the biosurveillance domain will facilitate distributed coordination as well as communication of critical shared SA information requirements. Taken together, well-designed user-centered systems and tools coupled with training targeted at essential SA skills can lead to improved decision-making performance and effective team coordination and, ultimately, ensure timely and accurate outbreak detection and management in biosurveillance.

References

Centers for Disease Control and Prevention (CDC). 2003, March. Update: Outbreak of severe acute respiratory syndrome—worldwide. *Morbidity and Mortality Weekly Report (MMWR)* 52(12): 241–48 [March 28, 2003], http://www.cdc.gov/mmwr/preview/mmwrhtml/mm5212a1.htm (accessed November 19, 2008).

Centers for Disease Control and Prevention (CDC). 2007. Public health needs for BioSense, http://www.cdc.gov/biosense/background.htm (accessed November 19, 2008).

Centers for Disease Control and Prevention (CDC). 2009. H1N1 Flu (Swine Flu), http://www.cdc.gov/h1n1flu/ (accessed May 29, 2009).

CNNHealth 2009. Earliest case of swine flu tucked away in Mexico, officials say, http://www.cnn.com/2009/HEALTH/04/8/swine.flu/index.html#cnnSTCText, (accessed April 29, 2009).

Cooper, D.L., N.Q. Verlander, G.E. Smith, A. Charlett, E. Gerard, L. Willocks, et al. 2006. Can syndromic surveillance data detect local outbreaks of communicable disease? A model using a historical cryptosporidiosis outbreak. *Epidemiology and Infection* 134: 13–20.

Endsley, M.R. 1993. A survey of situation awareness requirements in air-to-air combat fighters. *International Journal of Aviation Psychology* 3(2): 157–68.

Endsley, M.R. 1995. Toward a theory of situation awareness in dynamic systems. *Human Factors* 37(1): 32–64.

Endsley, M.R., B.Bolte, and D.G. Jones. 2003. *Designing for situation awareness: An approach to human-centered design*. London: Taylor & Francis.

Endsley, M.R., and W.M. Jones. 2001. A model of inter- and intrateam situation awareness: Implications for design, training and measurement. In *New trends in cooperative activities: Understanding system dynamics in complex environments*, ed. M. McNeese, E. Salas, and M.R. Endsley, 46–67. Santa Monica, CA: Human Factors and Ergonomics Society.

Fricker, R.D., Jr., B.L. Hegler and D.A. Dunfee. 2008. Comparing syndromic surveillance detection methods: EARS' versus A CUSUM-based methodology. *Statistics in Medicine* 27 (17): 3407–29.

Garrett, S.K., and B.S. Caldwell. 2009. Human factors aspects of planning and response to pandemic events. *Proceedings of the 2009 Industrial Engineering Research Conference*, 30 May–3 June 2009, in Miami, Florida.

Gibbs, S. 2009. Mexico economy squeezed by swine flu. *BBC News*, April 30, 2009, http://news.bbc.co.uk/2/hi/americas/8026113.stm (accessed June 7, 2009).

Gilmore, G.J. 2002. DoD database provides global tripwire for bio-terror. *American Forces Press Service*, December 2002, http://www.defenselink.mil/news/newsarticle.aspx?id=42379 (accessed June 17, 2009).

Heymann, D.L., and G.R. Rodier. 2001. Hot spots in a wired world: WHO surveillance of emerging and re-emerging infectious diseases. *Lancet Infectious Diseases* 1: 345–53.

Kass-Hout, T. 2008. What is biosurveillance? What is InSTEDD's role?, http://kasshout.blogspot.com/2008/01/biosurveillance.html (accessed November, 19, 2008).

Mac Kenzie, W.R., N.J. Hoxie, M.E. Proctor, M.S. Gradus, K.A. Blair, D.E. Peterson, et al. 1994. A massive outbreak in Milwaukee of cryptosporidium infection transmitted through the public water supply. *The New England Journal of Medicine* 331(3): 161–67.

Marley, C.T., M.E. Levsky, T. S. Talbot, and C.S. Kang. 2004. SARS and its impact on current and future emergency department operations. *The Journal of Emergency Medicine* 26(4): 415–20.

Mnatsakanyan, Z.R., S.P. Murphy, R.J. Ashar, and H. Burkom. 2007. Hybrid probabilistic modeling and automated data fusion for biosurveillance applications. *Advances in Disease Surveillance* 2: 58, http://www.isdsjournal.org/article/view/822/709 (accessed April 2, 2009).

National Public Radio. 2008. SARS timeline, http://www.npr.org/news/specials/sars/timeline.html (accessed November 17, 2008).

Rodman, J.S., F. Frost, and W. Jakubowski. 1998. Using nurse hot line calls for disease surveillance. *Emerging Infectious Diseases* 4: 329–32, http://www.cdc.gov/ncidod/eid/vol4no2/rodman.htm (accessed April 9, 2009).

Salas, E., C. Prince, D.P. Baker, and L. Shrestha. 1995. Situation awareness in team performance: Implications for measurement and training. *Human Factors* 37(1): 123–36.

Strater, L., S. Scielzo, M. Lenox-Tinsley, C.A. Bolstad, H.M. Cuevas, D.M. Ungvarsky, et al. 2009. Tools to support ad hoc teams. *Proceedings of the Advanced Decision Architectures Final RMB Workshop*, July 22–23, 2009, in Washington, DC.

Wagner, M.M., A.W. Moore, and R.M. Aryel. 2006. *Handbook of biosurveillance*. St. Louis, MO: Elsevier Science & Technology Books.

World Health Organization (WHO). 2009, June. World now at the start of 2009 influenza pandemic. Statement to the press by WHO Director-General Dr Margaret Chan, http://www.who.int/en (accessed June 11, 2009).

5

The Role of Zoos in Biosurveillance

Julia Chosy, PhD
Davee Center of Epidemiology and Endocrinology
Lincoln Park Zoo
Chicago, Illinois

Janice Mladonicky
Davee Center of Epidemiology and Endocrinology
Lincoln Park Zoo
Chicago, Illinois

Tracey McNamara, DVM
College of Veterinary Medicine
Western University of Health Sciences
Pomona, California

CONTENTS

5.1 Introduction

If you were to log onto YouTube and type in "moonwalking bear," a very interesting video would pop up. It shows two teams of people dressed in either white or black tossing around a basketball. You are asked to count the number of passes made by the white team. Many people focus intently on the video and get the correct answer, but when asked to review the tape again, they are shocked to find that a guy in a bear suit moonwalked across the crowd and they missed this entirely. How is it possible not to have seen something so obvious? How could something in plain sight be overlooked? Bombarded with information, the viewers had narrowed their focus on the ball alone. The voice-over ends with "It is easy to miss something you are not looking for."

One can draw parallels between this example of selective attention and the events surrounding the discovery of the West Nile virus (WNV) in the summer of 1999. Crows were dropping out of the sky, and yet it took an astonishing 2½ months before the link between the human and avian deaths was achieved. Many factors contributed to this delay, including the relative insensitivity of state wildlife agencies to animal die-offs, the paucity of diagnostic capabilities at the state wildlife lab level, the fact that the zoo birds that were critical to the investigation fell between jurisdictional cracks of federal agencies and so on. However, most of all, the diagnosis was missed because the key to the mystery lay not in people but in captive and free-ranging birds.

The WNV outbreak underscored the absolute need to look for disease threats across species. It highlighted our vulnerabilities when it comes to surveillance of free-ranging wildlife and pointed out the unfortunate exclusion of the private sector in biosurveillance efforts. Analyses of the outbreak emphasized the need to work across agencies, across species, at the local, state, and federal level, and the need to develop partnerships with nontraditional health partners.

Zoos, it turns out, are ideal long-term urban biosurveillance monitoring sites and are of great value to public health. Zoos have "situation awareness" of the biological threats in their area. They house a captive collection of animals that can serve as sentinels for many zoonotic threats at a known point source location. The valuable animals in their care are evaluated on a daily basis by zoo professionals and/or veterinarians. Medical records are maintained. Zoos also do active and passive disease surveillance of local wildlife that may be found on zoo grounds because they represent the threat of disease introduction. Because of their commitment to conservation efforts, zoos maintain serum and tissue banks that can prove critical to disease investigations. Necropsies are performed on all collection animals in accredited institutions. Most important of all, zoo surveillance is *sustainable* as disease surveillance is part of their everyday activities. Recent examples of the value of zoos in public health surveillance include the discovery of the first plague outbreak since 1968 in metropolitan Denver when the zoo submitted five squirrels and one rabbit for diagnostic evaluation in May 2007. Another example is the discovery that felids are susceptible to H5N1 influenza, known only because the zoo in Thailand performed necropsies and submitted tissues for diagnosis on dead tigers and leopards (Keawcharoen et al. 2004).

In this chapter, we describe a number of zoo initiatives that have proved to be beneficial to public health efforts. These programs leverage the activities routinely done in zoos, and, in doing so, they close at least one of the many surveillance gaps between human, agricultural, and nonagricultural species. There are too many proverbial balls in the air to have any level of comfort that the next emerging zoonotic threat will not be missed as has been the case in the past. It makes sense for public health entities to partner with the zoo community. As Laura Kahn stated in "Animals: The World's Best (and Cheapest) Biosensors" (Kahn 2007), "those of us who are truly concerned about early identification of emerging infectious diseases and bioterrorism should promote and encourage funding of programs such as the national zoo surveillance network and other programs that focus on the surveillance of nonagricultural species. Time and time again, they've proven to be the best and cheapest environmental biosensors around."

5.2 Association of Zoos and Aquariums (AZA) Ungulate Tuberculosis Monitoring Program

5.2.1 Infectious Agent

Tuberculosis (TB) is a chronic disease of mammals caused by bacteria of the genus *Mycobacterium*. The organisms can be found worldwide, generally living in water and food sources. There are many species of *Mycobacterium*, each with its own preferred hosts. For example, the reservoirs for *M. bovis* include cattle, dogs, and pigs, while *M. avium* is found most frequently in birds, pigs, and sheep. Humans are most often infected with *M. tuberculosis*, though this species can also be passed to nonhuman primates, cattle, dogs, pigs, and psittacine birds.

Transmission occurs through aerosol droplets or contact with infected animals or contaminated surfaces. TB can also be transmitted through ingestion of contaminated food, often unpasteurized milk, and products made from unpasteurized milk. Human-to-human transmission mostly occurs through aerosol droplets that are expelled into the air by coughing, sneezing, laughing, or talking. According to the World Health Organization (WHO), an untreated person with an active TB infection will infect an average of 10 to 15 people. Cases can be treated with approved antimicrobials. However, the course of treatment can take 6 to 12 months, and the emergence of extensively drug-resistant TB (XDR-TB) threatens the ability to treat the infection. The global mortality rate for TB is 1,577 per 100,000 persons. It is the most common bacterial cause of human death in the world (Colville and Berryhill 2007).

TB can cause asymptomatic infections in humans and animals if their immune systems are able to suppress bacterial replication. This is referred to as latent TB because the host remains colonized and symptoms can occur later if the immune system is no longer able to prevent replication. Approximately, 5% to 10% of people with latent TB will develop an active infection at some point in their lives. In people with active TB, symptoms often involve the pulmonary system and may include a productive cough, fever, bloody sputum, and chest pain. Some infections in humans are extrapulmonary, involving the central nervous system, vascular system, or other organs.

In cattle, TB can either be chronic or acute, depending on the host immune system and the dose of bacteria. Active infections are characterized by low fever, decreased milk production, weakness, anorexia, and progressive emaciation. There may also be respiratory symptoms and enlarged lymph nodes. Just as with humans, latently infected animals may become symptomatic if their immune system fails to control bacterial replication.

TB is a concern for zoological institutions primarily because it can cause morbidity and mortality in the animals in their collections, many of which represent endangered or threatened species (Lacasse et al. 2007). Additionally, the zoonotic nature of the disease presents a risk to zoo employees handling potentially infected animals. There is also concern among zoological institutions that strict regulatory measures for TB could be imposed. In the agricultural system, animals testing positive for TB are culled. This is not a favorable option for zoos. Further, restrictions may be placed on the transfer of animals across states lines due to concerns of introducing the disease to the agricultural industry. These apprehensions call for a reliable method of diagnosing TB in zoo species, which requires more information about the tests currently being used and their results.

5.2.2 Creation of the System

In 1996, several zoo elephants were diagnosed with active *Mycobacterium tuberculosis* infections (Michalak et al. 1998, Mikota et al. 2001). This led the Tuberculosis Committee of the United States Animal Health Association (USAHA) to recommend the creation of a working group to address the issue of tuberculosis in exotic animals. The result was the formation of the National Tuberculosis Working Group for Zoo and Wildlife Species, which brought together an interdisciplinary group representing the zoological, wildlife, regulatory, and diagnostic fields. This working group created two documents: *Guidelines for the Control of Tuberculosis in Elephants*, and the *Tuberculosis Surveillance Plan for Non-Domestic Hoofstock*.

The surveillance plan was meant to estimate the incidence and prevalence of the *Mycobacterium tuberculosis* complex (a group of mycobacteria including *M. tuberculosis, M. bovis,* and *M. avium paratuberculosis*; henceforth referred to as "TB") in zoological collections, gather prospective data on diagnostic tests for TB in order to establish sensitivity and specificity of the tests in exotic ungulate species, and provide guidance to state and zoo veterinarians in the case of exposure to tuberculosis-infected animals. The working group established a set of criteria for the system, including that it be Web-based and user friendly, and that it provide assurance of confidentiality, real-time summaries of data entered, and easy integration with other data/record keeping systems.

In order to obtain baseline information, a survey was sent to all AZA-accredited zoological institutions that currently or previously held ungulates. The survey was aimed at examining TB testing practices and establishing the prevalence of TB in zoo ungulate populations. The results demonstrated a prevalence of less than 5% (Ziccardi et al. 2000). However, testing practices varied across institutions. Given this variation and the fact that the diagnostic tests for TB are not validated for exotic species, it is difficult to accept this prevalence estimate with much certainty.

As a result of the survey findings, the AZA Ungulate Tuberculosis Monitoring Program was developed to create a mechanism by which long-term prospective data on testing methods and results could be collected across AZA institutions. Lincoln Park Zoo's (LPZ) Davee Center for Veterinary Epidemiology (now the Davee Center for Epidemiology and Endocrinology) constructed a Web site to house data from this surveillance and monitoring system. The goal was not only to collect the information laid out by the working group but also to establish a tool for the long-term monitoring of other diseases of importance to captive and free-ranging wildlife.

5.2.3 Structure and Implementation of the System

The AZA Ungulate Tuberculosis Monitoring Program was a voluntary program offered to all 210 AZA-accredited zoological institutions from 2003 until 2006. In order to make the system known to potential participants, announcements were made at the Animal Health Committee meeting at the annual AZA conference and at the general session and Infectious Disease Committee meeting at the annual conference of the American Association of Zoo Veterinarians (AAZV; Travis et al. 2003). Additionally, information about the program, including how to participate, was listed on both the AZA and the AAZV Web sites.

There were two ways to participate in the program. Information could be collected through a Web-based interface or by paper format that could be mailed or faxed to LPZ. The online database was secured with multiple firewalls and data encryption; access required a username and password acquired from LPZ. Confidentiality was an important part of the program as the consequences of announcement of TB found in a zoo could significantly affect gate receipts as well as the institution's ability to transfer animals to other zoos, as is often called for by AZA's Special Survival Plans (SSP) in order to maximize genetic diversity among zoo animals. Only two parties had access to all the data within the system: the project manager at LPZ and the system technical manager responsible for maintaining the Web site and database.

The intradermal tuberculin test is the primary screening test for TB in domestic hoofstock. However, no standard TB testing protocols were in place for zoological institutions, even though AZA and AAZV recommend testing for TB in zoo animals. The AZA Ungulate Tuberculosis Monitoring Program was designed to collect information on all possible test types for TB, including bacterial culture, PCR, histopathology, ELISA, and acid-fast testing. An additional open-ended data collection sheet allowed for descriptions of any other testing methods used.

5.2.4 Results

In its 3 years of operation, 17 zoological institutions representing 14 states participated in the monitoring system. These zoos submitted data on a total of 326 TB testing events for 278 animals, which represented 56 different species of ungulates.

The primary intradermal tuberculin test was by far the test of choice for TB, accounting for 87% of the test data submitted to the system. That percentage rises to 99% if secondary confirmatory intradermal tuberculin tests are included. The other test results submitted to the system were from histopathology examination and acid-fast testing.

Of the 278 animals, 4 (1.4%) reacted to the primary intradermal test, and 23 (8.3%) were suspect positive. Secondary confirmatory test data were submitted for 14 of the 23 suspect animals; 13 (93% of the confirmatory test results) were negative on the second test and one (7.1%) remained suspect positive. This suggests a low specificity for the tuberculin test in exotic ungulates, but additional data supporting this relationship are required to make this conclusion with certainty.

5.2.5 Evaluation of the System

In order to assess the degree in which the AZA Ungulate TB Monitoring Program met its objectives, a comprehensive evaluation was performed in 2008. As part of the evaluation, a survey was offered to all AZA institutions, regardless of their participation in the program. The survey was designed to collect relevant information suggested by a protocol designed by the National Animal Health Surveillance System (NAHSS) to evaluate animal health systems initiated by the U.S. Department of Agriculture (USDA; NAHSS 2006).

The results of the survey provided insight into the attitudes of zoo veterinarians about TB as a public health and regulatory concern, the perceived disease risk to zoo animals, and the importance of TB monitoring in zoos. A major part of the survey dealt with examining the reasons that contributed to or prohibited zoo veterinarians from participating in the program.

The survey drew 81 respondents, but only 74 of those had been employed at an AZA-accredited institution from 2003 until 2006. The data from the remaining seven were not included in the analysis. The 74 respondents represented 68 institutions. Overall, the survey results suggest that zoo veterinarians are concerned about TB as a public health and regulatory concern. They also expressed unease about the disease risk to zoo animals, especially when transferring animals to and from different institutions. However, according to the results, the importance of monitoring for TB in zoos was their greatest concern. If zoo veterinarians feel that TB monitoring is of value, why was participation in the Ungulate TB Monitoring Program so low?

According to the survey results, 34% (25/74) of respondents were unaware of the program. These respondents did report lower attendance at AZA and AAZV annual conferences (where information about the system was reported), yet 80% of these individuals were members of AAZV. Of the survey participants who were aware of the program, 69% (33/48) chose not to participate. The two primary reasons these respondents gave for not participating were lack of time and lack of resources. Additional reasons included animal safety concerns (the injection site for the tuberculin test must be palpated 72 hours after administration, requiring two separate handlings of the animal), confidentiality concerns, and the lack of an incentive. Similar reasons were given by the 32% (8/25) of respondents who were unaware of the program but reported they would not have participated anyway.

Among the survey respondents, 20% (15/74) had participated in the Ungulate TB Monitoring Program. The main reasons they cited for participating were that they felt it was an important objective to the AZA community, and they wanted to support AZA-sponsored health initiatives. Participants also indicated that they felt the objectives were important to their individual zoological institutions.

5.2.6 Lessons Learned

As the first national zoo-wide attempt to gather centralized information on a zoonotic disease, there were many lessons to learn from the TB Ungulate Monitoring Program and its evaluation. Perhaps the most important is why participation was so low. Approximately 66% of the target audience became aware of the program through fairly passive means (announcements at meetings and information on Web sites). This was all that was possible given the limited resources at LPZ. With greater funding, a person dedicated to communicating with the zoological institutions could have been hired. A more direct recruitment approach would have raised awareness and allowed for an opportunity for potential participants to have their individual questions answered. According to the evaluation, one recommendation for improving the system was to clarify the roles of government and private sectors in the regulation of TB control. Having a person committed to the role of "communicator" or "zoo-program liaison" would also have allowed for additional follow-up with participating institutions. This kind of support would have made the system easier to use and clarified its importance.

The two main reasons survey respondents said they did not participate in the program were lack of resources and lack of time. Though it is unlikely that funding would allow zoos to be paid for their participation, incentives such as free diagnostic testing might have encouraged more zoos to join the system. An additional benefit of offering testing at no cost would be data collection from a larger sample, thus adding power to the analysis of the sensitivity and specificity of available TB tests for exotic hoofstock. In order to reduce the time necessary to participate, collaborations with existing zoological data recording systems could be explored. Currently, many zoos use ARKS (Animal Record Keeping System) and MedARKS (medical record keeping). If the relevant information could be extracted from one of these systems for each institution, data entry on the part of the institution would be greatly reduced or possibly rendered unnecessary.

One issue that turned out to be a problem was the use of outside contractors to design, maintain, and host the Web site. When collaboration with the initial contractor was no longer possible, a second company had to be found to take over the maintenance and hosting of the Web site. The result of this transition was a period of 2 months during which the Web site was unavailable. Ideally, the project would have a dedicated programmer who would be responsible for this aspect of the system. Having someone on site would allow for a more tailored Web interface that could be rapidly updated or changed. This would also provide an additional layer of security for the data, as previously the companies maintaining and hosting the Web site had access to all the information in the database, though contracts in place detailed LPZ's ownership of the data and the code.

Another important lesson learned with this program was to establish sampling strategies to acquire the necessary sample size for analysis. Several survey respondents recommended increasing participation and devising sampling schemes for institutions with few hoofstock. Others suggested making the program mandatory, perhaps through collaboration with the AZA's SSPs, which recommend breeding pairs across institutions to maximize the genetic diversity of endangered species.

5.3. West Nile Virus Zoological Surveillance Project

5.3.1 Infectious Agent

West Nile virus (WNV) is a member of the *Flaviviridae* family of viruses. Like most members of this family, WNV relies on an arthropod vector, namely, the mosquito, to transmit infection from host to host. Over 60 separate species of mosquitoes have been found to be positive for WNV in the United States. However, not all are competent vectors. Members of both the *Culex* and *Aedes* genera of mosquitoes have been found to be proficient at transmitting WNV (Kilpatrick et al. 2005; Molai and Andreadis 2006). Birds are the most common host of WNV, though morbidity and mortality varies greatly across avian species (O'Donnell and Travis 2007). Mammals infected with WNV are considered "dead-end hosts" since viremia does not reach high enough levels to pass on the infection via mosquito bite.

The majority of humans infected with WNV show no observable clinical symptoms. Approximately 20% develop a mild, self-limiting illness known as "West Nile fever," whose symptoms include fever, headache, fatigue, muscle ache, and lymphadenopathy. In less than 1% of human infections, a more serious neuroinvasive condition develops that is characterized by meningoencephalitis with a mortality rate of almost 10%. This severe form of the disease is most commonly seen in persons over 50 years of age.

WNV was originally isolated from a febrile woman in Uganda in 1937. Over time, it was found to be a widely distributed across Africa, Asia, Europe, and the Middle East. Prior to 1999, the virus had never been seen in the Western Hemisphere. In August of that year, New York City began to observe unusual cases of encephalitis in humans (Briese et al. 1999). The initial diagnosis was St. Louis Encephalitis virus (SLE), a member of the *Flaviviridae* virus family commonly found in North America that occasionally causes illness in humans. However, at the same time, an abnormally high rate of bird mortalities was detected in the same area (Ludwig et al. 2002). While SLE does not generally cause disease in birds, necropsies performed on deceased animals showed pathology similar to that produced by SLE (Steele et al. 2000; Hansen et al. 2001). Dr. Tracey McNamara, the pathologist at the Bronx Zoo, performed these necropsies and sent tissue samples to the National Veterinary Diagnostic Laboratory (NVSL) in Ames, Iowa, for further testing. The virus was isolated and forwarded to both the Centers for Disease Control and Prevention (CDC) and the Armed Forces Institute of Pathology (AFIP). After sequencing and PCR analyses, the isolate was determined to be West Nile virus (McNamara 2007). Subsequent testing on isolates from human encephalitis patients demonstrated the presence of the same isolate (Lanciotti et al. 1999; Nash et al. 2001).

As WNV spread across the country, surveillance for the virus in zoological institutions became tremendously important. With some zoos having already lost valuable birds to the virus, anxiety grew at zoological institutions about how to protect the birds in their collections. Diagnostic testing for WNV in zoos was hindered by testing limitations in exotic species and the financial burden of having samples analyzed. Zoo veterinarians needed access to affordable, reliable diagnostic testing in order to assess and protect the health of animals in their collection, animals that often represent endangered or threatened species.

At the same time, public health officials were recognizing the potential value of zoos as sentinels for monitoring the spread of zoonotic infectious diseases. Reliable data gathered from this system could be a useful addition to national WNV surveillance. A further benefit would be the strengthening of the relationship between public and animal health agencies. A 2000 report to Congress from the Government Accountability Office (GAO) on the West Nile virus outbreak emphasized "the value of communication between public and animal health communities, the latter including those dealing with domestic animals, wildlife, and other animals such as zoo animals." The report went further to state that one of the five lessons learned from the outbreak so far was that "links between public and animal health agencies are becoming more important" (GAO 2000).

5.3.2 Creation of the System

In June 2001, LPZ in conjunction with the CDC hosted the National Zoological West Nile Virus Surveillance Working Group to discuss the design and implementation of a nation-wide surveillance system for WNV in zoological institutions. The meeting brought together zoo professionals with human and veterinary public health experts from local, state, and federal agencies. The result of the workshop was a set of guidelines entitled Surveillance for West Nile Virus in Zoological Institutions and the implementation of a 1-year pilot study. The system was endorsed by the CDC, the AZA, and the AAZV.

The pilot began in 2001 with six AZA-accredited zoos and aquariums with outdoor exhibits. However, as WNV continued to move west across the United States, zoos and other wildlife-related organizations became increasingly concerned about the safety of their animals. By 2003, the surveillance system had expanded to 130 participants. At its conclusion in 2006, nearly 180 zoological institutions, wildlife sanctuaries, private veterinarians, and animal rehabilitation centers had submitted samples as part of the system.

5.3.3 Structure and Implementation of the System

The WNV surveillance system for zoological institutions was a voluntary program that offered free WNV diagnostic testing for participants. It was initially offered only to AZA-accredited zoos and aquariums. As concern over the virus grew, the system was opened up to any zoo, regardless of accreditation. Eventually, the system began accepting samples from other groups with wildlife under their care. In addition to free diagnostic testing, the system was designed to increase communication between zoological institutions and their local public health departments, a benefit to both parties.

The WNV surveillance system included sampling for both active and passive surveillance components. Active surveillance consisted of obtaining blood samples from healthy collection animals during routine physical exams, preshipment quarantine, or other situations in which the animal was already being handled (e.g., banding, examination for injury).

For the passive surveillance component, samples were taken from sick or deceased outdoor birds and mammals that were part of the zoological collection. This piece of the surveillance methodology also included sampling of deceased wild birds found on zoo grounds. This was an important part of the system since the most sensitive surveillance tool for tracking the spread WNV had been the examination of dead wild birds (McLean et al. 2001). Zoos are in a unique position to test wild birds as many free-ranging animals utilize zoo grounds for seasonal or permanent habitat. This testing not only offers additional information regarding the presence of WNV but also provides zoological institutions with important information about health risks to the animals in their collection. For many outdoor exhibits, it is nearly impossible to prevent all free-ranging wildlife from accessing the interior.

In order to sample wild birds found on zoo grounds, permits must be acquired from the U.S. Fish and Wildlife Services (USFWS) under the Migratory Bird Treaty Act (MBTA).* In addition to this federal permit, some states require further permits in order to handle migratory birds. The MBTA, which was originally enacted into law in 1918, establishes broad restrictions to protect more than 800 species of migratory birds, their feathers, eggs, and nests. Even birds that are already deceased are protected under the MBTA. Originally, each institution had to acquire their own permits in order to test injured, sick, or dead wild birds found on zoo grounds. However, as WNV continued to spread and anxiety rose, a unique blanket permit was granted that allowed all participating institutions to sample deceased wild birds found on their grounds.

An additional component of the surveillance system consisted of a retrospective serosurvey for healthy outdoor animals that were part of the zoological collection. Participating institutions were asked to bank sera from healthy at-risk animals for later testing. These longitudinal data allowed an examination of seroconversion rates and susceptibility to WNV. Additionally, WNV-positive animals could be followed up to evaluate any potential long-term sequelae of infection.

The National Animal Health Laboratory Network (NAHLN) laboratory at Cornell University served as the primary diagnostic laboratory for the

* The Migratory Bird Treaty Act: http://www.fws.gov/laws/lawsdigest/migtrea.html.

system. This choice was optimal not only for the interest and willingness of the lab to participate but also because they had expertise in WNV testing and the ability to provide full-service diagnostic testing. Sample types requested by the diagnostic laboratory included blood (preferably serum) and tissue, including kidney, heart, and brain.

A major concern of participants was the privacy of the information gathered from their institution. When the media reported that WNV was found at the Bronx Zoo, gate receipts fell 30% (T. McNamara, pers. comm.). As most zoos rely heavily on their gate receipts for funding, it was understandable for institutions to have trepidation about testing for WNV on their grounds. As such, it was crucial to the system that data flow be precisely delineated so participants were ensured their data would remain confidential. The first step to protecting the data came from requiring the diagnostic laboratory to report test results directly to the submitting institution. Those data were also sent to a secure centralized database at LPZ.

The second step was to require the submitting institution to relay results to their local public health agency. This was meant to strengthen the relationship between zoos and their local public health authorities. An important aspect of this relationship was the sense of trust that would allow zoos to report results to public health agencies without fear of inappropriate release. This step was also essential as the response to an outbreak is much timelier if initiated at the local level.

The third step was to de-identify any data made available to the public. De-identified data from the LPZ database were summarized and made available to animal and public health agencies. In keeping with the goal of providing additional data to national WNV surveillance, the de-identified results from the surveillance system could also be uploaded into ArboNet, a cooperative database for WNV surveillance maintained by the CDC.

5.3.4 Results

The WNV surveillance system was well received by the zoological community, as well as rehabilitation centers, animal hospitals, and wildlife centers. Nearly 180 organizations representing 45 states and U.S. territories submitted samples to the system during its 5 years of operation. The response was so great that the NAHLN laboratory at Cornell University where the testing was taking place surpassed its maximum capacity. Many submissions had to be stored temporarily while the lab continued to process WNV samples. More than 17,800 samples were submitted for testing. This represented more than 14,000 individual animals, including approximately 10,600 birds, 3,300 mammals, and 150 reptiles. Furthermore, the system received multiple samples from more than 3,700 animals, providing an opportunity for longitudinal analysis.

Although virus isolation was the gold standard for confirmed WNV infection, the CDC later expanded the diagnostic case definition to include positive PCR results for the virus (CDC 2004). Of the animals tested, 1.8% were positive for WNV by virus isolation. An additional 3.7% were positive by WNV PCR. These combined results show that 5.5% of individual animals tested through the system were actively infected at the time of sampling. Furthermore, 12% of the animals tested were sero-positive, suggesting either exposure to the virus at some previous time or a history of WNV vaccination.

5.3.5 Lessons Learned

There were many lessons learned from the WNV surveillance system for zoological institutions that can be used to make future zoonotic disease surveillance in zoos more efficient and successful. The majority of these lessons revolved around data collection and entry. Each institution was instructed to complete two forms after sampling, (a) the standard sample information sheet for the lab, and (b) a short individual animal form, which collected demographic and clinical information about the animal that was sampled. Both of these were sent to the laboratory with the samples, at which point the lab would fax or mail the individual animal form to LPZ where it would be manually entered into an Access database. At Cornell, information about the sample was entered into their Laboratory Information Management System (LIMS). Once results were obtained, they would be entered into LIMS and then faxed to LPZ where they would be added to the Access database. As the program grew and system administrators no longer had the capacity, Cornell took over all data entry. Once all the samples had been tested, an attempt was made to join the two databases. Unfortunately, the merge was not smooth. An extensive amount of work was required to compile the information from both systems. This was a very clear lesson that data entry should take place at one location only.

Perhaps one of the largest difficulties with the database involved the institutional ID for the animals. Each zoological institution has its own format for assigning IDs to animals in their collection. These can range from fairly simple (e.g., "wallaby") to quite complex (e.g., 992201 N2002279). One issue that complicated data collection was slight variations in the way IDs were recorded across the submitted sheets and over time. For example, on the sample submission sheet, one zoo employee may write "Flaming 128" while another may write "128 Flamingo." Yet another may write "Flamingo_128." The database sees these as three separate animals. A great deal of work went into identifying entries that represented the same animal. In a similar regard, if the animal moved to a different institution, it was assigned a new ID according to the format used by the receiving zoo. Both zoos had to be contacted to get the old and new IDs in order to link records representing the same animal. This problem may be solved once the Zoological Information Management System (ZIMS) is complete. This system is meant to standardize data collection and animal records across zoological institutions.

Another problem encountered by the WNV surveillance system is one common to long-term disease studies: changes to the case definition of infection. At the start of the surveillance system, the CDC defined virus isolation as the sole means to identify WNV infection. As time progressed, PCR tests for WNV became more accepted and the case definition expanded (CDC 2004). Where possible, laboratory results had to be revisited to maintain a consistent case definition across the study period. Data collection for the surveillance system also suffered from other problems commonly seen in survey-based studies, namely, missing data, inconsistent interpretation of questions across institutions, and loss of information due to open text fields.

A very important lesson learned was to remember the capacity of the diagnostic lab before opening the system to too many participants. In the case of WNV where fears were stoked as the virus continued to expand its geographic range, the system grew quickly and the diagnostic lab became overwhelmed. In a less urgent situation, it would be easier to keep sampling to a minimum or to incorporate more diagnostic labs to help with the testing.

Finally, the importance of following up with participating institutions was made clear by the fact that many institutions did not report their test results to their local public health agency. When asked about this later, many participants said they did not realize it was their responsibility to report these results. Intermittent follow-up with the institutions would have ensured that they knew their responsibilities. Additionally, this would have allowed participants to have questions answered that they may have had about the system. At the time this system was operating, LPZ did not have the resources to provide follow-up contact to submitting institutions. However, in the future, this will be an important aspect of a successful surveillance system.

5.4. USDA APHIS AZA Management Guidelines for Avian Influenza: Zoological Parks and Exhibitors Surveillance Plan

5.4.1 Infectious Agent

Originally isolated in Hong Kong in 1999, highly pathogenic H5N1 avian influenza virus (HPAI H5N1) has since spread to 63 countries in Asia, Africa, and Europe. It is of concern because of its extremely high mortality rate in domesticated birds—mostly, chickens, ducks, and turkeys—and its ability to cause fatal infections in humans. As of August 2009, there have been 438 human cases of HPAI H5N1, 262 of which have resulted in death, representing a mortality rate of nearly 60% (WHO 2009). Though the highly pathogenic form of the virus has yet to be isolated in the Western Hemisphere, it could arrive via migratory birds or through the importation (legal or illegal) of infected birds (Kilpatrick et al. 2006).

HPAI H5N1 is an influenza A virus belonging to the *Orthomyxoviridae* family of viruses. Influenza A viruses can be classified by the combination of two separate surface antigens present on the virion: hemagglutinin (H) and neuraminidase (N). There are 16 different types of the H antigen and 9 types of the N antigen, providing for a broad range of possible viral strains. Because of the large number of different isolates and the interchangeability of these antigens, influenza A viruses are known to undergo antigenic shift, a process in which at least two different strains combine to form a new strain. In addition to this shift, the viruses undergo antigenic drift, the accumulation of random mutations resulting in an antigenic change. These processes give influenza A viruses the ability to mutate rapidly in a relatively short amount of time, a quality that is central to the concern over HPAI H5N1 becoming the next influenza pandemic.

Wild aquatic birds are the natural host for nearly all of the influenza A viruses, though they can occasionally be transmitted to other species. The natural host often shows no clinical signs of infection but can secrete large quantities of the virus in its feces for several weeks (Hulse-Post et al. 2005). Thus, the normal means of bird-to-bird transmission in the wild is through contact with contaminated water sources. With a highly pathogenic virus such as HPAI H5N1, the virus can appear in a flock of domestic poultry and rapidly kill 90% to 100% of the birds (OIE Avian Influenza Fact Sheet 2008). Bird-to-bird transmission in these cases occurs through direct contact with feces, respiratory secretions, and contaminated surfaces.

Transmission of HPAI H5N1 to humans appears to depend on close exposure to sick or dead poultry or, in a few cases, exposure to raw poultry products from infected birds (Perdue and Swayne 2007). The majority of the human cases were reported to have slaughtered or defeathered sick or dead poultry in the week prior to developing flu-like symptoms. Though a few family clusters of infections have shown some evidence of human-to-human transmission of the virus, it was limited and nonsustained (Writing Committee of the WHO Consultation on Human Influenza A/H5 2005, 2008). This is an important finding as the concern about HPAI H5N1 is that it will mutate to a form as easily spread from person-to-person as the seasonal flu, which could spark the beginning of another influenza pandemic. This pandemic would be of special concern if the mutated influenza isolate retained its high human mortality rate.

Surveillance for avian influenza in zoological institutions is important for the continual assessment of the health and safety of the animals in the collection. Many free-ranging birds, often waterfowl and shorebirds, find the grounds of zoological institutions to be an advantageous place to live. Plentiful food availability and protected areas offer the birds an ideal locale, and interaction between these free-ranging birds and zoo animals in outdoor habitats is inevitable. Therefore, it is critical to monitor for diseases transmissible by birds, as well as other free-ranging animals or insects that may come into contact with zoo animals.

For H5N1 avian influenza viruses, it is especially important for zoological institutions to be prepared. Current H5N1 vaccines have not been validated in exotic species and, since no set of standards currently exists for the future transport or release of vaccinated animals, the vaccine is not being offered to zoological institutions in the United States. Because of this, zoos will need to rely on maximum biosecurity measures balanced with the welfare of the animals (Redrobe 2007). This makes surveillance for H5N1 avian influenza viruses all the more critical for zoological institutions.

5.4.2 Creation of the System

In January 2006, LPZ hosted the National Avian Flu Surveillance Planning Meeting for Zoos. Organized and hosted by Dominic Travis, Vice President of Conservation and Science at LPZ, and Tracey McNamara, Professor of Pathology, Western University of Health Sciences, the 4-day meeting brought together representatives from the CDC, the USDA, the U.S. Department of the Interior (DOI), the AZA, state and local public health departments, zoo and university researchers, local wildlife experts, and human health professionals. The group drafted a plan to provide AZA zoos with standardized guidelines for the collection and testing of samples and to direct the distribution of data to researchers looking for signs of H5N1 in the United States.

The meeting highlighted the value of establishing a surveillance system for avian influenza across zoological institutions nationwide. With support from the USDA Animal and Plant Health Inspection Services (APHIS) and the backing of the AZA, LPZ created the Zoo Animal Health Network (ZAHN). The first initiative of ZAHN was to draft the USDA APHIS AZA Management Guidelines for Avian Influenza: Zoological Parks and Exhibitors, which would lead to the construction of a surveillance system for avian influenza in AZA institutions across the United States.

Building on the foundation established by the Ungulate Tuberculosis Monitoring Program and the West Nile Virus Zoological Surveillance Project, ZAHN is creating the infrastructure for a long-term disease surveillance system across zoological institutions. Though the initial system is designed to detect avian influenza viruses, it is being built with sufficient flexibility such that it can be easily and quickly adapted to other diseases of concern. This is an important aspect of the system given that 60.3% of emerging infectious disease events between 1940 and 2004 were zoonotic in nature, and the percentage of the events with wildlife as a source has increased from 43% to 52% over time (Jones et al. 2008). This is likely due to the increase in human–wildlife contact as the human population and agricultural demands expand.

5.4.3 Structure and Implementation of the System

The USDA APHIS AZA Management Guidelines for Avian Influenza Surveillance Plan will initially be open only to AZA-accredited institutions, though, if necessary, the program could be made available to other zoological institutions and animal exhibitors as defined by the Animal Welfare Act.* Participation in the system is voluntary and will offer several benefits to zoological institutions. In addition to free sampling materials and diagnostic testing, participating zoos will be integrated into the system framework such that they can easily participate in surveillance for future diseases of concern, providing them with an early warning of local disease introduction. Furthermore, the surveillance system is only one of three components of these management guidelines. The two others include outbreak management and vaccination plans. By participating in the surveillance component, zoological institutions will also be given assistance in creating an outbreak management plan tailored to their facility and will be eligible to apply to their State Veterinarian for avian influenza vaccination.†

The surveillance system combines both active and passive surveillance methods to detect avian influenza viruses in zoo birds. The active component is based on a statistically derived sample number to ensure with 95% confidence that the disease would be detected if it were present. For this system, a maximum of 25 birds per month could be sampled at each institution. Consistent with the disease ecology of avian influenza, sampling of Anseriformes, Charadriiformes, and Ciconiiformes are preferable, though the choice of birds to sample is at the individual zoo veterinarian's discretion. The passive component includes sampling of sick and dead birds in the zoo's animal collection. Additionally, if the participating zoological institution acquires the appropriate permits required by the Migratory Bird Treaty Act,‡ samples could be taken from sick, injured, or dead wild birds found on zoo grounds.

Sampling methodology for avian influenza follows that of the NVSL of the USDA, including oropharyngeal and cloacal swabbing. Additionally, intermittent serum collection is requested in order to allow for longitudinal data collection on seroconversion events. Diagnostic testing will be performed by laboratories in the NAHLN system of the USDA.

Data collection and storage will take place through a password-protected online data entry portal on the ZAHN Web site. The data will be housed in a secure server at LPZ. Each participating institution will have its own username and password to log on and enter the basic information for each sample sent to the NAHLN laboratory. Data entry screens will also be present

* An overview of the Animal Welfare Act: http://www.aphis.usda.gov/publications/animal_welfare/content/printable_version/animal_welfare4-06.pdf.

† Per the current draft of the USDA APHIS Vaccination Plan for HPAI for AZA Zoos, institutions must be conducting surveillance prior to being given permission to vaccinate animals in their collection for avian influenza.

‡ The Migratory Bird Treaty Act: http://www.fws.gov/laws/lawsdigest/migtrea.html.

to collect more in-depth information about the bird sampled and details about its enclosure environment at the zoo. If the institution does not have Internet access, data forms can be faxed or mailed to LPZ. By collecting these additional details, the system hopes to perform epidemiological analyses to determine whether certain characteristics correlate with the presence of avian influenza viruses.

Diagnostic results from the NAHLN laboratories will be sent to the database in real time via Health Level 7 (HL7) messaging. This is a technology of growing popularity among diagnostics labs, hospitals, doctors, and pharmacies that allows health information to be shared instantly among relevant parties. As such, participating zoological institutions will have the ability to log onto the ZAHN Web site and retrieve their sample test results as soon as they are known. Though each institution will have access to their results only, quarterly reports will be sent to all participants summarizing the findings to date, with identifying information removed prior to distribution.

5.4.4 Current Status

At the time of this writing, the USDA APHIS AZA Management Guidelines for Avian Influenza: Zoological Parks & Exhibitors Surveillance Plan is nearing the launch of its pilot operation. For the system, the country has been divided into three geographic regions, each with its own coordinator and NAHLN lab. For the pilot, one institution in each of the three regions is scheduled to begin sampling and submitting to their regional NAHLN lab for testing. Once the system is running efficiently, it could be opened up to all AZA-accredited facilities.

5.4.5 Future Directions

Once the pilot for the USDA APHIS AZA Management Guidelines for Avian Influenza: Zoological Parks & Exhibitors Surveillance Plan has launched and the system has been improved, it may be expanded to additional zoological institutions and NAHLN laboratories. The objective is to have enough participating institutions such that geographic coverage of the United States is sufficient to detect a disease wherever it may be introduced. If this infrastructure is already in place when the next zoonoti c disease of concern emerges, then the system will be swiftly modified in order to conduct surveillance for this disease. With a database and communication system already in place, the transition should be relatively smooth. Outbreak management guidelines for any new disease will be facilitated by the relationship each zoo has made with its animal and public health agencies at both the local and state level as a result of the AI Surveillance Plan.

While both the AI Surveillance Plan and the AI Outbreak Management Plan are in place, ZAHN will soon be working with the USDA and AZA to improve the current *USDA APHIS Vaccination Plan for HPAI for AZA Zoos*. This document will outline important information regarding vaccination efficiency and administration. Little is known about the effectiveness of AI vaccines in exotic animals or any risks that may be involved in the vaccination process. At present, no AZA-accredited zoological institutions are using an AI vaccine because the current Vaccination Plan states that zoos must be conducting surveillance in order to vaccinate.

In addition to progressing and improving the AI surveillance system, ZAHN will be working on a foreign animal disease initiative with the support of the USDA and the backing of the AZA. The goal is to create educational modules to teach paraprofessionals at zoological institutions how to recognize and prevent foreign animal diseases in the zoo. In the long-term future, ZAHN will continue to work toward strengthening the relationship between animal and public health experts in the hopes of protecting the health of humans and of wild and captive animals.

References

Briese, T, X Jia, C Huang, LJ Grady, and WI Lipkin. 1999. Identification of a Kunjin/West Nile-like flavivirus in brains of patients with New York encephalitis. *Lancet* 354:1261–1262.

CDC. 2004. Neuroinvasive and non-neuroinvasive domestic arboviral diseases. http://www.cdc.gov/ncphi/disss/nndss/casedef/arboviral_current.htm. Last accessed August 17, 2009.

Colville, JL and DL Berryhill. 2007. *Handbook of Zoonoses: Identification and Prevention*. St. Louis, MO: Mosby Elsevier Press.

GAO/HEHS-00-180-2000. 2000. *West Nile Virus Outbreak: Lessons for Public Health Preparedness*. http://www.gao.gov/archive/2000/he00180.pdf. Last accessed August, 2009.

Hansen, GR, J Woodall, C Brown, N Jaax, T McNamara, and A Ruiz. 2001. Emerging zoonotic diseases. *Emerg Infect Dis* 7(suppl. 3):537.

Hulse-Post, DJ, KM Sturm-Ramirez, J Humberd, P Seiler, EA Govorka, S Krauss, et al. 2005. Role of domestic ducks in the propagation and biological evolution of highly pathogenic H5N1 influenza viruses in Asia. *PNAS* 102(30):10682–10687.

Jones, KE, NG Patel, MA Levy, A Storeygard, D Balk, JL Gittleman, et al. 2008. Global trends in emerging infectious diseases. *Nature* 451(21):990–994.

Kahn, L. 2007. Animals: The best (and cheapest) biosensors. *Bulletin of Atomic Scientists* March 13.

Keawcharoen, J, K Oraveerakul, T Kuiken, RAM Fouchier, A Amonsin, Payungporn, et al. 2004. Avian influenza H5N1 in tigers and leopards. *Emerg Infect Dis*. [serial on the Internet]. 2004 Dec [date cited]. Available from http://www.cdc.gov/ncidod/EID/vol10no12/04–0759.htm.

Kilpatrick, AM, AA Chmura, DW Gibbons, RC Fleischer, PP Marra, and P Daszak. 2006. Predicting the global spread of H5N1 avian influenza. *PNAS* 103(51): 19368–19373.

Kilpatrick, AM, LD Kramer, SR Campbell, EO Alleyne, AP Dobson, and P Daszak. 2005. West Nile virus risk assessment and the bridge vector paradigm. *Emerg Infect Dis* 11(3):425–429.

Lacasse, C, K. Terio, MJ Kinsel, LL Farina, DA Travis, R Greenwald, et al. 2007. Two cases of atypical mycobacteriosis caused by *Mycobacterium szulgai* associated with mortality in captive African elephants. *J Zoo Wildlife Med* 38(1):101–107.

Lancioota, RS, JT Roehrig, V Deubel, J Smith, M Parker, K Steele, et al. 1999. Origin of the West Nile virus responsible for an outbreak of encephalitis in the northeastern United States. *Science* 286:2333–2337.

Ludwig, GV, PP Calle, JA Mangiafico, BL Raphael, DK Danner, JA Hile, et al. 2002. An outbreak of West Nile virus in a New York City captive wildlife population. *Am J Trop Med Hyg* 67(1):67–75.

McLean, RG, SR Ubico, DE Docherty, WR Hansen, L Sileo, and TS McNamara. 2001. West Nile virus transmission and ecology in birds. In West Nile Virus: Detection, Surveillance, and Control. *Ann New York Acad Sci* 951:54–57.

McNamara, T. 2007. The role of zoos in biosurveillance. *Int Zoo Yb* 41:12–15.

Michalak, K, CA Austin, S Diesel, JM Bacon, P Zimmerman, and JN Maslow. 1998. *Mycobacterium tuberculosis* infection as a zoonotic disease: transmission between humans and elephants. *Emerg Inf Dis* 4(2):283–287.

Mikota, SK, L Peddie, J Peddie, R Isaza, F Dunker, G West, et al. 2001. Epidemiology and diagnosis of *Mycobacterium tuberculosis* in captive Asian elephants. *J Zoo Wild Med* 32(1):1–16.

Molaei, G and TG Andreadis. 2006. Identification of avian- and mammalian-derived bloodmeals in *Aedes vexans* and *Culiseta melanura* (Diptera: *Culcidae*) and its implication for West Nile virus transmission in Connecticut. *J Med Entomol* 43(5):1088–1093.

Nash, D, F Mostashari, A Fine, J Miller, D O'Leary, K Murray, et al. 2001. The outbreak of West Nile virus infection in the New York City area in 1999. *NEJM* 244:1807–1814.

National Animal Health Surveillance System (NAHSS). 2006. Surveillance and data standards for USDA/APHIS/Veterinary Services. http://www.aphis.usda.gov/vs/nahss/docs/surveillance_standards_chapter1_planning_surveillance_systems_v1.0_july_2006.pdf. Last accessed on August 17, 2009.

O'Donnell and D Travis. 2007. West Nile virus. *Int Zoo Yb* 41:75–84.

OIE Avian Influenza Fact Sheet. 2008. http://www.oie.int/eng/ressources/AI-EN-dc.pdf. Last accessed on August 17, 2009.

Perdue, ML and DE Swayne. 2005. Public health risk from avian influenza viruses. *Avian Dis* 49:317–327.

Redrobe, SP. 2007. Avian influenza H5N1: a review of the current situation and relevance to zoos. *Int Zoo Yb* 41:96–109.

Steele, KE, MJ Linn, RJ Schoepp, N Komar, TW Geisbert, RM Manduca, et al. 2000. Pathology of fatal West Nile virus infections in native and exotic birds during the 1999 outbreak in New York City. *Vet Pathol* 37:208–224.

Travis, DA, RB Barbiers, and MH Ziccardi. 2003. An overview of the national zoological tuberculosis monitoring system for hoofstock. American Association of Zoo Veterinarians. Minneapolis, MN.

WHO. 2009. Confirmed human cases of avian influenza A(H5N1). http://www.who.int/csr/disease/avian_influenza/country/en/. Last accessed August 17, 2009. Figures are from the August 11, 2009, report; case counts are updated regularly.

Ziccardi, M, SK Mikota, RB Barbiers, TM Norton, PK Robbins, and the National Tuberculosis Working Group for Zoo and Wildlife Species. 2000. Tuberculosis in zoo ungulates: survey results and surveillance plan. Proceedings of the AAZV and IAAAM Joint Conference. pp. 438–411.

6

HealthMap

Amy L. Sonricker, MPH
Children's Hospital Boston
Computational Epidemiology Group
Children's Hospital Boston Informatics Program
Boston, Massachusetts

Clark C. Freifeld
Children's Hospital Boston
Computational Epidemiology Group
Children's Hospital Boston Informatics Program
Boston, Massachusetts

Mikaela Keller, PhD
Children's Hospital Boston
Computational Epidemiology Group
Children's Hospital Boston Informatics Program
Department of Pediatrics, Harvard Medical School
Boston, Massachusetts

John S. Brownstein, PhD
Children's Hospital Boston
Computational Epidemiology Group
Children's Hospital Boston Informatics Program
Department of Pediatrics, Harvard Medical School
Boston, Massachusetts

CONTENTS

6.1 Introduction

A freely accessible, automated electronic information system, HealthMap was developed in 2006 for organizing data on outbreaks according to geography, time, and infectious disease agent (Brownstein et al. 2008). This organization of data provides a structure to information flow that would otherwise be overwhelming or would obscure important elements of a disease outbreak (Keller et al. 2009). HealthMap relies on a variety of electronic media sources, including online news sources through aggregators such as Google News, expert-curated discussion such as ProMED-mail, and validated official reports from organizations such as the World Health Organization (WHO) (Brownstein et al. 2008).

6.2 Data Acquisition

Currently, the HealthMap system collects reports from 21 sources, which in turn represent information from more than 20,000 Web sites, every hour, 24 hours a day allowing for real-time intelligence. An average of 300 reports per day are collected, with approximately 85.1% acquired from news media sources. Internet search criteria include disease names, symptoms, keywords, and phrases (Brownstein et al. 2008). Fully automated, the system uses text-mining algorithms to determine the disease category and location of the outbreak. Alerts, defined as information on a previously unidentified or currently ongoing outbreak, are geocoded to the country scale with province-, state-, or city-level resolution for select countries. Surveillance is conducted in several languages, including English, Spanish, French, Russian, Chinese, Portuguese, and Arabic (Keller et al. 2009).

In order for the system to organize alerts by infectious disease agent, it draws from a continually expanding dictionary of pathogens (human, plant, and animal diseases) (Brownstein et al. 2008). Since words may have multiple spellings, for example, the American "diarrhea" and the British "diarrhoea," this dictionary is continuously expanding with multiple patterns (Freifeld et al. 2008).

As shown in Figure 6.1, the HealthMap system gathers alerts, classifies them by location and disease, stores them into a database, and then displays them to the user. As raw data are loaded from the Web, it is converted into a standard "alert" format. This standard format consists of a headline, alert issue date, brief summary of the alert, and text that is fed into a parsing engine for an initial classification. The classification engine determines the principal diseases and locations associated with an alert. Upon being classified by disease and location, the alerts are stored within a database designed primarily to support features of the HealthMap Web application, however, also remain readily accessible for retrospective epidemiological studies, public health risk mapping, and other research applications (Freifeld et al. 2008).

More simply put, the HealthMap system characterizes disease outbreak reports by utilizing a series of text mining algorithms, including the disease and location extraction described previously, in addition to algorithms that determine the relevance of the alert (whether a report refers to a current disease outbreak), and groups together similar alerts while also removing duplicates (Figure 6.2) (Brownstein et al. 2008). After categorization by location and disease, articles are automatically tagged according to their relevance. Tags include (1) breaking news (e.g., a newly discovered outbreak), (2) warning (initial concerns of disease emergence, e.g., in a natural disaster area), (3) old news (reference to a

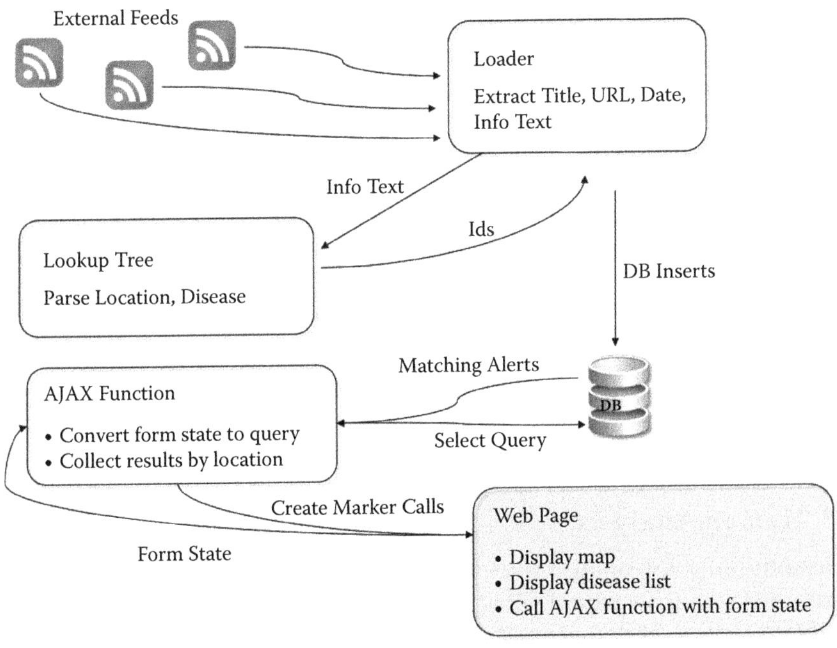

FIGURE 6.1
HealthMap System Architecture.

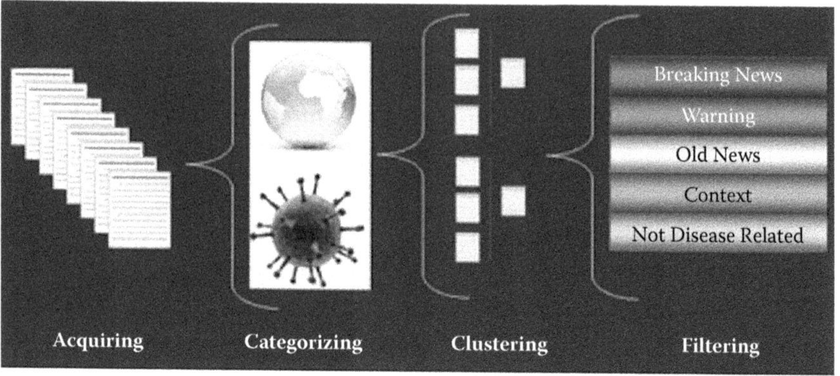

FIGURE 6.2
Stages of HealthMap surveillance. (1) Web-based data are acquired from a variety of Web sites every hour, 7 days a week (ranging from rumors on discussion sites to news media to validated official reports). (2) The extracted articles are then categorized by pathogen and location of the outbreak in question. (3) Articles are then analyzed for duplication and content. Duplicate articles are removed; while those that discuss new information about an ongoing situation are integrated with other related articles and added to the interactive map. (4) Once classified, articles are filtered by their relevance into five categories. Only articles tagged as "breaking news" or "warning" are added as markers to the map. (From Brownstein, J. et al. 2008. Surveillance Sans Frontieres: Internet-Based Emerging Infectious Disease Intelligence and the HealthMap Project. *PLoS Med* 5 (7):6. With permission.)

past outbreak), (4) context (information on disease context, e.g., preparedness planning), and (5) not disease-related (information not relating to any disease [3–5 are hidden from the main HealthMap user interface]) (Brownstein et al. 2008; Keller et al. 2009). Another category recently added is applied to alerts that may constitute a public health event of international significance per the WHO Interim Guidance for the use of Annex 2 of the International Health Regulations (2005) (WHO 2008). Alerts tagged as internationally significant are automatically e-mailed to HealthMap users who have opted to receive these notifications. Finally, once the automated process is complete, an analyst corrects misclassifications where necessary (Brownstein et al. 2008).

6.3 Human Analysis

Currently, only one analyst works to review and correct the posts; however, additional resources would allow for more detailed multilingual curation of collected reports (Brownstein et al. 2008). Misclassifications such as incorrect tagging (e.g., "breaking" versus "context"), incorrect geographic location, and/or incorrect disease classifications occur occasionally, and are manually amended. At a basic level, the accuracy of the HealthMap classifier can be measured by the percentage of reports entering the system that need not have their classifications corrected in any way. In more detailed analysis, the number of alerts requiring a correction of disease classification as compared with the number requiring a location correction can be examined. These analyses of manual corrections allows for the overall accuracy of the system to be continuously studied (Freifeld et al. 2008).

In addition to correcting misclassifications, the human analyst adds precise location information when that level of information is available within a given alert. In summary, although HealthMap currently relies on significant manual curation, one future objective of the system is to maximize automation, in order to minimize laborious classifications and leverage the human contribution (Freifeld et al. 2008).

6.4 Data Dissemination

Reducing information overload and providing users with news of immediate interest is of particularly high importance to HealthMap. The filtering and visualization features of HealthMap serve to bring structure to an otherwise overwhelming amount of information, enabling the user to quickly and easily find those elements pertinent to his or her area of interest. Since not all information collected has relevance to every user, only articles classified as "breaking" and "warning" are posted to the HealthMap Web site in order to provide focused news of immediate interest (Brownstein et al. 2008; Keller et al. 2009; Freifeld et al. 2008).

After being collected, the data are aggregated by source, disease, and geographic location and then overlaid on to an interactive map (Keller et al. 2009). The user controls within the interactive map include the ability to select which data feeds (sources), diseases, and geographical regions are displayed (Keller et al. 2009). Clicking on a country name zooms the map view to that country for easy viewing of alerts in that specific location. A date slider below the map allows the user to control the date range of displayed alerts. The user can set a start and end date at any point in the previous 30 days. "Full Screen" mode expands the map to cover the full browser window, allowing for richer visual display and navigation. Lastly, the color of each marker on the map indicates the "Heat Index" value for the location, with the deeper red color indicating more intense recent activity as contrasted by the paler yellow color (Freifeld et al. 2008). This "Heat Index," or composite activity score, is calculated based on both the reliability of the data source and the number of unique data sources. Alerts from governmental agencies (e.g., CDC, EuroSurveillance), international organizations (e.g., WHO), and expert-moderated services (e.g., ProMED-mail, CIDRAP) typically provide

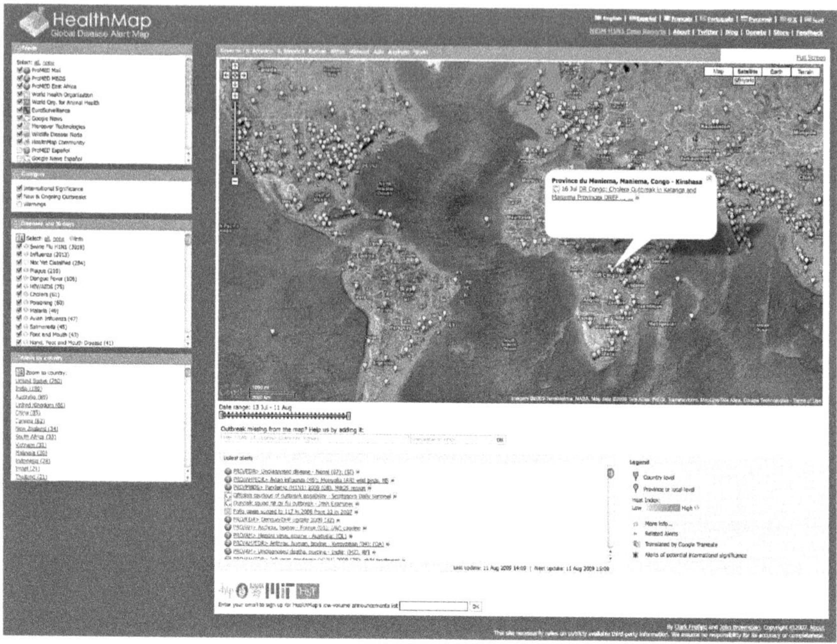

FIGURE 6.3
HealthMap main page user interface. (From http://www.healthmap.org. Clark Freifield and John Brownstein. 8/21/2009. With permission.)

more reliable information, and are therefore more heavily weighted than local media alerts in the composite activity score. This "meta-alert" score is based on the idea that multiple sources of information about a particular incident provide greater confidence in the reliability of the report than any one source alone (Brownstein et al. 2008).

In addition to an interactive map, the main page of HealthMap (Figure 6.3) features an interface with a variety of information boxes. Details such as the number of active alerts in each country and a list of the most recent alerts in reverse chronological order are given. Finally, as shown in Figure 6.4, each alert is linked to a related information window with details on reports of similar content as well as recent reports concerning either the same disease or location and links for further research (Keller et al. 2009).

6.5 Goals of HealthMap Program

A primary goal of the HealthMap program is to deliver real-time intelligence on emerging infectious diseases to a diverse audience (Brownstein et al. 2008). While some projects such as GPHIN and ProMED work more specifically

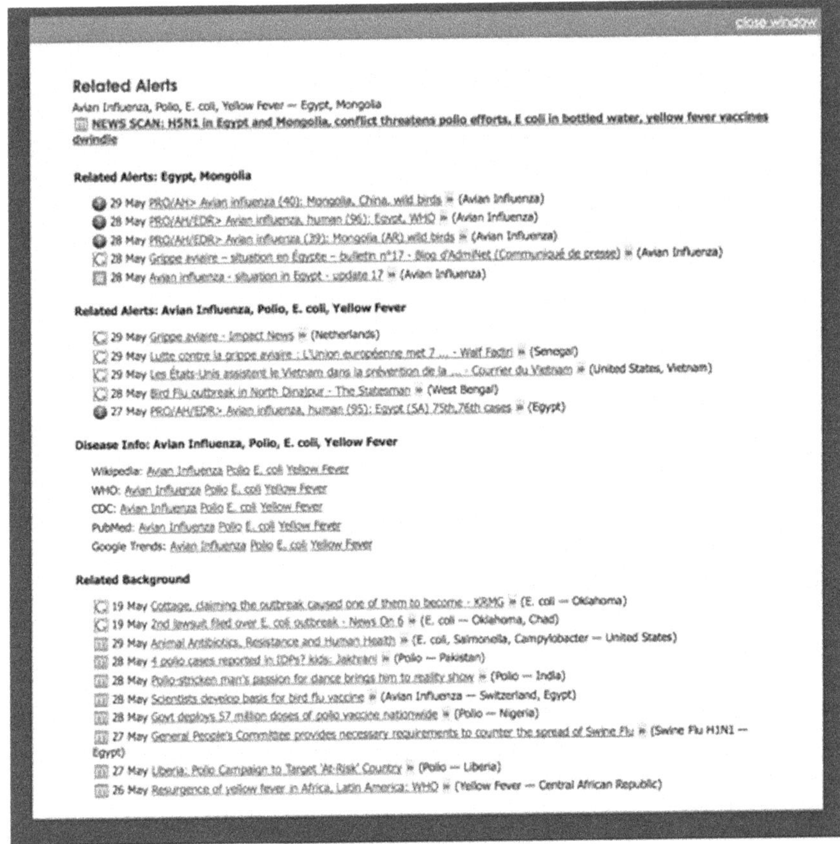

FIGURE 6.4
HealthMap Situation Awareness Window. (From http://www.healthmap.org. Clark Freifield and John Brownstein. 8/21/2009. With permission.)

All articles related to a given outbreak are aggregated by text similarity matching in order to provide a situation awareness report. Furthermore, other outbreaks occurring in the same geographic area or involving the same pathogen are provided. The window also provides links to further research on the subject. In this example, we show pertinent information relating to the diseases (arian influenza, polio, e.coli, and yellow fever) and locations (Egypt and Mongolia) in original alert.

to serve public health authorities, infectious disease Web sites that serve the general public are increasing in popularity. These sites are helping to increase awareness of public health issues, especially for international travelers. As part of this new generation of online resources, HealthMap brings together automated processing of a broad range of Internet data sources and rich, accessible visualization tools for laypeople and public health professionals alike (Freifeld et al. 2008). The HealthMap system is currently utilized as a direct information source for libraries, schools of public health, local health departments, governments, and multinational agencies (Brownstein et al. 2008).

Another goal of the HealthMap program is to leverage nontraditional sources of surveillance data. An enormous amount of valuable information about infectious diseases is found in nontraditional Web-accessible information sources such as discussion sites, disease reporting networks, and news outlets. These resources often support situation awareness by providing current, highly localized information about outbreaks, even from areas relatively invisible to traditional global public health efforts. The availability of Web-based news media thus provides an alternative public health information source in under-resourced areas. In addition, these data sources hold tremendous potential to initiate epidemiologic follow-up studies, provide complementary epidemic intelligence context to traditional surveillance sources, and support increasing public awareness of disease outbreaks prior to their formal recognition. Ultimately, the use of nontraditional sources of surveillance data can provide an integrated and contextualized view of global health information (Brownstein et al. 2008).

A third important goal of the system is to cover as broad a range of geography and disease as possible, without bias toward particular regions or pathogens. Since HealthMap currently relies heavily on the United States edition of Google News for reports, the system is biased toward the United States and Canada as well as other English-speaking countries around the world. However, to address this problem, HealthMap has expanded to other languages and data sources as resources have permitted (Freifeld et al. 2008). Information is now also monitored in Chinese, Spanish, Russian, French, Arabic, and Portuguese, with additional languages under development (Brownstein et al. 2008). Through HealthMap's multistream approach, integrating outbreak data from multiple electronic sources, HealthMap is able to present a unified and comprehensive view of global infectious disease outbreaks in space and time (Keller et al. 2009).

In regard to the range of pathogens, HealthMap was designed to obtain comprehensive coverage of disease activity, encompassing diseases of animals and plants, as well as some insect pests and other invasive species. This broad disease coverage is of particular importance, as many infectious diseases of public health concern are zoonotic, naturally circulating among wildlife reservoir hosts before emerging in the human population (Freifeld et al. 2008).

6.6 System Benefits

One important benefit of the HealthMap system is that it is a freely accessible, automated resource. Whereas some systems are currently closed, requiring either paid subscription or approved access, HealthMap is freely available to the public without subscription fees (Freifeld et al. 2008; Brownstein et al. 2008). The system has even been featured in mainstream media publications, such as Wired News and Scientific American, indicating the broad utility of such a system that extends beyond public health practice (Keller et al. 2009).

Additionally, the system is fully automated, acquiring data every hour and utilizing text-mining algorithms to characterize reports. With full automation, minimal staff are needed to accomplish the primary aims of HealthMap, and focus can be placed on system-wide improvements and ongoing research (Keller et al. 2009).

The ability of HealthMap to organize data according to geography, time, and infectious disease agent is yet another benefit to this system. The system automatically queries, filters, integrates, and creates a visualization of Web-based reports on infectious disease outbreaks. This structured visualization of outbreaks onto an interactive map gives users the ability to quickly and easily focus in on specific areas of interest.

6.7 Limitations

One limitation to the HealthMap system is that sources that are currently freely available may not always be accessible. As business models change, news sources may begin to charge an online subscription fee. Currently, operational costs remain minimal for HealthMap, as reports are acquired solely from free sources. In addition to potential increases in cost, the format that online news has taken may change and develop in the upcoming years, which would require a retooling of the system in order to continue to capture the appropriate information (Brownstein et al. 2008).

The use of international news media for public health surveillance has a number of potential biases that warrant consideration. While local news sources may report on incidents involving a few cases that would not be picked up at the national level, such sources may be less reliable, lacking resources and public health training, and may report stories without adequate confirmation. Other biases may be more intentional such as those introduced for political reasons through disinformation campaigns or state censorship of information relating to outbreaks (Brownstein et al. 2008). There may also be economic incentives for countries to not fully disclose the nature and extent of an outbreak (Wilson and Brownstein 2009). Through a 43-week evaluation of HealthMap data, it was found that the frequency of reports about particular pathogens was related to the direct or potential economic and social disruption caused by the outbreak versus the associated morbidity or mortality impact (Brownstein et al. 2008).

In addition, there is a clear bias toward increased reporting from countries with higher numbers of media outlets, more developed public health resources, and a greater availability of electronic communication infrastructure (Brownstein et al. 2008). Surveillance capacity for infectious disease outbreak detection can be costly, and many countries lack the public health infrastructure to even identify outbreaks at their earliest stages (Wilson and Brownstein 2009). Critical gaps exist, for example, in media reporting in tropical and lower-latitude areas, including major parts of Africa and South America—the very regions that have the greatest burden and risk of emerging infectious diseases (Brownstein et al. 2008).

Another limitation with HealthMap's current system is in its use of a dictionary of known locations and diseases. This dictionary limits the system to what is already known. Enhancing the system consists of augmenting the database by capturing correct locations and disease names, often involving careful manual data entry. The system must also be manually updated to reflect new geography, albeit infrequently, as national borders shift and names of places change (Freifeld et al. 2008).

One final important limitation is HealthMap's use of unstructured, free text information. While Web-based electronic information sources are potentially useful, information overload and occasional difficulties in distinguishing "signal from noise" pose substantial barriers to fully utilizing this information. In addition, public awareness of these "signals," if they are openly accessible, could create problems in terms of risk communication for public health officials. While HealthMap works to address the computational challenges of utilizing such unstructured data by generating meta-alerts of disease outbreaks, further in-depth evaluation is required with respect to false positives and gaps in coverage (Brownstein et al. 2008; Wilson and Brownstein 2009).

6.8 System Utilization during a Disease Outbreak (Novel Influenza A (H1N1))

In early April 2009, HealthMap's Spanish-language system collected and disseminated a local media report describing evidence of an epidemic of acute respiratory infections in La Gloria, Veracruz, Mexico (April 1, 2009, see Figure 6.5) (Brownstein, Freifeld, and Madoff 2009). It was estimated in the report that 60% of the town's 3000 inhabitants had been infected and that two had died since early March 2009 (Morales 2009). This was followed by a second report on April 2, 2009, which discussed the possible role of a United States–owned pig farm in the epidemic (Martinez 2009). Reports of this outbreak did not appear in English-language media until weeks later (April 21, 2009) when two unrelated children in California were confirmed to have Influenza A, H1N1 without prior exposure to pigs. The timeline of reports of this emerging novel infection emphasizes the importance of surveillance of

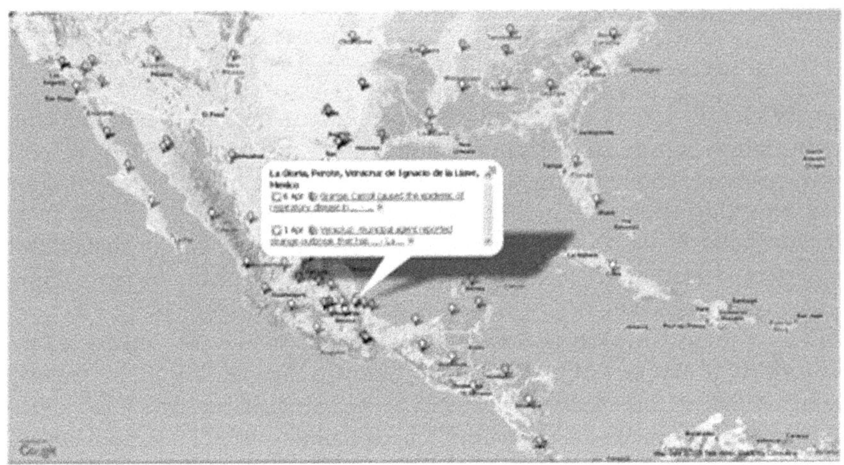

FIGUZRE 6.5
The balloon shows the initial reports from La Gloria, Veracruz. The markers represent locations where there have been unofficial reports about suspected or confirmed cases of novel influenza A (H1N1) (not the individual cases themselves) as well as other reports of influenza and other respiratory illness. Darker markers indicate increased recent report volume. (From http://www.healthmap.org. Clark Freifield and John Brownstein. 8/21/2009. With permission.)

local-level information in local languages (Brownstein, Freifeld, and Madoff 2009).

In addition to being among the first organizations to pick up Spanish-language reports of novel influenza A (H1N1), HealthMap used social networking tools to disseminate information regarding the rapid development of the outbreak. Twitter (http://twitter.com), for example, provides a real-time messaging service that allows people to follow the sources most relevant to them and to access information as it is posted. HealthMap utilized Twitter as a tool to inform HealthMap "followers" of news updates and alerts regarding the outbreak as they occurred. In addition to Twitter, HealthMap relayed messages to Facebook (http://facebook.com) "fans" regarding the outbreak's developments. A special version of the HealthMap main page was also created, which showed only the worldwide reports of "swine flu," influenza, and respiratory illness, as opposed to all infectious disease alerts.

Finally, HealthMap partnered with the New England Journal of Medicine's H1N1 Influenza Center to create an interactive map (http://healthmap.org/nejm/) showing worldwide cases of novel influenza A (H1N1) as reported by both media outlets and official sources, including the World Health Organization, the Centers for Disease Control and Prevention, and the Public Health Agency of Canada. This map was updated daily with media reports and official reports as they became available. Both confirmed and suspect novel influenza A (H1N1) deaths and cases were shown, and an interactive timeline progression tool offered an animated view of the spread of the disease from the inception of the outbreak.

6.9 Conclusions

Rapidly identifying an infectious disease outbreak is critical, both for effective initiation of public health intervention measures and for timely alerting of government agencies and the general public. The Internet is revolutionizing how this epidemic intelligence information is gathered. Freely available Web-based sources of information have allowed for earlier detection of outbreaks with reduced cost and increased reporting transparency (Wilson and Brownstein 2009).

While mining the Web is a valuable new approach, these sources cannot replace the efforts of public health practitioners and clinicians. Information overload, false reports, lack of specificity of signals, and sensitivity to external forces such as media interest may limit the realization of their potential for public health practice and clinical decision making. Ultimately, the Internet provides a powerful communications channel, but it is health care professionals, and the public who can best determine how to use this channel for surveillance, prevention, and control of emerging diseases (Brownstein, Freifeld, and Madoff 2009).

6.10 Future Work

In an effort to improve coverage, HealthMap is exploring the use of other Internet-based sources, including additional news aggregators—such as Yahoo! News, Factiva, and LexisNexis—blogs, and veterinary news sources such as the World Organization for Animal Health (OIE) (Freifeld et al. 2008). Social-networking sites for clinicians, patients, and the general public also hold potential for harnessing the collective wisdom of the masses for disease detection. Eventually, mobile phone technology, enabled by global positioning systems and coupled with short-message service (SMS) messaging and "microblogging," might also come into play (Brownstein, Freifeld, and Madoff 2009). This is especially relevant in developing countries where Internet access is frequently unreliable at best. The use of hand-held devices and mobile phones that connect to the Internet and have SMS capability can help fill technology gaps in resource-poor settings (Wilson and Brownstein 2009). Further, user search queries aggregated across Internet users, such as those used by Google Flu Trends (http://www.google.org/flutrends/), may provide additional important insights into public health trends. It has recently been shown that search query data can be harnessed as a form of collective intelligence where patterns of population-level searching mirror and may even predict disease outbreaks (Wilson and Brownstein 2009). The addition of automated analysis of online video materials and radio broadcasts will also add to HealthMap's list of sources for early detection (Brownstein, Freifeld, and Madoff 2009).

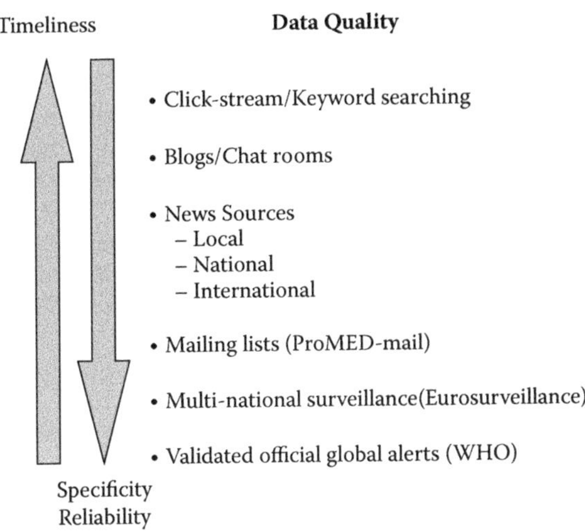

FIGURE 6.6
Quality of data scaled by timeliness and specificity/reliability.

In an effort to further develop data filtering, HealthMap is working to improve natural language processing capabilities for additional automated data processing, such as distinguishing discrete outbreaks from endemic activity, the spatial resolution of location extraction, and identifying reports indicating the absence of disease or the end of a previously identified outbreak (Freifeld et al. 2008).

Continued system evaluation is another essential part of future work for HealthMap. The sensitivity, specificity, and timeliness of different news source types need to be quantified and considered (see Figure 6.6). Integrating unstructured online information sources with other health indicator data needs to be considered as well to provide a broader context for reports. Finally, in an effort to define populations at risk and predict disease spread, the integration of additional pertinent data sets such as mortality and morbidity estimates, laboratory data, field surveillance, environmental predictors, population density and mobility, and pathogen seasonality and transmissibility need to also be considered (Brownstein et al. 2008).

References

Brownstein, John S., Clark C. Freifeld, and Lawrence C. Madoff. 2009. Digital Disease Detection—Harnessing the Web for Public Health Surveillance. *N Engl J Med* 360 (21):5.

Brownstein, John S., Clark C. Freifeld, and Lawrence C. Madoff. 2009. Influenza A H1N1 Virus, 2009—Online Detection and Monitoring. *N Engl J Med* 360 (21):1.

Brownstein, John S., Clark C. Freifeld, Ben Y. Reis, and Kenneth D. Mandl. 2008. Surveillance Sans Frontieres: Internet-Based Emerging Infectious Disease Intelligence and the HealthMap Project. *PLoS Med* 5 (7):6.

Freifeld, Clark C., Kenneth D. Mandl, Ben Y. Reis, and John S. Brownstein. 2008. HealthMap: Global Infectious Disease Monitoring through Automated Classification and Visualization of Internet Media Reports. *J Am Med Inform Assoc* 15 (2):8.

Keller, Mika, Michael Blench, Herman Tolentino, Clark C. Freifeld, Kenneth D. Mandl, Abla Mawudeku, Gunther Eysenbach, and John S. Brownstein. 2009. Use of Unstructured Event-Based Reports for Global Infectious Disease Surveillance. *Emerging Infectious Diseases* 15 (5):7.

Martinez, Regina. 2009. Extraño brote epidemiológico causa la muerte a dos bebés en Veracruz. *Proceso*, April 2, 2009.

Morales, Andrew. 2009. Veracruz: reporta agente municipal extraño brote epidémico que ha cobrado dos vidas. *La Jornada en linea*, April 1, 2009.

WHO. 2008. WHO Interim Guidance for the use of Annex 2 of the INTERNATIONAL HEALTH REGULATIONS (2005). Edited by W. H. Organization.

Wilson, Kumanan, and John Brownstein. 2009. Early Detection of Disease Outbreaks Using the Internet. *Canadian Medical Association Journal* 180 (10):1.

7

The Role of SMS Text Messaging to Improve Public Health Response

Elizabeth Avery Gomez, PhD
New Jersey Institute of Technology
Newark, New Jersey

CONTENTS

7.1 Introduction

Timeliness and early detection are critical in controlling a disease outbreak. Recognizing each case of an outbreak has unique characteristics that influence transmission dynamics, controlling the spread of infectious disease remains a challenge. Early indications (syndromes or symptoms) of disease outbreak in a new area (community) are important for containment. Information dissemination at the local community level, which is closest to the public, plays a critical role and an area of scant research. One viable lowest-common denominator is "free text" exchange through SMS text messaging, which has received little attention. Moreover, how training could improve "free text" use through plain language training and situation awareness has not been studied in relation to biosurveillance initiatives.

Two-way communication during an outbreak or in a crisis provides the exchange of essential information that can aid in the distribution and allocation of resources. Along the same continuum is the opportunity to intercept messages through an automated system and triage accordingly with role-based agents. Dov Te'eni (2006) notes that "the complexity of implementing communicative action grows with the need for coordination, the contextual demands (norms and values) and the use of scarce resources." The introduction of role-based agents (automated triage) could mitigate the contextual demands between the sender and receiver. How systems can log copies of "free text" for communication exchange could be another option for early outbreak detection and to ensure timely and effective response. A monitoring system could then leverage data mining techniques to identify patterns within log files in preparation of future crisis. The same log files could be analyzed for plain language training improvements. At present the next steps of this research have been expedited with the novel influenza A (H1N1) pandemic and preparedness initiatives for the fall of 2009.

To collect a sample of "free text" responses and establish a baseline for use with different responder roles and different levels of ICT experience, a Web-based training application was developed. The emphasis of the application was to study user behavior, response, and training effectiveness (refer to Section 7.4. Simulating SMS Text Messaging for Training) when using "free text" in 160 character chunks to mirror the SMS exchange limit. The training application, which was field tested in the spring of 2007, used a bottom-up approach and proposed to increase community responder readiness and improve message response (accuracy/content) when using SMS text messaging to communicate from a mobile device. The study participants within the community were in a role that is considered a "feeder" to public health systems. At present, the output of each training task is being analyzed for patterns that could translate into triage options for the community responder role. With plain language training, similarities can be identified and assessed over time the more plain language is used. The task responses are based on a crisis scenario that runs from start to finish for the entire training session. The study revealed that with minimal training, practitioner's (community responders) use of plain language did show significant improvement. The inter-rater reliability and coding of "free text" responses also revealed the importance and need for situation awareness training. Data mining methods and feeder systems with accumulated data such as over-the-counter (OTC) medicine purchases, emergency room visits, ambulance responses, and absenteeism have also been investigated for use in biosurveillance and early outbreak detection.

With respect to biosurveillance systems, the exchange of "free text" to identify early/potential cases and its impact to create panic should not be overlooked. Jurisdictional authorization, such as state legislatures in the United States must also be considered (Halperin, Baker, and Monson 1992). So as to expand on the premise of surveillance, which "was restricted, in public health practices, to watching contact of serious communicable diseases, such as smallpox, to detect early symptoms so that prompt isolation could be instituted," to now include chronic diseases, occupational safety, and health, environmental health, injuries, personal health practice, and preventive health technologies (Halperin et al. 1992), we discuss the potential of plain language training to systematically "triage" biosurveillance threats that could improve timeliness and situation awareness details for response readiness.

The goal of this discussion is to present findings from the spring 2007 study that could be applicable for biosurveillance initiatives where early detection and just-in-time training are needed. We step through the Web-based application and the potential to offer more detailed training for biosurveillance. The contribution of this discussion is to introduce conditions that could be leveraged for the triage of role-based agents who take the role of a community responder in a crisis. Examples of SMS text message responses from the initial study participants are presented to support the direction of this research. The benefits of simulation through an Internet browser before extending to an actual mobile device are also discussed. Through a combination of actual and perceived measures, user profile is evaluated for effective training and user behavior before and after training.

7.2 Information and Communication Technology (ICT) Training for Community Needs

Increased use of information and communication technology (ICT) can improve communication exchange between community responders, and between community responders and citizens in a local community. Communication messages from community responders can also be used for feeder systems, such as biosurveillance. Public health in the 21st Century depends on technology for information delivery and communication through multiple technologies to:

- Support the critical role of preparing public health professionals to function effectively toward improved population health
- Increase Internet and e-mail access and usage by state and local agencies
- Teach employees how to apply the use of information and data to the public health practice (Cingular Wireless 2006)

Individual and community preparedness should also improve and benefit efforts associated with homeland security, independent of the knowledge domain within the public health infrastructure. For example, the Centers for Disease Control and Prevention (CDC) (Foundations for Recovery 2006) will help identify the most effective tools and actively encourage their international use, applying expertise and resources in laboratory research, public health policy, program management, and health communications to overcome scientific, financial, and cultural barriers. The impacts technology imposes are rapidly changing and have become a challenge for the current public health infrastructure (Federal Emergency Management Agency [FEMA] 2005).

A current example of ICT training for community needs is the novel influenza A (H1N1) virus that has now reached the World Health Organization (WHO) level 6 of pandemic alert. While one might hypothesize that in reaching level 6, mass media notifications would be prevalent; instead, in the United States, the control and containment of the virus has been managed at the local level through memorandums sent via backpack mail and similar local distributions. While some schools have phone alert systems in place, the schools did not choose to disseminate the information with phone alerts. School nurses also were carefully screening students in class and the absentee confirmations included additional questions on the details of the absence. At the turning point of confirmed cases by county (within a state), one use of SMS would have been for each home (physical address) to respond to a request for confirmation of "healthy" families. This would allow the community to at least identify which homes were certain there were no cases for the given address.

7.3 Communication Protocols

The convergence of computing and communication technologies in lieu of face-to-face meetings can challenge communication theories. Crisis response places emphasis on the individual responding in a call for assistance, based on a request to respond that has taken place. Communication theory plays an important role in crisis response when two or more responders must communicate from the field with limited use of ICT. The responder's communicative action draws upon goal-oriented behavior from Habermas' Theory of Communicative Action (Te'eni 2001, Te'eni 2006), and focuses on communication to achieve and maintain mutual understanding (Ngwenyama and Lee 1997). The communication exchange in a request to respond between the sender and receiver of information varies based on the uniqueness of the incident creating an element of uncertainty. Increased communication device options (i.e., QWERTY keypad vs. alpha use of a numerical keypad on cell phones; 160 character exchange limit for SMS text messages) also challenge the sender–receiver exchange of information.

7.3.1 SMS Text Messaging

SMS text messaging is a form of written communication that exchanges packets of information between information communication technologies (McAdams 2006). The versatility and high reliability of SMS text messaging offers promise for disease outbreak or crisis response, especially for community responders who have limited access to ICT resources. SMS text messaging can be used between two mobile devices or between a mobile device and stationary computer (desktop, laptop). The caveat when communicating with someone who is using a small device is the limitation of reading and responding across the small device, in addition to the 160-character message exchange limit. Individualized training for each device that exists also challenges training.

Being able to adapt to the size and capacity of the communication device and platform when communicating with SMS text messaging takes practice for effective use. Practice writing a 160 character message in lieu of a lengthy message that could be exchanged via e-mail for example is one action that can be practiced on both a stationary device and mobile device. Moreover, recognizing that some devices allow the device user to send more than 160 characters at one time, the receiving service could arbitrarily break the message into 160 character units regardless of if the break falls between words or in the middle of a single word. Some cellular services, such as Cingular Wireless (Gomez et al. 2006), do label each message (i.e., 1 of 2, 2 of 2, etc.) while others do not. Some agent-based services will provide one message with hyperlinks within the message to allow navigation to each part of the message in sequence, as seen with Google SMS (2006).

SMS text messaging is a simple low-cost technology that is durable because of its small packet exchange technology. SMS has begun inroads as an SOS equivalent due to the alternate delivery route to voice channels. During Katrina, SMS text messages got through when other communication methods failed. Coast Guard officials used the technology for direct life saving helicopter rescues during the Gulf Coast hurricanes. SMS text messaging can be considered a simple technology. For example, the ability to send small packets that sit in a message queue outweighs the use of voice calls that require you to continuously redial. There are approximately 190 million Americans with text messaging functionality on their cell phones. The use of text messaging won't overload the telecommunication systems (Strong Angel 2006a). The federal government is currently piloting its use with four major wireless carriers. Mass text messaging could be problematic if not carefully tested. The preferred design is for smaller distributions resembling that of a community of interest. Local public health organizations could also fit the criteria of a community of interest. "There is no doubt SMS has the ability to save lives in an emergency" (Strong Angel 2006b).

7.3.2 Plain Language across Organizations

Independent of device medium, the use of plain language across organizations is an interoperability focus for FEMA's National Incident Management System (NIMS), and associated agencies, such as the National Institutes of Health (NIH). Plain language is becoming a standard (FEMA 2005) for interoperable communication in emergency response, and dates back to at least May 2005 when a directive on new procedure codes was issued phasing out agency and jurisdiction specific codes with the use of standard language. Plain language initiatives in emergency preparedness are being realized at the international, national, and local levels. FEMA (2005), for example, states that plain language must be used with interoperable communication systems (enabling fire, police, EMS/medical to collaborate and communicate) replacing the use of 10 codes (Table 7.1).

Each speech act type is introduced (Table 7.2) through a prompt that requests an SMS text message response, allowing for the assessment of each speech act type based on the communication responses for the specified prompt. Each Speech Act Type can be categorized for the crisis incident coordinator, improving timeliness to respond. For example, if the role-based agent intercepts a response that has been identified as "ask for," branching could occur to only notify the coordinator when a long lapse of time and no "ask for" response has been received (Table 7.3). This would reduce the management of messages received by the coordinator allowing them to focus on messages of higher urgency. An algorithm accessing a list of word choices for illocutionary speech act type can be developed and associated with the most common word choices and word placement in a sentence as displayed in Task Response 2 (Table 7.3) denotes the use of the word "need directions" by study participants 1, 2, and 3. Study participant 4 uses the word "cannot locate," which is not indicative that help is needed ("ask for" speech act type). You will also note that participant 3 replies with "need directions," but the request does not contain any content that could be used by the crisis incident coordinator. For example, there was no location to allow the coordinator to assist the community responder.

The use and practice of plain language is also proposed to bring the use of words, such as "proceeding" and "arrived" closer together by reducing the vocabulary used by responders. The current field study takes a baseline measure and then introduces plain language training that parallels each

TABLE 7.1

Role-Specific Terminology

Terminology for crisis response roles	
Type	**Essential rule definition**
Police	Police 10 codes
Fire	Fire 10 codes
EMS/medical	Medical terminology
Disaster relief	Humanitarian-specific terminology
Specialty teams	Specialty-/task-specific terminology
Community responder (volunteer)	Organization-specific terminology

TABLE 7.2

Illocutionary Speech Acts

Illocutionary speech acts—task assignments		
Illocutionary acts	**Essential rule**	**Task assigned**
Asking or answering a question	Performance of an act in saying something where a certain effect is achieved.	
Assert (confirm)	Counts as an undertaking to the effect that *p* represents an actual state of affairs.	Pretrain Task 1
		Posttrain Task 3
Warn	Counts as an undertaking to the effect that E is not in H's best interest.	
Advise	Counts as an undertaking to the effect that A is not in H's best interest.	Pretrain Task 2
		Posttrain Task 4
Question (ask for)	Counts as an attempt to elicit this information from H.	
Thank	Counts as an expression of gratitude.	Pretrain Task 2b
		Posttrain Task 5
Request	Counts as an attempt to get H to do A.	

Source: Adapted from Austin/Searle (AMCIS 2009, Austin, J.L. (1962). How to do things with words. J.O.Urmson and Marina Sbiba, Editors. Harvard University Press, Cambridge, Massachusetts; Searle, J.R. (1969). Speech acts: An essay in the philosophy of language. Cambridge University Press.

speech act type as a way to begin measuring the reduction in vocabulary and word placement within a sentence for algorithm development. Alike, task prompt 4 continues to "advise" with a status. The status for three of the four study participants also uses the word "arrived."

Task Prompt 2

1. Advise about Route 80 road closure.
2. Ask for detour directions from your current location to your assigned neighborhood.

Task Prompt 4

1. Advise that you are now at the last house of your assigned neighborhood.
2. Ask for medical resources to help a resident with breathing difficulties. (Table 7.4)

TABLE 7.3

Pretraining Task Responses

Participant number	Participant response for task prompt 2	Response level
1	I am a bit lost here. I had to make a detour-route 80 is closed. I am sitting at the corner of Broad st and Karen dr in Clifton. I need directions from here	4
2	I-80 closed, detoured onto Rte 19, now at Broad and Karen in Clifton, need directions to assignment.	4
3	Joe I need instructions	1
4	Rt. 80 is closed and the location you are you cannot locate the street number so he can help you get to your assigned neighborhood.	1

Source: Adapted from Austin/Searle (AMCIS 2009, Austin, J.L. (1962). How to do things with words. J.O.Urmson and Marina Sbiba, Editors. Harvard University Press, Cambridge, Massachusetts.

TABLE 7.4

Posttraining Task Responses

Participant number	Participant response for task prompt 4	Response level
1	At last house. Send ambulance for resident having breathing difficulties. Flooding intensifying, wind picking up, darkening skies.	4
2	At last assigned house. Need medical help for resident with breathing problem.	4
3	I will try to work with them. I will call for help while we wait for someone, I will try to make her feel well.	1
4	Approached last house on Orchard Street. Enter house, notice elderly alone with son. Indicates son having trouble breathing. Need medical resources to aid.	4

Source: Gomez, E.A. (2009). Improving ICT Use within the Underserved Community: Empowering the Non-Native English Speaker, AMCIS 2009.

Each cell phone device offers a different user interface and different features. The differences also depend on the service provider. Offering training directly on a mobile device limits training for a wider audience. Using an actual mobile device for initial training either narrows the training by making it device dependent or forces the training attendee to adapt to an unfamiliar device.

7.4. Simulating SMS Text Messaging for Training

A Web-based application was designed to simulate a cell phone interface with SMS text messaging's 160 character limitation. The Web-based application uses a PHP/HTML design to facilitate the modular approach of the application and extend portability for the targeted study participant. A MySQL database collects the actual task performance measures while the delivery of both the crisis scenario (including individual episodes) and the plain language training are presented with multimedia movie clips of streaming video and voiceovers.

Speech acts and plain language protocols are one mechanism that could improve information exchange and were utilized for this research. Two-way communication exchange, especially when timeliness of information is at stake, can benefit from role-based agents that intercept a message and serve as a triage to the message recipient. The queuing of messages between a sender and receiver ultimately become event logs of written communication and can also serve as an enabler for agent-based information exchange (Zhu 2006; Zhu, Zhou, and Seguin 2006).

In our research, e-readiness encompasses both the message form (contents) and the ability to use the technology to send and receive the message. Increasing readiness of information communication technologies (ICT) through training and practice places emphasis not only on the communication protocol but also on the message adaptiveness for the crisis. The ability to communicate using more than one medium is essential, and data redundancy is often encouraged (Austin 1962). In a crisis, one communication medium cannot be predetermined. Most devices used with biosurveillance and early detection have text-based capabilities.

Interactive text-based training and simulations can aid individual responders based on their role and level of experience. For example, increased use of SMS text messaging has demonstrated high reliability for one-way communication. For the spring 2007 study, the use of SMS text messaging was proposed as the lowest-common denominator to reach community responders who have limited resources for mobile information technology and who find themselves responding in the field when a crisis occurs. Findings revealed the importance of a baseline to establish different levels of plain language training and also to introduce training for situation awareness, which was not addressed in the spring 2007 study. Moreover, training is needed before varying the multiple modes of communication and before varying mobile communication options. Mobile technologies have become an integral part of everyday life for many people, providing ubiquitous information access, entertainment, and helping people stay connected to work, friends, and families.

While the focus of this research is on the message exchange with a mobile device, the message form is the focus of this discussion rather than the device itself. Te'eni (2001) notes that effective communication could be adapted for communication technology and how "recommending to the sender the optimal amount of context information in the message" can be achieved. Moreover, Habermas (1998) defines communicative action as "the interaction of at least two subjects capable of speech and action who establish interpersonal relationships. The actors seek to reach an understanding about the action situation and their plans of action in order to coordinate their action by way of agreement" (Te'eni 2001; Habermas 1984).

Reaching our targeted audience of community responders who have limited ICT resources, the platform and the resources needed to run the training application were also a consideration. Recognizing other software applications may provide a level of sophistication and savvy a esthetics greater than PHP/HTML, the unknowns and lack of ICT resources for many of our study participants would be compromised, increasing the risk of problems during the study while participating from a remote location. Post-study statistics and system log files, also confirmed that the application design did accomodate the participant ICT resources. The findings reflect that study participants did not encounter any performance issues or interface issues. The study participants were located in five states and two countries with participation from rural, suburban, and urban areas.

To initiate the training, one continuous crisis scenario was introduced. As the crisis scenario unfolded, the participant was prompted to respond to a task (request for information). The crisis scenario was designed for the role of a community volunteer who has been requested to respond in an early storm warning. A series of five episodes (six tasks) were introduced. Responder pretraining assessment measures serve as a baseline before training is introduced and the focus of our discussion. Two episodes with three tasks are performed before training is introduced as a way to obtain a pretraining baseline communication exchange message and capture three task responses. Three short training modules with associated communication episodes and tasks are then introduced. This one-to-one relationship of task prompt type with an associated episode and tasks allows for the task prompt type to parallel the speech act invoking the SMS text message response. To conclude the training session, posttraining assessment measures are collected. Moreover, pretraining and posttraining tasks have parallel task prompts (Figure 7.1).

7.4.1 Web-Based Application Participant Role

The Web-based training application that was field tested leverages Searle's Speech Act Theory, and Ruth and Murphy's Writing Task Assessment Model to obtain written SMS text message responses that can be objectively assessed based on the 160 character per text-message exchange limit. Figure 7.2 depicts the role of the study participant as an action team volunteer where the action team coordinator is a simulated role.

The community responder role (community volunteer), which feeds the public health system, is the focus of this research. The community responder

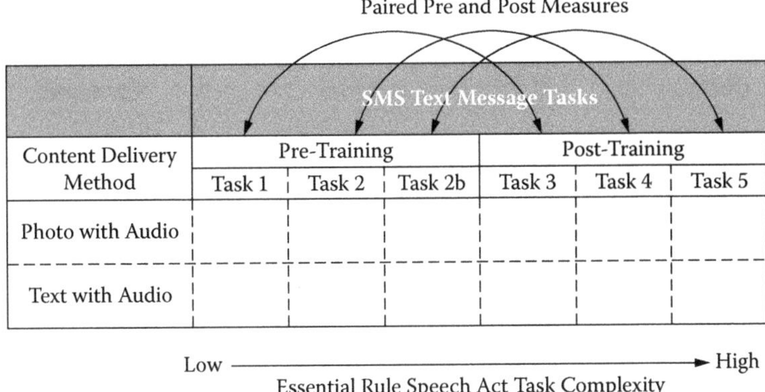

FIGURE 7.1
Parallel pretraining and posttraining measures.

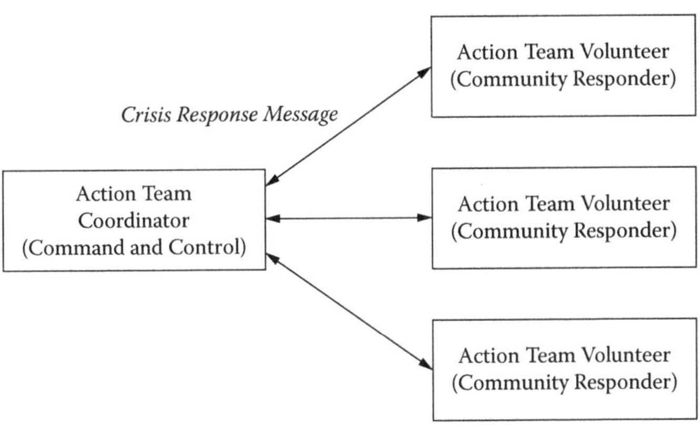

FIGURE 7.2
Two-way communication exchange.

is a member of a local community who is not trained as a first responder (fire, police, EMS/medical) but is responding to a crisis (Gomez, Passerini, Hare 2006). The frequency of quick-response tactics is limited because the community responder is not called upon to respond as frequently as a first responder. Biosurveillance crises are among those less frequently performed tasks. Zhu and Zhou (2006) note that "attention has been paid to roles in different areas relevant to systems such as modeling, software engineering, access control, system administration, agent systems, database systems, and collaborative systems. Roles can help team members avoid being inundated by overwhelming information." Turoff et al. (2004) also discuss the role transferability and availability of responders in disaster response. Roles can also

TABLE 7.5

Roles per Category as a Community Responder

Question	Categories	N	Percentage
I have been working/ volunteering in the field of crisis response for:	Less than 1 year	4	8.0%
	From 1–2 years	5	10.0%
	3–5 years	5	10.0%
	6–10 years	1	2.0%
	More than 10 years	4	8.0%
	I do not work/ volunteer in crisis response	31	62.0%
On average, how frequently do you use the Internet for job-related work?	About once a day	7	14.0%
	Several times a day	33	66.0%
	A few times a week	4	8.0%
	Less than once a month	5	10.0%
	Once a month	0	0%
	A few times a month	1	2.0%

Note: N = 50.

TABLE 7.6

Pretraining mobile device usage

Pretraining usage	N	Percent
Use text messaging	23	46%
Use camera and movie recordings	19	38%

Note: N = 50.

assist in collaboration and when undertaking responsibilities than can duplicate efforts.

7.4.2 Study Participants

A total of 50 study participant's were recorded as of April 11, 2007. The descriptive statistics for this study placed emphasis on ICT frequency of use, and demographics related to crisis response, age, and gender (Table 7.5). Pretraining and posttraining factor loadings and tests of normality are also discussed at this time before additional results are introduced.

The demographic information presented a balance between genders (25 male and 25 female), and a significant difference between responder roles was noted. The Responder Role categories from the study are noted and include (1) community responders; (2) practitioner with crisis response responsibilities, (3) academic researcher; (4) student, citizen; and (5) none (please specify).

Of the 50 study participants, approximately 46% currently use text messaging (Table 7.6). Findings also reflected 38% use camera and movie recordings presenting a contrast between graphics and text.

If we review the user pretraining profile in closer detail, focusing on the findings of survey question #19 "I know how to send text messages from my computer (0 = yes, use SMS), (2 = no, use SMS)." Approximately 63% of participants who use SMS text messaging can send a message and another 17.5% are neutral, an indicator on awareness of SMS capabilities from a stationary computer.

Comparing question #19 to question #20 "I know how to send text messages from my cell phone (0 = yes use SMS), (2 = no use SMS)." It can be noted that 63% of participants who use SMS text messaging can send a message and another 11.1% are neutral, an indicator for future research that perhaps suggests limited comfort when sending an SMS text message from a cell phone. Findings from questions #19 and #20 suggest Web-based applications could benefit community responders before field training on a mobile device.

7.5 Conclusions

This chapter presents a modular Web-based application design to reach a wider audience with limited resources and assesses the potential for triage with role-based agents, beginning with the role of community responders who do not have specific terminology for their respective role. Leveraging plain language written communication exchange of community responders offers a potential baseline for this ongoing research. The task design built upon the Ruth and Murphy Writing Assessment Model suggests delineation for triage both based on the task and the word choice. Observations from the pilot study suggested further alignment of the five task prompts to better assess the responses and use of clear and concise (plain language) language. The intent is to deliver training that focuses on communication protocols portable to any ICT device increasing interoperable communications. The application itself was also designed to reach a wider audience with limited ICT skills, lowering the need for human intervention while providing them with a simulated experience within their reach with their own resources in the hope that they would begin practicing, once the training was completed. Research is currently under way to extend the training into practice with actual mobile devices in the field and capturing succinct SMS text messages and also those requiring some fluency (descriptive in nature). Being able to implement a scorecard for feedback is an essential part of the long-term goal that enhances the user experience and also helps the user improve their communication protocols.

References

Austin, J.L. (1962). *How to Do Things with Words*. J.O. Urmson and Marina Sbiba, Eds. Harvard University Press, Cambridge, Massachusetts.

CDC (Centers for Disease Control and Prevention). (2002). Protecting the Nations Health in an Era of Globalization: CDC's Global Infectious Disease Strategy. www.cdc.gov/globalidplan.htm.

Cingular Wireless. (2006). www.cingularwireless.com.

FEMA. (2005). FEMA Promotes Plain Language Radio Response. http://www.impact-information.com/impactinfo/newsletter/plwork18.htm September 2005.

Foundations for Recovery. (2006). Need for FEMA and Red Cross to Coordinate more effectively with Local and Faith-Based Organizations Identified. http://www.foundationsforrecovery.org/, June 19, 2006.

Gomez, E.A. (2009). Improving ICT Use within the Underserved Community: Empowering the Non-Native English Speaker, AMCIS 2009.

Gomez, E.A., Passerini, K., and Hare, K. (2006). Public Health Crisis Management: Community Level Roles and Communication Options, *Proceedings of the 3rd Annual ISCRAM*, Newark, NJ.

Google Mobile (2009). http://www.google.com/mobile/products/sms.html#p=default.

Halperin, W., Baker, E.L., and Monson, R.R. (1992). *Public Health Surveillance*. Van Nostrand Reinhold, New York.

Institute of Medicine. (2003). *The Future of the Public's Health in the 21st Century*. Washington, DC: The National Academies Press.

McAdams, J. (2006). SMS for SOS: Short Message Service earns valued role as a link of last resort for crisis communications. http://www.fcw.com/article92790-04-03-06-Print April 3, 2006.

Ruth, L. and Murphy, S. (1988). *Designing Writing Tasks for the Assessment of Writing*. Ablex Publishing Corporation. Norwood, NJ.

Searle, J.R. (1969). *Speech Acts: An Essay in the Philosophy of Language*. Cambridge University Press.

Strong Angel III (2006a). Integrated Disaster Response Demonstration. http://www.strongangel3.net/files/SAIII_working_report_20061106.pdf, October 1, 2006.

Strong Angel III. (2006b). Press Release: At Strong Angel III Disaster Response Demonstration, Internews Advises on Information Dissemination. http://www.internews.org/prs/2006/20060905_us.shtm, September 5, 2006.

Te'eni, D. (2001). Review: A cognitive effective model of organizational communication for designing IT. *MIS Quarterly*, (25)2, p. 251.

Te'eni, D. (2006). The language-action perspective as a basis for communication support systems. *Communications of the ACM*, (49)5, pp. 65–70.

Turoff, M., Chumer, M., Van De Walle, B., and Yao, X. (2004). The design of a dynamic emergency response management information system (DERMIS). *Journal of Information Technology Theory and Application (JITTA)*, (5)4, pp. 1–35

Zhu, H. (2006). Separating Design from Implementations: Role-Based Software Development, *Proceedings of the 5th IEEE International Conference on Cognitive Informatics*, Beijing, China, July 17–19, 2006, pp. 141–148.

Zhu, H. and Zhou, M.C. (2006). Supporting software development with roles, *IEEE Transactions on Systems, Man and Cybernetics*, Part A, 36(6), pp. 1110–1123.

8

Using Prediction Markets to Forecast Infectious Diseases

Philip M. Polgreen, MD, MPH
Carver College of Medicine
University of Iowa
Iowa City, Iowa

Forrest D. Nelson, PhD
College of Business
University of Iowa–Tippe
Iowa City, Iowa

CONTENTS

8.1 Introduction

Until recently, forecasting health-related events has been uncommon compared to other fields, such as metrology, finance, and geology. One reason is that traditional forecasting approaches require reliable data for long periods of time, and these data generally need to be updated quickly. Unfortunately, in comparison to other fields, health data is almost always old by the time it becomes available. The absence of timely disease data has motivated several syndromic surveillance efforts using alternative information such as drug sales (Hogan et al. 2003, Welliver et al. 1979, Magruder et al. 2003, Davies at al. 2003), emergency department visits (Irvin et al. 2003, Yaun et al. 2004, Suyama et al. 2003), absentee data (Lenaway et al. 1995) and Internet search query log data (Polgreen et al. 2008, Ginsberg et al. 2009). In the case of seasonal influenza, these approaches have provided improved lead-time over traditional disease activity reports (Dailey et al. 2007). However, all of these approaches rely on quantitative data that can produce "false alarms" or miss abrupt changes. Often the addition of human interpretation can supplement such quantitative data streams, but it is difficult to aggregate subjective data. In this chapter we propose a relatively new method for gathering and aggregating disease information. This method involves operation of specialized futures markets called *prediction markets* and inviting health experts to trade in these markets. The prices generated in these markets can provide a consensus view regarding the likelihood of future disease-related events. After a brief discussion of futures markets and prediction markets, we present data from a pilot novel influenza A (H1N1) prediction market.

8.2 Futures Markets

In traditional futures markets, traders buy and sell contracts that specify the quantity and quality of commodities to be delivered by a certain date. In some cases, these contracts are associated with crops that have not yet been planted or oil that is still in the ground. These markets exist to help producers and consumers of commodities plan for the future. For example, they enable farmers to lock in prices for their crops before those crops are planted. On the other side of the market, food processors use futures markets to ensure a steady supply of raw materials at a specific price. Widespread adoption of futures markets have led to dramatic stabilization of agricultural prices.

The prices in futures markets change because they incorporate information that might affect the supply and demand for goods in the future. For example, geopolitical events can dramatically affect oil futures prices. It is not surprising that these prices change according to expectations of future events, but what is surprising is how fast new information is incorporated into futures prices. Orange juice futures markets provide a classic example. In these markets, commodity traders buy and sell contracts for the future delivery of orange juice. The prices they pay for these contracts reflect traders' beliefs about the future price of orange juice. Because the size of the orange crop is affected by the weather, orange juice prices are also influenced by the weather. A severe frost can decimate the U.S. orange crop in Florida. Therefore, the price of futures contracts should be, and is, influenced by weather forecasts. If a heavy freeze is predicted, traders anticipate that orange juice prices will go up and, therefore, they bid up the price of orange juice futures. Interestingly, an analysis of the timing of the changes in orange juice futures prices demonstrated that the changes in the price of futures seemed to precede, and thus anticipate, the weather forecasts released by the National Weather Service (Roll 1984). Apparently, commodity traders with large sums of money at stake effectively seek out and use information that is not yet available to, or not yet used by, the National Weather Service.

8.3 Prediction Markets

In recent years, markets in more "unusual" commodities have been developed solely for their utility in predicting future events. These markets are designed exclusively to exploit the information contained in the prices of the financial instruments, or contracts, traded. No tangible "commodity," such as a crop or raw material, is attached to the contracts that participants buy and sell. They are based instead on the outcome of some future event. We call these markets prediction markets rather than futures markets; this name implies their intended use and helps to distinguish them from traditional financial futures markets. They have also been called decision markets, event markets, and information markets.

One can think of prediction markets as specialized futures markets in which artificial financial instruments are traded. The instruments (i.e., contracts) are defined by the operators of the market to have a value to be determined by the outcome of the event of interest. Participating traders in the market are experts with information regarding that event. They are motivated to trade by the prospect of making profits. Thus, traders buy contracts that are undervalued by the market, according to their beliefs, and sell those which are overvalued. The prices at which these instruments trade reflect a consensus belief about their future value, and thus can be used as a prediction of the future event.

8.3.1 How Do Prediction Markets Work?

Prediction markets are effective because they aggregate the disparate and diffuse information held by different participants. A simple example, patterned after one provided by Eisenberg and Gale (Eisenberg et al. 1958), illustrates how markets aggregate information. Suppose there are two traders and three possible outcomes to an event: A, B, C. Only one outcome will occur 6 months from now. With no other information, each trader might regard each outcome as equally likely to occur and thus be willing to pay the same amount for contracts linked to those outcomes. Suppose, instead, that each trader has access to different information. Trader 1 knows that event A will not occur, and trader 2 knows that event B cannot occur. Each trader is still is uncertain about the outcome. However, trader 1 believes that events B and C each have a 50% chance of occurring, and trader 2 believes that events A and C each have a 50% chance of occurring. On the basis of their privileged knowledge, trader 1 pursues contracts based on events B and C, and trader 2 pursues contracts based on events A and C. Competition drives the price of contract C higher, while the lack of competition drives the price of contracts A and B toward zero. Thus, the prices investors are willing to pay for the contracts will reveal the actual outcome.

In general, prediction markets work because they: (1) aggregate information from all participants, each of whom has different information about the issue in question; (2) provide incentives that encourage participants to reveal their knowledge in their trades; (3) provide feedback to participants—through market prices, traders learn about the beliefs of other traders and are motivated to collect more information; and (4) allow traders to share their knowledge anonymously, thereby, encouraging traders to signal information through the market that they might not state publicly.

8.3.2 Requirements for Prediction Markets

Prediction markets are commonly compared to surveys since both tools ask questions of participants, and both are designed to aggregate information. However, the number of potential applications for prediction markets is smaller than for surveys. First, unlike surveys, a successful application of a prediction market requires both uncertainty about an outcome and differing opinions about the outcome probabilities. If all participants have the same information and the same opinions, then no one will trade, no prices will be generated, and no information will be aggregated. Second, also unlike surveys, prediction markets need to be based on an outcome that can be verified after the fact. Consider, for example, the question of the reemergence of SARS. A feasible prediction market contract might be based on a question such as "Will at least one case of human-to-human transmission of SARS occur in Hong Kong by January of 2012, as documented by the World Health Organization?" A contract based on a question such as "Will there be several unreported cases of SARS in Hong Kong by January of 2012?" would not be successful. The outcome of the event is inherently unobservable, so ultimate liquidation of the contracts would be in dispute and traders would have no reason to buy or sell those contracts. Surveys, on the other hand, could ask either question.

There are several other important considerations for successful prediction markets. First, successful markets require data from diverse sources. Specifically, traders must have different information and opinions. Thus, for a local seasonal influenza market, the goal would be to enlist a diverse group of traders from a variety of healthcare professions and geographical locations. For example, physicians, nurses, pharmacists, clinical microbiologists, teachers, administrators, and public health practitioners all have some knowledge about influenza activity in their communities. Second, an active trading base is needed. We know from both theory and experience that increasing the number of traders increases the accuracy of the predictions. While the minimum number of traders needed for an accurate prediction is still an open research question, the empirical data from prediction markets designed to forecast elections suggests that the number of participants need not be as large as the number required to obtain comparable accuracy with surveys. For example, election prediction markets with 200 active traders routinely yield predictions with smaller errors than those from opinion polls involving ten times as many respondents. And predictions markets designed to predict sales for a company have performed well with as few as a dozen traders. In general, prediction markets with at least 20 or 30 traders can yield good results, but accuracy tends to improve as the number of traders increases.

Finally, there must be incentives to trade; transactions made for the purpose of maximizing profits are the means by which traders reveal their private information to the marketplace. However, the use of money involves two problems. First, current gambling laws and financial market regulations prohibit the operation of prediction markets in which traders put their own money at risk. And, second, use of money to motivate traders might have negative connotations in some health care settings.

A "funny money" market solves both of those problems; it was the solution adopted for the novel influenza A (H1N1) prediction markets described below. Specifically, trading takes place in an artificial currency, some amount of which is endowed to each trader at the beginning of the market. After the market closes, the balances remaining are worthless, but during the course of the market, the account balances serve as a measure of the trading and prediction success of individual traders. Those balances can, for example, be posted, either anonymously or with the traders identified, and the standing on this "leader board" might itself provide motivation for active and careful market participation. The efficacy of funny-money markets has not yet been completely resolved. Some experimental evidence, however, shows that accurate results can be achieved, though the variance around predictions seems to be greater than with markets in which traders earn real profits and losses (Servan et al. 2004).

A second solution is to operate the markets with real money, but the money used is provided by the market managers rather than by the participants. As with funny-money markets, traders are given a trading account endowed with some amount of an artificial currency, but at the end of the market, the balance in the account—the original endowment plus trading profits and less trading losses—is converted to U.S. dollars and paid to the trader. Traders thus realize real monetary rewards in exchange for their participation, much like respondents are sometimes paid for their completion of a survey instrument. The difference, however, is that the size of the reward depends on the success of the participant, both in accurate assessment of the likelihood of event outcomes and in successful market actions. To minimize any adverse reactions, the payments at the end of the market can be in the form of educational grants to traders for use in paying for reference books, journal subscriptions, conference fees, education-related travel costs, and so forth. Most of the health-related markets our group has run have operated in this fashion.

8.3.3 Examples of Prediction Markets

The concept of a prediction market was first developed by investigators at the University of Iowa's Tippie College of Business; the original prediction market, the Iowa Electronic Market (IEM), opened in 1988 and still operates today. Unlike other prediction markets, the IEM's mission is not financial gain, but research and teaching. Currently, it is the only prediction market authorized by the Commodity Futures Trading Commission to permit traders to invest their own money. That authorization is in the form of a "no-action letter," which spells out strict conditions regarding the size of investments permitted, the number and nature of traders allowed, and the topics on which the markets can be based. Since 1988, the IEM has run markets for currency prices, stock options, elections around the world, and movie box office receipts, and it has achieved a prediction record superior to alternative methods such as opinion polls (Forsythe et al. 1992, Forsythe et al. 1991, Forsythe et al. 1997). In his acceptance speech after winning the Nobel Prize in Economics in 2002, Vernon Smith cited the IEM as providing one of the best demonstrations of how markets efficiently aggregate information about future events (Smith 2003).

Experimental prediction markets have been used successfully to forecast future events in several settings. For example, Hewlett-Packard has used experimental markets to forecast sales of its printers, and those markets outperformed the company's own statistical sales forecasts (Plott 2000). Similarly, The Hollywood Stock Exchange has accurately predicted Oscar winners and opening-weekend movie box-office receipts (Pennock et al. 2001). The Foresight Exchange operated markets to predict a variety of events such as whether specific mathematical conjectures will be proved (Pennock et al. 2001). More recently, Google has used internal prediction markets with employees as traders to help guide business decisions (Cowgill et al. 2008). One set of contracts, for example, served to predict how many people would sign up for their free e-mail service. Similarly, Best Buy has used these markets to predict what consumer electronic products will be in high demand (Dvorak 2008). Indeed, a small industry has evolved to provide software and consulting to businesses seeking to use prediction markets as a management tool. NewsFutures and Inkling are two examples of such firms.

8.3.4 Prediction Markets for Public Health

Most prediction markets currently focus on helping businesses make decisions, and not surprisingly, most health applications of prediction markets involve the pharmaceutical industry. Applications include, for example, predicting demand for their drugs. To investigate other public health applications for prediction markets, we started a seasonal influenza market in the state of Iowa and have been operating that market since 2004. Even the original market with only 20 or so active traders successfully predicted the start, peak and end of the influenza season in Iowa between 2, and 4 weeks in advance (Polgreen et al. 2007). We have since generated similar results in other states. We subsequently experimented with prediction markets to investigate emerging infectious diseases. To determine whether prediction markets could accurately forecast events related to the spread of H5N1 influenza, we collaborated with the Program for Monitoring Emerging Diseases (ProMED-mail). In this market, the prices were designed to represent the real-time aggregate view of our traders regarding the probability of different avian influenza events. Contracts were based on public policy decisions or numbers and locations of human and animal H5N1 cases. The majority of the events (whether new human or animal cases of H5N1 appeared in particular regions within particular time periods and whether WHO announced H5N1 pandemic levels 4 or 5) did not come true. Our market prices predicted each of these outcomes months in advance. We were also able to predict ranges on the number of human cases worldwide months in advance (Polgreen et al. 2009).

8.4 Novel Influenza A (H1N1) Case Study

One advantage of prediction markets is that once a trading system and a pool of traders are in place, contracts for new events can be introduced with very short notice. As soon as trading starts, the market provides probability estimates for those events. In late April of 2009, the international public health community learned of a novel strain of H1N1 influenza that had reportedly caused multiple deaths in Mexico, and it appeared to be spreading quickly among humans as new reports occurred in new locations on a daily basis. As information about the cases in Mexico increased so did the confusion surrounding the early clinical future of the disease. For example, in late April there seemed to be a discrepancy between the severities of the cases in Mexico compared with cases in the United States. Also, the outbreak started in the spring, when seasonal influenza seasons tend to end. Thus, there was a great deal of uncertainty regarding the likely duration of the outbreak, its geographic spread, how many cases would arise, and the severity of the infections.

To help resolve some of the uncertainty about this new emerging disease, we quickly opened a novel influenza A (H1N1) prediction market. Since the short notice provided little opportunity for securing funding for trader accounts, it was determined to operate the markets using funny money. Thus, in addition to gaining information about the progression of the disease, we used the novel influenza A (H1N1) market to test the feasibility and accuracy of a "funny money market" for emerging infectious diseases. We had four general questions: (1) How many cases would occur in the United

States? (2) What geographic areas would be infected in the United States and worldwide? (3) Would the morbidity and mortality in the United States be similar to the early reports from Mexico? and (4) How long into the summer would the 2009 novel influenza A (H1N1) outbreak last?

As of late April, we were unsure of what type of novel influenza A (H1N1) surveillance would be conducted, for how long it would continue, and at what granularity the data would be reported. Thus, we designed contracts that we thought would be easy to verify over subsequent months. The full list of contracts appears in Table 8.1. All contracts were designed to be worth 1.00 H1N1 dollar if the specified event occurred and 0 H1N1 dollars if it did not.

On April 27, 2009, we opened five contracts, and we sent a single e-mail to current and previous participants in our other health prediction markets inviting them to join (see Table 8.1). We specified that all U.S.-based contracts would be resolved using data from the Centers for Disease Control and Prevention, and World Health Organization (WHO) data would be used for international-based contracts.

Each participant who signed up received 100 H1N1 dollars with which to trade in any of the novel influenza A (H1N1) related contracts. In addition to serving as the medium of exchange for the market, this valueless currency also provided a measure of the trading and prediction success of individual traders. All trading occurred on our Web site, and the market was open 24 hours each day. Figures 8.1a,b show the beginner and advanced trading interface. We sent only one reminder to trade on May 11, 2009.

Signing up for accounts were 160 individuals. However, only 64 participated. Traders from a variety of backgrounds participated, including physicians, epidemiologists, nurses, pharmacists, and health administrators. From Tuesday, April 29, to Wednesday, July 1, 2009, a total of 6,753 shares were traded. The number of orders per trader ranged from 1 to 400, and on July 2, trading balances range from H1N1$1.66 to H1N1$137.10.

As traders bought and sold contracts over the Internet, in accordance with their individual expectations regarding novel influenza A (H1N1) activity, a price was generated for each transaction. Because all contracts were to have liquidation values of either H1N1$0.00 or H1N1$1.00, these prices generated by the market can be interpreted as the consensus probability that the event specified by the contract would occur. For example, if a contract trades for H1N1$0.90, this translates into a 90% probability of the event occurring.

Figures 8.2–8.6 show how consensus emerged very quickly among traders for each of our contracts. For example, almost as soon as the market opened, traders predicted that the mortality rate in the United States would be less than 1% (Figure 8.2) and that there would be more than 1,100 confirmed cases within a month (Figure 8.3). The market also predicted within a day of opening that more than 40 states and 50 countries would have confirmed cases by the end of May (Figures 8.4 and 8.5a,b). All of these events occurred. Traders also predicted, but with a bit less certainty, that

TABLE 8.1

Iowa Electronic Health Market Novel Influenza A (H1n1) Markets and Contracts

How many cases of novel influenza A (H1N1) will be confirmed in the United States by end of May 2009?	
	200 or fewer cases
	201 to 350 cases
	351 to 600 cases
	601 to 1100 cases
	1101 or more cases
How many states in the United States will have at least one confirmed case of novel influenza A (H1N1) by the end of May 2009?	
	1 to 10 states
	11 to 20 states
	21 to 30 states
	31 to 40 states
	41 to 50 states
What will the mortality rate for novel influenza A (H1N1) be by the end of July 2009?	
	Lower than 1%
	1% to 2.5%
	2.5% to 5%
	5% to 10%
	Higher than 10%
How long will the novel influenza A (H1N1) outbreak last?	
	Before May 31
	June 1 to June 30
	July 1 to July 31
	After July 31
How many countries will have at least one confirmed case of novel influenza A (H1N1) by the end of July 2009?	
	25 or fewer countries
	26 to 50 countries
	51 to 75 countries
	76 to 100 countries
	101 or more countries

the novel influenza A (H1N1) outbreak would last for more than 2 months in the United States (Figure 8.6).

We were pleased with the performance of our market. Despite a limited number of active traders, we were able to aggregate information and make reasonably accurate predictions. Our recruitment efforts were minimal. For example, unlike for our H5N1 market, we did not recruit traders using the ProMED-mail Listserv. In addition, unlike for our previous infectious disease markets, we sent only one e-mail reminder to trade, that e-mail coming after we opened two

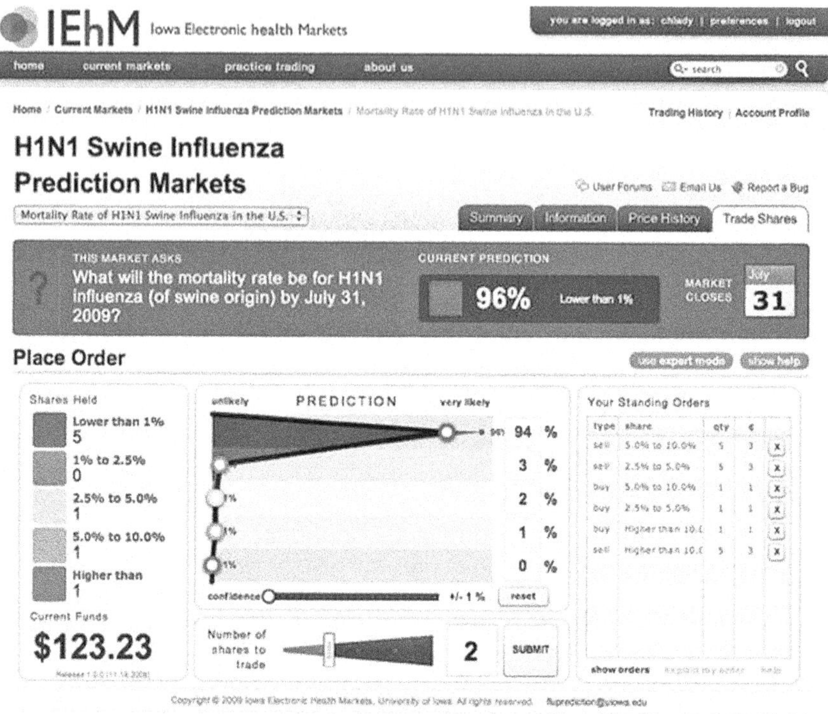

FIGURE 8.1a
Beginning trading interface.

new contracts. In other markets, our practice has been to send weekly e-mail reminders to all traders. One of the new contracts we opened was related to novel influenza A (H1N1) vaccine availability during the next influenza season and the other regarded the likelihood of the return and the extent of the return of novel influenza A (H1N1) during the next influenza season.

Some of our market's limitations were related to the availability of underlying surveillance data. We considered opening additional contracts to predict the total number of cases in the United States, but some states decided after a few weeks not to attempt confirmation of all suspected novel influenza A (H1N1) cases. Thus, we did not open new case-number contracts. We also found that the variance around some of our predictions seemed higher than that of previous markets. This is likely because we did not use real money in this market. In addition, the volume of trading decreased over time. In the past, we have demonstrated that trading levels are higher with reminder e-mails. Thus, in future projects, we would advocate sending weekly reminders for trading. Interpretation of prices also depends upon active trading. Because prices change with each trade, one trader can greatly affect the short-term price of a contract. In an active market, this is less likely. Our country contract shows how volatile markets can be and underscores

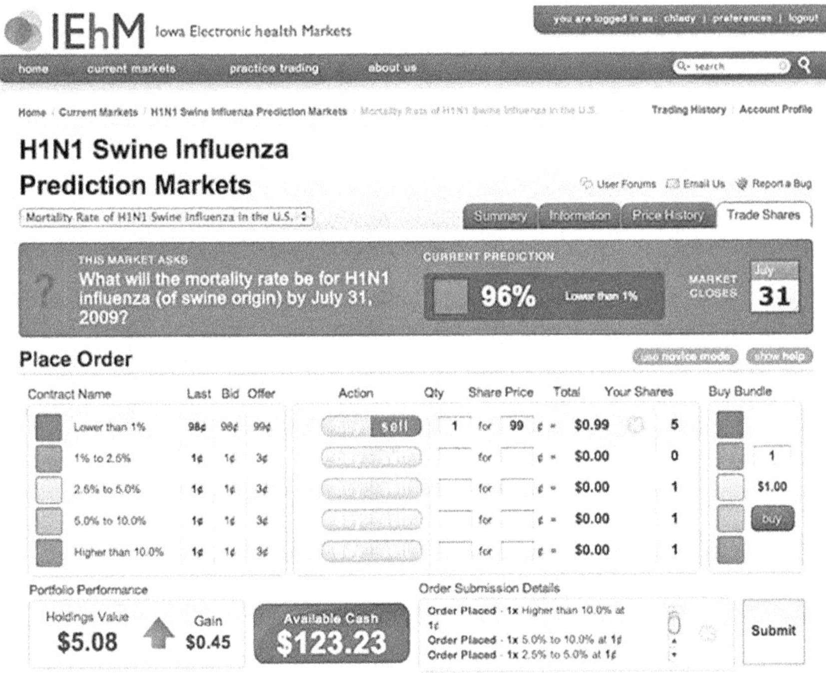

FIGURE 8.1b
Advanced trading interface.

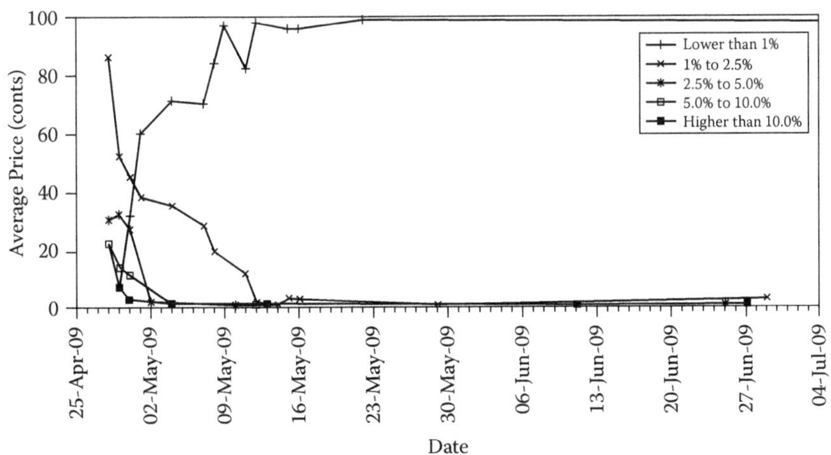

FIGURE 8.2
Price graph for the contract "What will the mortality rate for novel influenza A (H1N1) be by the end of July 2009?"

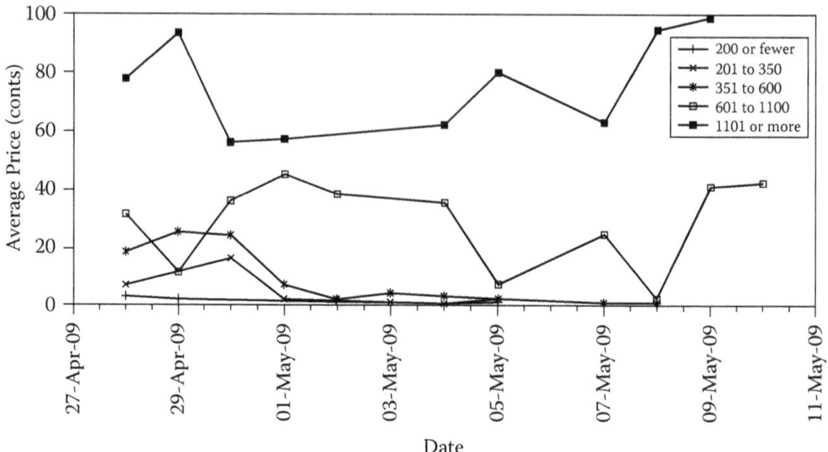

FIGURE 8.3
Price graph for the contract "How many cases of novel influenza A (H1N1) will be confirmed in the United States by end of May 2009?"

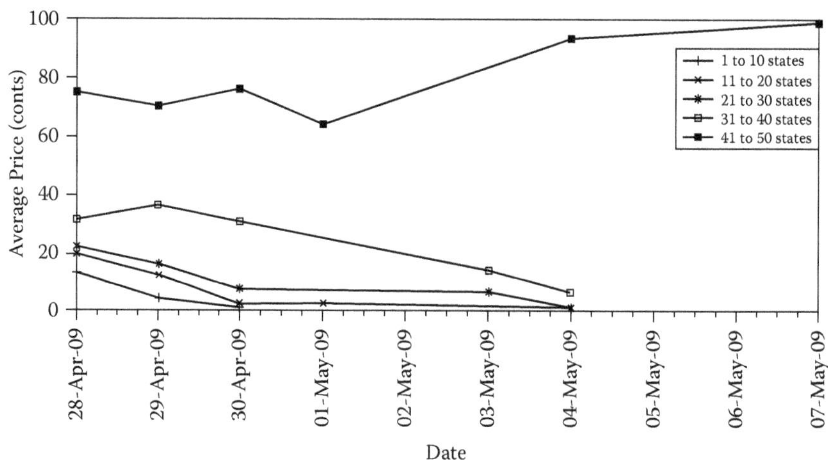

FIGURE 8.4
Price graph for the contract "How many states in the United States will have at least one confirmed case of novel influenza A (H1N1) by the end of May 2009?"

this limitation. For many weeks, the market consensus was that novel influenza A (H1N1) would affect more than 100 countries. However, for a number of days in June, the number of countries affected seemed to level off at fewer than 90 countries. Subsequently, a few trades caused the price of the contract based on "between 76 and 100 countries" to increase dramatically. A few days later, more than 100 total countries were reported affected. Did the market miss it? Yes and no. Technically, yes, however, the general trend of

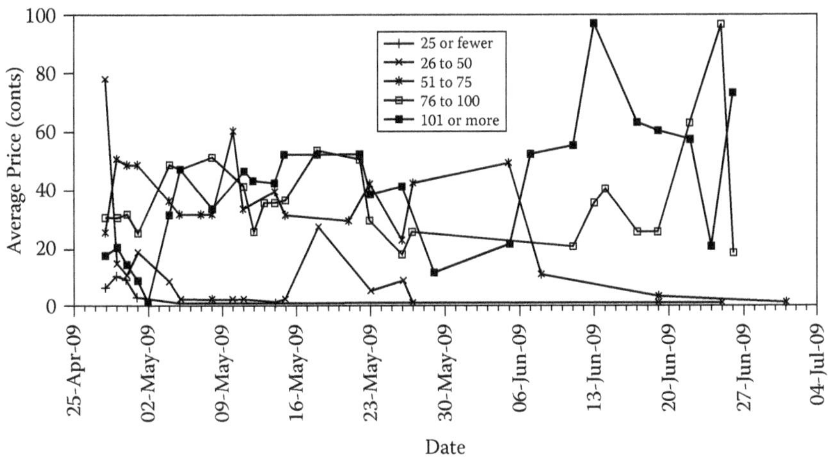

FIGURE 8.5a
Price graph for the contract "How many countries will have at least one confirmed case of novel influenza A (H1N1) by the end of July 2009?"

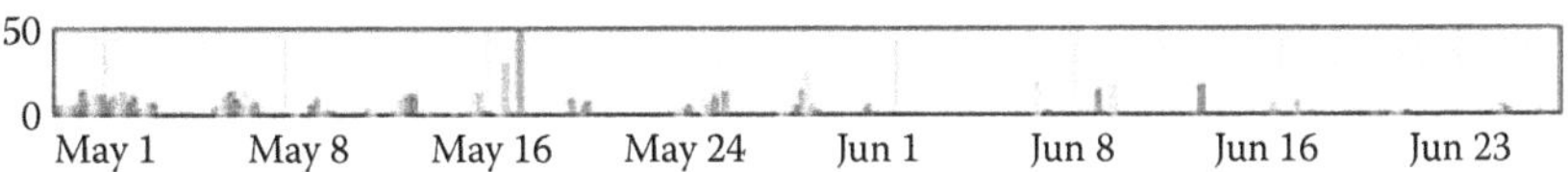

FIGURE 8.5b
Trading volume for market in Figure 8.5a.

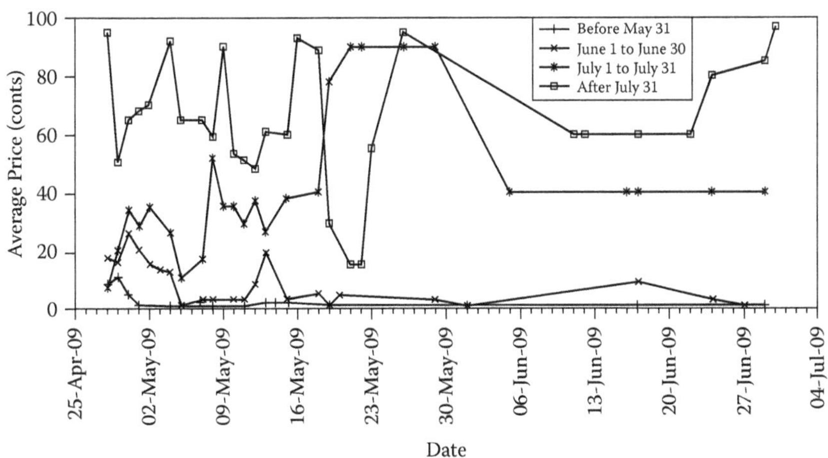

FIGURE 8.6
Price graph for the contract "How long will the novel influenza A (H1N1) outbreak last in the United States?"

the market still demonstrates that the traders collectively thought that novel influenza A (H1N1) would travel quickly around the world and would affect a very large number of countries. Nevertheless, this example shows how volatile prices in lightly traded markets can be and signals the importance of carefully considering dramatic price changes caused by a very limited number of trades. In some situations, in thinly traded markets, it might be more accurate to look at moving-average prices. For example, a "three-day moving average" or a weekly average (if most traders only trade once per week).

Ultimately, though, our pilot novel influenza A (H1N1) market did show that a diverse group of participants could accurately predict a series of novel influenza A (H1N1)–related events using a prediction market based on a valueless currency. Thus, we think that prediction markets may provide a flexible and effective way to aggregate both objective and subjective information about emerging infectious diseases, even without monetary incentives. Given a pool of informed participants willing to trade in a market, one can envision that probabilities generated by the market could help public health officials plan for the future and coordinate resources.

8.5 Conclusions

Prediction markets might seem like a very academic or impractical approach to forecasting disease activity. However, consider the alternative. Currently, the public health community does not have any convenient way to ask a diverse group of experts about the likelihood of the occurrence of disease-related events. Public health officials can ask their co-workers questions or sponsor conference calls, but these are difficult to arrange across different time zones. Surveys could also be distributed, but there are several limitations to running surveys to aggregate information about emerging infectious diseases. In fact, prediction markets have several advantages over surveys: (1) They are continuous and ongoing, allowing immediate revelation of new information. (2) While some surveys offer a small incentive in return for participation, the incentives earned by traders in a prediction market increase in proportion to the quality of the information provided. (3) Unlike surveys, a market provides immediate feedback to participants, allowing them opportunities to reassess their own information and to respond. (4) The market interface is interactive, in marked contrast to most surveys, providing further incentives for participation. (5) Furthermore, most surveys rely on random samples for validity and accuracy. In prediction markets, on the other hand, the best participants are those with the best information, and those are the very individuals who are most likely to self-select into the market. With surveys, this process would introduce a sampling bias, but with markets, the incentive structure tends to make the forecasts more accurate.

We do not think that prediction markets will replace existing influenza surveillance systems, nor will they eliminate the need for improvements to the existing systems. Instead, we propose prediction markets as a supplement to traditional surveillance approaches. Active prediction markets could act as a "barometer" for emerging infectious diseases. The probabilities generated by prediction markets could help policymakers and public health officials coordinate resources, facilitate vaccine production, manage stockpiles of medications, and plan for the allocation of personnel and other resources. Finally, once a broad group of traders are accustomed to using prediction markets for one disease, in many situations, they could be recruited to participate in markets for other infectious diseases, both emerging and reemerging.

References

Cowgill, B., Wolfers, J., and Zitzewitz, E. Using prediction markets to track information flows: Evidence from Google, Dartmouth College (2008); www.bocowgill.com/GooglePredictionMarketPaper.pdf.

Dailey, L., Watkins, R.E., and Plant, A.J. Timeliness of data sources used for influenza surveillance. *J Am Med Inform Assoc* 2007;14:626–31.

Davies, G.R. and Finch, R.G. Sales of over-the-counter remedies as an early warning system for winter bed crises. *Clin Microbiol Infect* 2003; 9:858–63.

Dvorak, P. Best Buy taps "prediction market." *Wall Street Journal*. September 16, 2008. Available at: http://online.wsj.com/article/SB122152452811139909.html.

Eisenberg, E. and Gale, D. Consensus of subjective probabilities: The pari-mutuel method. *Ann Math Stat* 1958; 30:165–8.

Forsythe, R., Berg, J., and Rietz, T. What makes markets predict well? Evidence from the Iowa Electronic Markets. In Alberts, W., Guth, W., Hammerstein, P., Moldovan, B., van Damme, E., Eds. *Understanding Strategic Interaction: Essays in Honor of Reinhard Selten*. Amsterdam, The Netherlands: Springer, 1997:444–63.

Forsythe, R., Nelson, F.D., Neumann, G.R., and Wright, J. Anatomy of an experimental political stock market. *Am Econ Rev* 1992; 82:1142–61.

Forsythe, R., Nelson, F.D., Neumann, G.R., and Wright, J. The explanation and prediction of presidential elections: A market alternative to polls. In: Palfrey, T.R., Ed. *Laboratory Research in Political Economy*. Ann Arbor, MI: University of Michigan Press; 1991:69–112.

Ginsberg, J., Mohebbi, M.H., Patel, R.S., Brammer, L., Smolinski, M.S., and Brilliant, L. Detecting influenza epidemics using search engine query data. *Nature* 2009 Feb 19; 457(7232):1012–4.

Hogan, W.R., Tsui, F.C., Ivanov, O., et al. Indiana-Pennsylvania-Utah Collaboration. Detection of pediatric respiratory and diarrheal outbreaks from sales of over-the-counter electrolyte products. *J Am Med Inform Assoc* 2003; 10:555–62.

Irvin, C.B., Nouhan, P.P., and Rice, K. Syndromic analysis of computerized emergency department patients' chief complaints: an opportunity for bioterrorism and influenza surveillance. *Ann Emerg Med* 2003; 41:447–52.

Lenaway, D.D. and Ambler, A. Evaluation of a school-based influenza surveillance system. *Public Health Rep* 1995; 110:333–7.

Magruder, S. Evaluation of over-the-counter pharmaceutical sales as a possible early warning indicator of human disease. *Johns Hopkins University Applied Physics Laboratory Technical Digest* 2003; 24:349–53.

Pennock, D.M., Lawrence, S., Giles, C.L., and Nielsen, F.A. The real power of artificial markets. *Science* 2001; 291: 987–88.

Plott, C.R. Markets as information gathering tools. *South Econ J* 2000; 67:1–15.

Polgreen, P.M., Chen, Y., Pennock, D.M., and Nelson, F.D. Using internet searches for influenza surveillance. *Clin Infect Dis* 2008 Dec 1; 47(11):1443–48.

Polgreen, P.M., Nelson, F.D., and Neumann, G.R. Use of prediction markets to forecast infectious disease activity. *Clin Infect Dis* 2007; 44:272–79.

Polgreen, P.M., Nelson, F.D., Neumann, G.R., Segre, A.M., Fries, J., and Madoff, L.C. Use of a prediction market to forecast H5N1 influenza. Presented at International Meeting on Emerging Diseases and Surveillance, Abstract 18.091, Vienna, Austria, February 13–16, 2009.

Roll, R. Orange juice and weather. *Am Econ Rev* 1984; 74, 861–80.

Servan-Schreiber, E., Wolfers, J., Pennock, D.M., and Galebach, B. Prediction markets: Does money matter? *Electronic Markets* 2004; 14:243–51.

Smith, V.L. Constructivist and ecological rationality in economics. *Am Econ Rev* 2003; 93:465–508.

Suyama, J., Sztajnkrycer, M., Lindsell, C., Otten, E.J., Daniels, J.M., and Kressel, A.B. Surveillance of infectious disease occurrences in the community: An analysis of symptom presentation in the emergency department. *Acad Emerg Med* 2003; 10:753–63.

Welliver, R.C., Cherry, J.D., Boyer, K.M., et al. Sales of nonprescription cold remedies: a unique method of influenza surveillance. *Pediatr Res* 1979; 13:1015–17.

Yuan, C.M., Love, S., and Wilson, M. Syndromic surveillance at hospital emergency departments—southeastern Virginia. *MMWR Morb Mortal Wkly Rep* 2004; 53(Suppl.):56–58.

9

The Role of Data Aggregation in Public Health and Food Safety Surveillance

Artur Dubrawski
Auton Lab, Carnegie Mellon University
5000 Forbes Avenue, NSH 3121, Pittsburgh, PA 15213, USA
awd@cs.cmu.edu

CONTENTS

9.1 Introduction

Data that can be used to support surveillance of public health are becoming available to the analysts at increasing volumes and varieties. Widening of the availability is accompanied by a rapid rise of the volume, specificity, and complexity of questions being asked about data. Those processes jointly exacerbate the challenges related to statistical reliability of the models used in the analyses, and to statistical significance of the findings. Efficient and effective implementations of data aggregation strategies can tackle several of such challenges, including those related to dealing with large volumes of high-dimensional data, or dealing with low density of useful evidence in data due to sparseness of patterns of interest and due to high specificity of analytic questions.

Data aggregation is a prominent component of the analytic processes that occurs naturally in multiple contexts and phases of data-driven biosurveillance (Burkom et al. 2004). For instance, it is relevant to the task of searching for the most interesting projections of multidimensional surveillance data, often encountered in adverse event detection or emerging pattern-tracking applications. Popular methods used to handle such tasks, such as temporal or spatial scanning methods (Kulldorff 1997, Kulldorff et al. 2007, Neill and Moore 2004, Naus and Wallenstein 2006, Dubrawski et al. 2007a, Neill and Cooper 2009), rely on more or less exhaustive screening of data for subsets that reveal unusual behaviors or that match tracked patterns, and on evaluating each subset using aggregate statistics such as, for instance, contingency tables or marginal distributions. That creates a requirement for scalable aggregation of data in order to support comprehensive surveillance in a computationally feasible manner. Another practical context, in which the need for data aggregation is apparent, involves exploiting corroborating evidence obtained from distinct sources. Aggregating multiple signals often leads to improved detectability of events, and it can boost statistical reliability of the involved models and findings.

This chapter discusses the utility of data aggregation and a few computationally efficient implementations of it using example applications in the areas of public health and food safety surveillance.

The next section introduces a data structure designed to efficiently represent large sets of multidimensional event data of the types often encountered in health surveillance. It is called T-Cube and it is an extension of the AD-Tree: an in-memory data structure that efficiently caches answers to all conceivable queries against multidimensional databases of categorical variables (Moore and Lee 1998). T-Cube extends the idea of AD-Tree toward an important task of very fast aggregation of multidimensional time series of counts of events. The attainable efficiencies support human users, who benefit from very fast responses to queries and from dynamic visualizations of data at interactive speeds. Fast querying also allows for large-scale mining of multidimensional categorical aggregates. Exhaustive searches for patterns in highly dimensional categorical data become computationally tractable. That minimizes the risk of missing something important by having to resort to a selective mode of surveillance.

Aggregation of evidence across multiple streams of data is the topic of the subsequent section. Exploiting corroborating evidence from separate sources has many practical applications. The approach used here as an illustration employs single-stream anomaly detectors and Fisher's method of p-value aggregation to construct powerful multi-stream detectors (Roure et al. 2007).

Section 4 deals with feature aggregation for cross-stream analysis. As the events of interest become sparser, it is typically more difficult to construct reliable models of correlations between streams of data. Data aggregation can sometimes come to the rescue, as in the example task of predicting the risk of occurrence of *Salmonella* at a food factory, given its recent history of sanitary inspections.

In many practical scenarios, sparse event data can be represented as a network of entities and links. Evidence pertaining to the individual entities can then be shared among their neighbors in the graph. It is shown in Section 5 that such an approach can boost predictive power of models built from sparse events data in practical applications (Sarkar et al. 2008, Dubrawski et al. 2009b, Dubrawski et al. 2007b).

9.2 Scalable Aggregation of Evidence in Multidimensional Event Data

Many data sets encountered in the practice of biosurveillance have the form of a record of transactions. Each entry in such data typically includes date/time of an event (such as a pharmacy sales transaction or an admission of a patient to a hospital) and a number of descriptors characterizing it (e.g., the brand, name, dose, and quantity of the pharmaceutical sold, or the age, gender, symptoms, and test results of the admitted patient). In order to understand and to monitor processes taking place in environments producing such data, one needs to track frequencies of events of various categories over time. This requires computing numerous different aggregations of data. For instance, when monitoring hospital records for indications of a possible local outbreak of a gastrointestinal ailment, the public health analysts may want to check daily counts of children reporting recently with bloody stools to hospitals in Pittsburgh, and compare these counts against the expectation derived from the analogical numbers observed over, for instance, the past 12 months. The number of possible count queries involving multiple multi-valued attributes that can be asked of such data can be actually very high. Given the large number of possibilities, answering all possible queries up to a certain level of specificity, as in exhaustive screening scenarios, poses a serious computational challenge.

One way of addressing that challenge is to precompute all counts of interest ahead of the time of analysis, for instance, upon loading the data. Database administrators do similar things routinely. They monitor frequencies of queries issued by the database users, and they cache the responses to the most popular ones in the server's operating memory, so that they are handy when the next predictable request comes along. This approach lessens the burden on the database system and often significantly boosts its throughput. Similarly, statisticians are used to construct contingency tables to represent distributions of multivariate discrete data. The cells in these tables store counts of events corresponding to all unique combinations of values of all involved dimensions. These counts, as soon as they are extracted from raw data and stored in the table, are readily available for very fast computations of estimates of all conceivable probabilities that can be derived from the data at hand. For instance, to compute today's estimate of the conditional probability of seeing a report of bloody stools given the young age of the triaged patient, and the recent admissions data, one needs to aggregate current counts from all cells at the intersection of *symptom* = "bloody stools" and *patients_age* = "child" and divide the result by the sum of the recent counts of patient visits retrieved from all cells matching *patients_age* = "child." The contingency table approach is very useful in facilitating data-intensive statistical mining. In its nutshell, it is more comprehensive than the standard database query caching strategy mentioned above in that it pays an equal attention to precomputing numbers needed to derive answers to all possible queries. Unfortunately, contingency tables may consume large amounts of memory, and they become infeasible to use in practice when the number of dimensions of data is not trivially small, and when the number of unique combinations of their values becomes very large.

T-Cube is an alternative data cache structure that addresses that challenge by memorizing a limited and controllable amount of information about data, which is sufficient for either direct retrieval or for rapid reconstruction of all conceivable aggregations (Sabhnani et al. 2007). It extends the idea of AD-tree (Moore and Lee 1998) to represent time series of counts. AD-tree is an in-memory data cache that leverages redundancies in the raw event data to represent it in a compact form. It enables rapid responses to all conceivable queries for counts of occurrences of events, and in that sense, it mimics the functionality of contingency tables. Its query-response time is independent of the number of records in the raw data, and it is typically orders of magnitude shorter than attainable with the state-of-the art database systems. AD-tree achieves that at substantially lower memory requirements than typically seen from contingency tables in multidimensional multi-valued data scenarios.

Figure 9.1 conveys the basic idea of T-Cube data representation and query retrieval applied to a simple public health data set. The top node of the tree represents the most general query, and it stores the cumulative time series of counts of all categories of events characterized by gender and two types of symptoms reported by patients (in this example, we focus on gastrointestinal and respiratory symptoms). Nodes at deeper levels of the tree store time series corresponding to increasingly more specific queries. Once the T-Cube is built, time series for any query can be retrieved in time independent of the number of records in the raw dataset. One example of such a query is "get me the time series by day for all males reporting with gastrointestinal but with no respiratory symptoms." The reply can be produced easily by navigating to the nodes of the tree, which represent exactly the conjunctive components of each query and by aggregating and/or subtracting time series stored in them as needed.

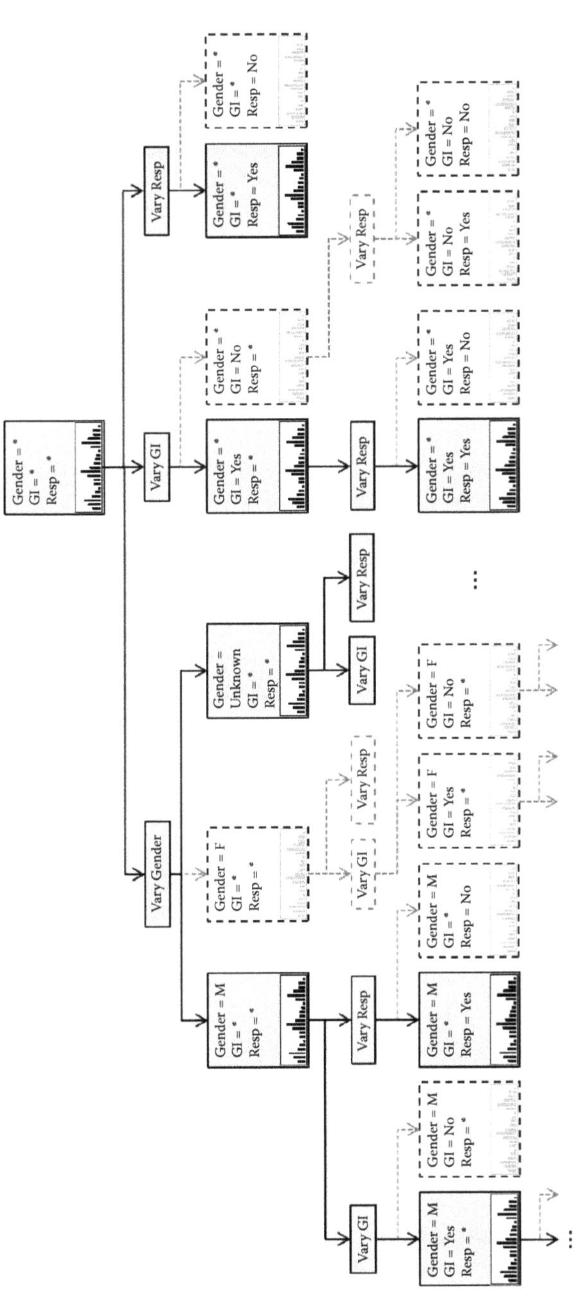

FIGURE 9.1
Simple example of a T-Cube structure built for data typical to the public health domain. Components shown in light gray can be pruned for large savings of memory at a marginal increase of computational costs.

A completely developed T-Cube may grow large when data have more than a few dimensions. But it can be severely pruned (using representational tricks originally developed for AD-trees) and still fully serve its purpose. Firstly, there is no need to store any nodes that correspond to time series of all zeros. Secondly, we can remove all sub-trees starting at the node corresponding to the most frequent value of the variable to be instantiated at each "vary" node in the tree diagram. This eliminates large portions of the tree (cf. Figure 9.1), and still the removed information can be cheaply recomputed on-the-fly with simple arithmetic operations using the data stored in the remaining nodes. Additional memory savings can be attained by not developing the tree to its full depth and instead terminating it at nodes corresponding to attribute-value combinations that occur less frequently in data with a set of pointers to the corresponding raw data records. This can reduce the memory requirements by another couple of orders of magnitude, with a trade-off in access time. Those tricks enable T-Cube to fit in memory and still retrieve time series substantially faster when compared to the current database technology. That helps in making many data-intensive analytic algorithms practical. It also enables user-level interactive visualization as well as real-time navigation through large sets of multidimensional temporal data.

Efficiencies offered by T-Cube enable large-scale mining of multidimensional bio event data. In general, the public health analysts may not know a priori which subsets of data require their immediate attention. Often, they resort to selective monitoring driven by intuition and experience, and therefore, they become exposed to the risk of missing less obvious patterns occurring outside of the scope of routine surveillance. This can be alleviated by implementing massive screening through multiple (ideally all possible) aggregations of data in search of those that contain the most statistically surprising abnormalities. T-Cube makes such tasks feasible when using popular temporal anomaly detection algorithms such as cumulative sum (Page 1954), temporal scan (Naus and Wallenstein 2006, Dubrawski et al. 2007a), or spatial scan (Kulldorff 1997, Kulldorff et al. 2007, Neill and Moore 2004, Neill and Cooper 2009).

Bi-variate temporal scan and Bayesian spatial scan are the analytic methods of choice in the Real-Time Biosurveillance Project (RTBP) (Dubrawski et al. 2009a). They are used for rapid and reliable detection of emerging outbreaks of diseases manifested in public health data collected in the country of Sri Lanka and, separately, in Tamil Nadu state of India. The RTBP consists of an information-gathering component based on mobile handheld devices and wireless networking, and of the data analysis and visualization component based on T-Cube. The latter enables geo-temporal visualization of syndromic data, navigation through different levels of data aggregation, as well as prospective and retrospective screening of data for patterns of public health interest.

Figure 9.2 presents results of an analytic scenario applied to the record of reportable diseases reported to the Sri Lankan Ministry of Healthcare

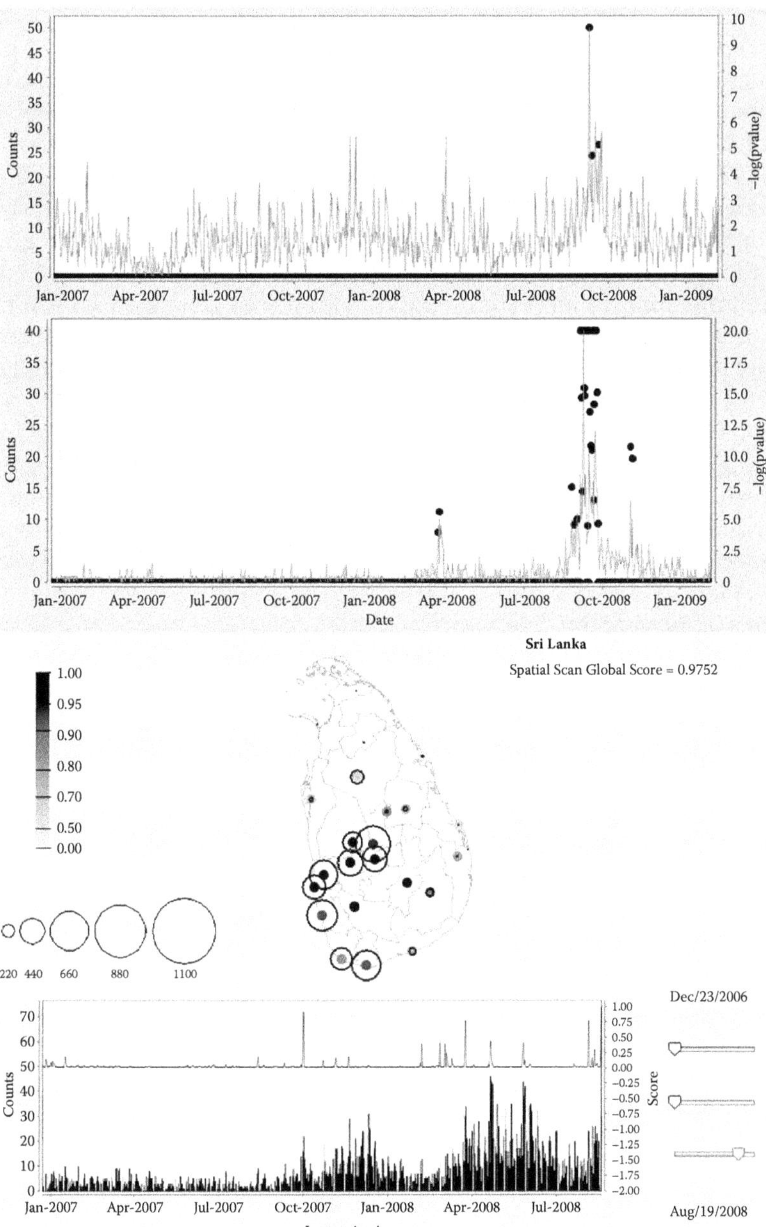

FIGURE 9.2
Within a couple of minutes from loading the data, the analysts found an emerging leptospirosis event in the southwestern and central provinces of Sri Lanka. Spatial scan algorithm tracks probabilities of leptospirosis outbreak anywhere in the nation for all days in the past data. On August 18, 2008, it went over 97%. Dark bars in the time-series plot and dark circles in the map depict the temporal and spatial distribution of the volume of patients diagnosed with the disease.

and Nutrition. The top graph depicts in gray time series of daily counts of all reportable disease occurrences in the region on Colombo, Sri Lanka. The alerts generated by the bi-variate temporal scan (shown as black dots) executed in the retrospective screening mode, indicate days in late summer of 2008 when the increases in these counts exceeded the nationwide trends. The analysts then run temporal scan screening against the data from Colombo. It identified that patients diagnosed with leptospirosis are the main contributing factor to the observed unusual trend (middle graph). Even though the disease outbreak escalated slowly over more than 45 days, the first meaningful alert from temporal scan was generated within three days of its onset. Further drill-down revealed that the leptospirosis event was not restricted to Colombo, but, as indicated by the Bayesian spatial scan analysis, it has shortly spread to seven other regions. High probability of the locations being affected by it is shown with large circles on the map in the bottom graph. Bayesian spatial scan tracked probabilities of leptospirosis outbreak anywhere in the nation for all days in the past data (plotted as the upper line in the plot under the map). On August 20, 2008, that probability exceeded 97%. Thanks to the efficiencies of T-Cube, the analysts could detect, identify, and geographically localize leptospirosis event within a few minutes of loading the data.

The RTBP system uses the T-Cube Web Interface (TCWI) as a platform to visualize and manipulate multidimensional time series. Variants of TCWI are also used elsewhere (Ray et al. 2008). Figure 9.3 presents a screenshot of a pane of the interface showing an overlay of spatiotemporal distributions of the results of food tests against *Salmonella* collected by the U.S. Department of Agriculture (USDA), and the counts of human cases of salmonellosis recorded by the Centers of Disease Control and Prevention (CDC). T-Cube Web Interface has enabled the USDA and CDC researchers to browse their data jointly. It allowed them to drill into details, to focus on specific *Salmonella* serotypes, to screen the data temporally and spatially as well as with respect to other dimensions in it, and to do all that on-the-fly in a fully interactive mode. This capability has led to discoveries of patterns in data that can be indicative of food-borne sources of human disease outbreaks. A generic variant of TCWI is also available for public evaluation (Auton Lab 2009).

T-Cube has emerged as an enabling technology that supports automated analyses as well as user manipulations of typical bio event data. By speeding up execution of evidence aggregation procedures, it enables more comprehensive and timelier surveillance of such data with virtually no additional burden on computing resources. It also enables closer-than-before interactions between users and their data. Thanks to rapid responses to ad-hoc queries, the analyst routine can be transformed from batch-mode processing of data into much more interactive and exciting real-time navigation through it.

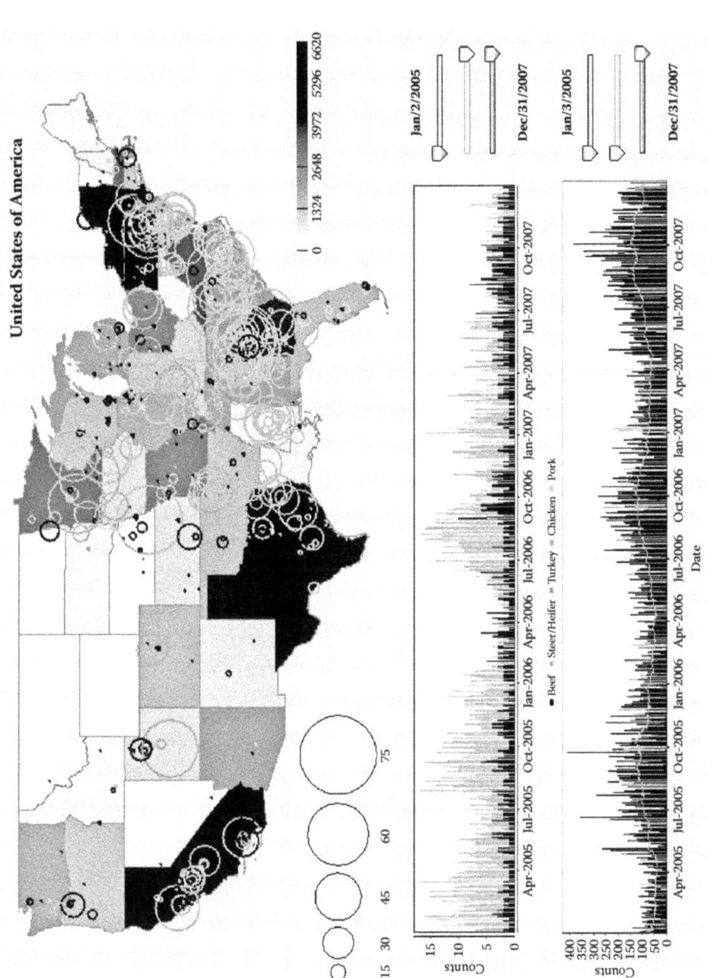

FIGURE 9.3
A screenshot of one pane of the T-Cube Web Interface showing spatial and temporal distributions of the USDA *Salmonella* tests data (circles: diameter indicates volume, location corresponds to the place of data acquisition, gray - negative results, black indicates positive results) and the CDC human salmonellosis data (aggregated statewide, the darker the background the higher the counts). The users can drill-down and roll-up through many dimensions of this data at fully interactive speeds thanks to the efficiency of the underlying T-Cube data structures.

9.3 Aggregation of Evidence across Multiple Streams of Data

Simultaneous monitoring of signals coming from distinct sources, or surveying diverse aspects of data even if it comes from a single source, can yield improvements in accuracy, sensitivity, specificity, and timeliness of event detection over more common single-stream analyses. That is possible if the individual streams contribute corroborating evidence to support determination of evaluated hypotheses. For instance, in public health domain, patient data collected at emergency rooms in hospitals can be used to corroborate epidemiological hypotheses derived by monitoring sales of certain classes of non-prescription medicines at nearby drugstores.

The best approach to handle multiple streams of such data is to model them jointly. However, it may not always be feasible in practice, given limited understanding of complex interactions of data between and within streams, and given limited amounts of data available for the joint model estimation. A typical way to overcome complexity is to develop a separate event detector for each individual stream and then raise an alert whenever either of them indicates abnormality (or, equivalently, to apply the *Minimum* operator to the set of single stream p-values, and to base the alert decision on its result). Unfortunately, information stemming from between-stream interactions is not used in this approach.

A useful alternative is the method that probabilistically aggregates p-values derived from anomaly detectors built for individual streams (Roure et al. 2007). The aggregated p-value represents the consensus estimate of strangeness. Since p-values follow a uniform distribution under the null hypothesis, Fisher statistic (the doubled sum of natural logarithms of the m independent p-values) has a χ^2 distribution with $2m$ degrees of freedom. There exists a closed form solution for the combined p-value, p_F:

$$p_F = k\sum_{i=0}^{m-1}\frac{(-\ln k)^i}{i!}, \quad \text{where} \quad k = \prod_{i=0}^{m-1} p_i.$$

Fisher's method is sensitive to situations where component p-values are just slightly greater than critical. That enables flagging cases in which the individual streams are of a marginal interest on their own, but they appear unusual when the corresponding pieces of evidence are combined. On the other hand, it is more conservative than the *Minimum* algorithm when either of the component p-values is substantially greater than critical. Conservative approach makes sense in many practical situations involving noisy data.

The example result shown in Figure 9.4 considers three streams of independently collected food and agriculture safety data involving records of daily counts of condemned and healthy cattle (Stream A), counts of positive and negative microbial tests of food samples (Stream B), and counts of

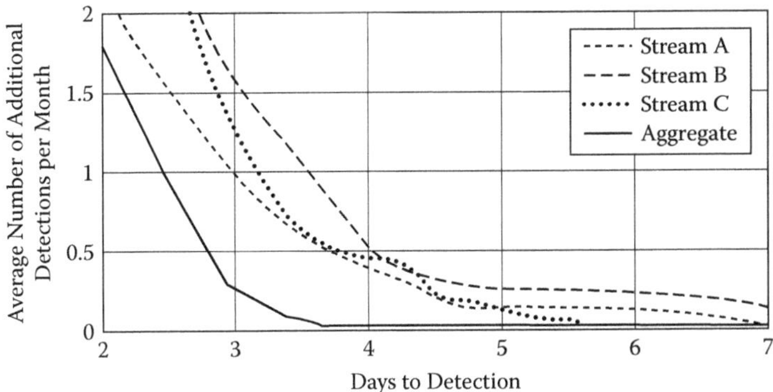

FIGURE 9.4
AMOC curves for univariate detectors (Streams A, B, and C) compared against the result of using Fisher's method of p-value aggregation. The vertical axis of the graph corresponds to the average frequency of detections outside of the duration of known events; the horizontal axis denotes the time to detection counted from the first day of the event.

passed and failed sanitary inspections conducted at the U.S. Department of Agriculture regulated slaughterhouses (Stream C). The task is to detect known patterns of increased activity synthetically introduced into the actual field data in order to measure power of the considered detectors. The synthetic activity manifests itself with the linearly increasing counts of events, induced independently but at the same date, over seven consecutive days. The average performance computed for univariate temporal anomaly detectors as well as the Fisher's aggregate on a sample of 100 synthetic injections are shown in Figure 9.4. The graph, showing Activity Monitoring Operating Characteristics (AMOCs), clearly depicts the benefits of aggregation of corroborating evidence across multiple streams of data. The aggregate detector is able to reliably call the event on the fourth day of its inception, two days ahead of the best of the univariate methods. Earlier detections are also possible at the cost of additional alerts generated outside of the scope of the known synthetic events. The average frequency of such alerts is substantially lower when using evidence aggregation, than with the use of the less informed alternatives.

9.4 Temporal Aggregation for Cross-Stream Analysis

Understanding relationships between disparate streams of event data can be difficult. The problems increase if the available data are sparse and if the events under consideration occur infrequently. In such cases, straightforward application of classical regression methods may not yield statistically reliable results due to the elevated risk of overfitting. Sometimes, simplification of

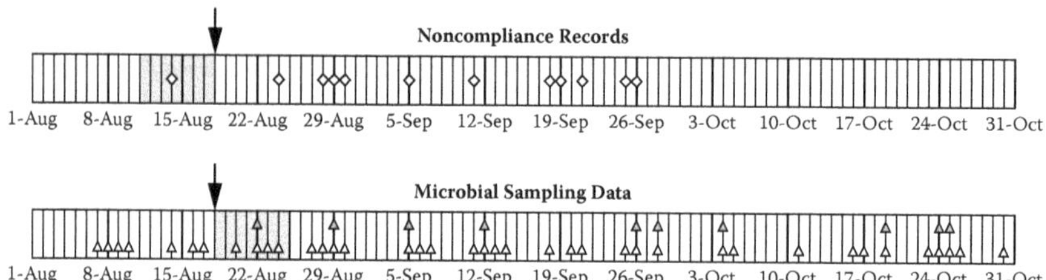

FIGURE 9.5
Temporal distribution of regulatory non-compliances and results of testing for *Salmonella* observed in one of the U.S. Department of Agriculture–regulated food factories.

the models combined with smart and purposive aggregation of data to produce informative features, can be the remedy.

An example can be drawn from a recent study into characterizing risk of a positive outcome of a test for *Salmonella* performed on a sample of food taken at a food factory, given the results of regulatory inspections conducted recently at the same factory. Applying regression directly to raw data does not yield useful outcomes. However, putting the problem into a temporal context followed by temporal aggregation of evidence, offers a more useful perspective. Figure 9.5 depicts temporal distributions of a certain class of failed regulatory inspections (labeled as non-compliance records) as well as passed and failed (marked with triangles) *Salmonella* tests of food samples, obtained for one of a few thousands of the U.S. Department of Agriculture regulated factories (note: this factory was particularly prone to violating regulations and was more intensively tested for *Salmonella* than the majority of its peers; the typical data from this kind of a source is sparser).

Let us pick one day in historical data, such as the one marked with arrows in Figure 9.5. The proposed retrospective data aggregation approach first checks whether, during a specific period in the future (typically one to a few weeks), the factory was subjected to any tests for *Salmonella* in food. If not, this particular day would be ignored and the algorithm would move on to the next day. Otherwise, the recent past is checked against regulatory violations and one of four possible outcomes can occur:

1. True Positive (period with at least one non-compliance followed by a period with at least one failed microbial test)
2. False Positive (ditto, but all the near-future microbial tests turned out negative)
3. True Negative (no recent non-compliances followed by negative test results)
4. False Negative (period with at least one non-compliance followed by negative microbial tests)

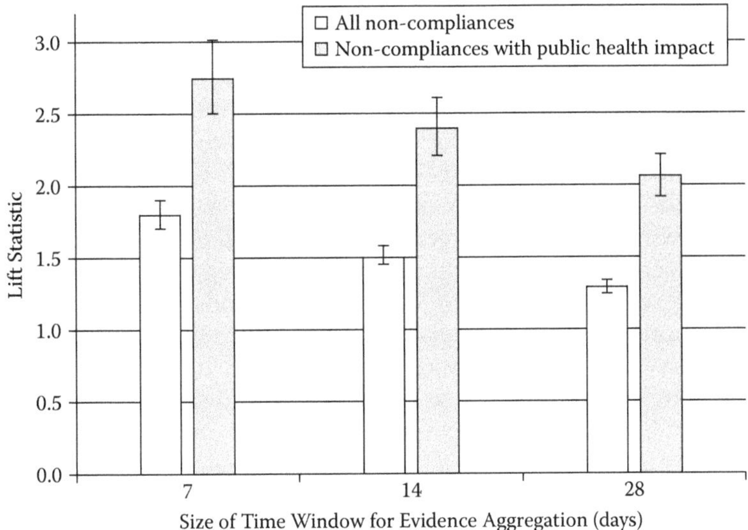

FIGURE 9.6
Results of lift analysis executed to characterize relationships between regulatory non-compliances and the outcomes of microbial testing of food samples for *Salmonella* at food factories.

These outcomes are accumulated in a 2-by-2 contingency table across multiple days and multiple factories. Then, a range of high-level statistics about the relationship between non-compliances and results of *Salmonella* tests, such as odds ratio, recall, false positive rate, lift, etc., can be derived from that table. Lift statistic estimates the ratio of conditional probability of observing a positive *Salmonella* test result in a randomly selected factory, given that it recently recorded non-compliances, to the prior probability of observing the *Salmonella* positive without taking non-compliances into consideration. Under null hypothesis of no relationship between non-compliances and *Salmonella* test results, lift should equal 1.0. Any lift value significantly greater than that suggests a positive correlation.

Figure 9.6 depicts results of computing lift statistic for two different subsets of non-compliances and three widths of temporal windows of evidence aggregation and the outcome window of seven days. The lift statistic characterizes here the utility of observing recent regulatory compliance records in order to predict the risk near future microbial problems. White bars depict performance attainable using occurrences of all kinds of non-compliances in making predictions. The gray bars correspond to using just a subset of non-compliances that are believed by the food safety experts to potentially bear public health consequences. Being more selective about data aggregation pays off, as the observed lift values exceed those obtained without discriminating between the different types of recorded non-compliances. Given that the data of public-health gravity is just a subset of the complete record of regulatory violations, we note a moderate increase in uncertainty about the lift estimates when using more specific information. Despite that, the use of public health–related non-compliances allows to consistently outperform the less specific alternative at a range of widths of windows of observation. At the shortest, a seven day observation interval, recording a public health–related regulatory violation increases the factory chances to record a positive for *Salmonella* during the next week 2.75 times on average, with respect to the model, which ignores the recorded non-compliances. As expected, the lift values decrease as the lengths of evidence aggregation periods increase. Observing a regulatory violation over longer periods of time becomes just more common and hence less useful in estimating the near future risk of microbial contamination of food. The presented approach provides an example of how a simple analysis combined with insightful aggregation of evidence can lead to useful discoveries (Food Safety and Inspection Service 2008).

9.5 Aggregating Evidence Using Graph Representations

In some application scenarios, due to either sparseness of the available data, infeasibility of independence assumptions, or presence of explicit or implicit notion of linkages between data elements, it makes practical sense to represent data objects as linked entities. Representing any data in such way can be useful in general as it usually allows leveraging a range of the existing algorithms originally developed for social network analyses.

One example comes from the food safety domain where predicting the risk of positive outcomes of microbial tests becomes harder when either such events happen to be naturally rare or if there is a need for a highly specific event designation (e.g., predicting the occurrence of one of hundreds of specific *Salmonella* serotypes as opposite to *Salmonella* in general), which substantially reduces the amount of available data per type of event. In such cases, it may be useful to consider methods that take advantage of either explicit (e.g., corporate membership, supplier-receiver relationship) or implicit (e.g., temporal co-occurrence of specific microbial serotypes) linkages between entities (e.g., food-processing plants) in data to boost predictability of the adverse events even if they are sparse. The approach takes advantage of similarities between entities to learn reliable models from evidence aggregated across multiple entities that are relatively close to each other in the resulting graph (Sarkar et al. 2008, Dubrawski et al. 2009b, Dubrawski et al. 2007b).

In one application scenario, food production facilities are modeled as one type of entities in a bi-partite graph that evolves over time. Another type of entity denotes various specific strains of *Salmonella*. Two entities are linked in the graph if a microbial test of food sample conducted at the specific food facility over a specific period of time turns out positive for the particular pathogen (Sarkar et al. 2008). The evolution of the graph over a sequence of discrete time steps is captured with the Dynamic Social Network in Latent space method (DSNL) introduced in Sarkar and Moore (2005). DSNL projects proximity between entities in the graph onto a low-dimensional Euclidean space so that images of pairs of closely connected entities end up near each other in the projection. The DSNL optimization algorithm combines the criterion of the fidelity of the projection with respect to the current graph topology, and the desire to maintain smooth transitions between projections computed for subsequent time steps. The results often produce meaningful visualizations of evolution of complex dynamic networks. Figure 9.7 depicts two consecutive embeddings of food factories obtained for microbial testing data collected over years 2005 and 2006. Each circle corresponds to a factory and its size to the observed frequency of positive results of tests against *Salmonella*. In 2005, factories A and B recorded some isolates, but ended up far apart in the Euclidean projection of the graph because the sets of serotypes of *Salmonella* positives found in them were not correlated. Moreover, a rare strain was found in factory A in 2005, and that pushed it into the periphery of the distribution of factories. The situation changed in 2006. Both A and B were then jointly exposed to a relatively popular *Salmonella Muenchen* and they ended up being projected close to each other and closer to the mainstream of the distribution of food factories.

It is also possible to use DSNL for link prediction. It then leverages link-entity-based aggregation of evidence available in historical data, to predict the probabilities of future occurrences of specific strains of *Salmonella* at specific food factories. One way to evaluate practical utility of such predictor is to measure for each factory the fraction of the top k% most likely serotypes predicted by the model that actually occur there. Table 9.1 presents

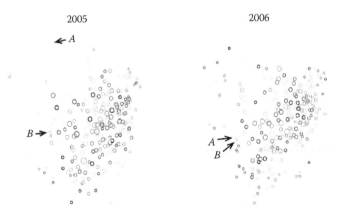

FIGURE 9.7
Mapping of the food factories obtained by embedding the bi-partite graph in a two-dimensional Euclidean space over two consecutive data collection cycles.

TABLE 9.1

Recall Scores of the DSNL Model Compared against the Baseline, Which Only Considers Histories of the Individual Food Factories Independently of Each Other

Fraction of the most likely serotypes	2.5%	5.0%	10.0%	15.0%	20.0%
DSNL	39.6%	53.7%	69.3%	80.4%	86.5%
Baseline	44.7%	52.9%	59.5%	61.9%	65.6%

such results averaged across all considered factories for varying values of the recall threshold (labeled in the table as the fraction of the most likely serotypes). The DSNL model result is compared against an alternative that takes into account only the individual factory histories in making predictions. The model leverages aggregation of data collected at factories that end up nearby in the graph significantly outperforms the baseline at recall thresholds of 10% and greater, and it correctly identifies more than 85% components of the top 20% of the ranking of predicted *Salmonella* serotypes. The differences in performance between DSNL and the baseline model observed at recall thresholds of 5% and lower are not statistically significant. These results show the benefits of relaxing the assumption of independence between factories, and they support the idea of combating sparseness of event data with link-entity based data aggregation.

Another approach uses Activity From Demographics and Links (AFDL) algorithm (Dubrawski et al. 2007b) in predicting likelihood of positive isolates obtained from microbial testing of food samples collected at food factories. AFDL is a computationally efficient method for estimating activity of unlabeled entities in a graph from patterns of connectivity of known active entities, and from their demographic profiles. The quantitative connectivity features are extracted from the topology of the graph using computationally efficient random walk algorithm and appropriate parameterization scheme, separately for each node in the graph. Then, each entity is represented by a data vector that combines together connectivity and demographic features, and the label of its status, if known. Such data can then be feed into a classifier for modeling and predicting probabilities of activity of unlabeled entities, and AFDL uses logistic regression to accomplish that.

Originally, AFDL algorithm has been developed for social network analysis and intelligence applications, but it has also been used to support analyses of food safety data. One possible usage scenario involves predicting positive outcomes of microbial tests of food samples taken at food factories based on historical records of microbial test results and on characteristic properties of these factories. Again, temporal co-occurrences of the same strain of bacteria

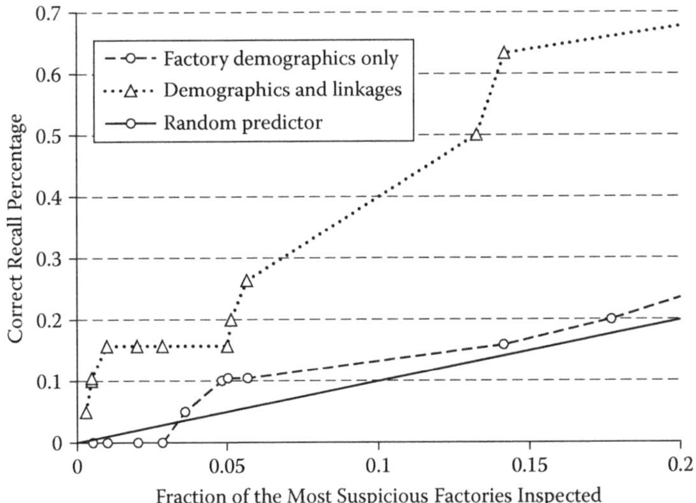

FIGURE 9.8
Recall characteristics obtained with AFDL using only factory profiles to estimate probability of future occurrence of *Salmonella Montevideo* (dashed line with circle markers) and when linkage features are added (dotted line with triangle markers) indicate benefits from aggregating evidence across entities with similar past behaviors.

(e.g., a particular serotype of *Salmonella*) in samples taken at different factories can be treated as phenomenological evidence of their potential relationship and put in as links of a uni-partite graph spanning all factories under consideration. Given profiles of factories, their historical patterns of linkage with other factories, and the information about the distribution of the currently observed microbial positives (which make the corresponding establishments "active" in the AFDL terminology), it is possible to predict which of the remaining establishments are likely to also report positive results of tests.

The AFDL's ability to predict which of the factories would record at least one positive for a specific strain, *Salmonella Montevideo,* has been tested over six months following two years worth of training data. Figure 9.8 presents lift charts that summarize the results. Using only demographic features of a factory to make predictions does not help much as the result is barely distinct from what can be obtained by randomly sampling the entities. But adding phenomenological linkage information improves percentages of correctly recalled "active" factories, in which in fact *Salmonella Montevideo* was found during the six-month test period. Using linkages derived from training data of co-occurrences of matching *Salmonella* serotypes substantially boosts the observed performance. It can be explained by the benefits of aggregating evidence across multiple factories sharing similar histories of microbial safety performance.

9.6 Conclusions

Data aggregation is a common subtask in many contexts and phases of biosurveillance. We have reviewed a few examples of its practical use. They were selected to show that it is sometimes possible to opportunistically structure the approach to biosurveillance in order to reap substantial benefits from data aggregation. Specific scenarios involve aggregating evidence across multiple subsets of the same stream of multidimensional data, or aggregating it across multiple separate streams of data, as well as across multiple distinct entities—the subjects of surveillance.

Aggregation can be the pragmatic strategy of choice when dealing with data that provides little support of useful evidence per individual hypothesis to be tested or per individual entity whose behavior is to be monitored. Sharing relevant information between similar entities and combining signals obtained from distinct sources can be used to boost reliability of the models used in surveillance and to improve statistical significance of the results.

In some applications, such as those involving spatial or temporal scan algorithms, data aggregation may put a serious burden on computational resources. One of the methods of mitigating such effects is to cache sufficient statistics of data ahead of the time of analysis. Caching reduces latencies due to information retrieval, and it allows data-intense algorithms to run faster. To illustrate that we used an example of T-Cube—a data structure that enables very fast aggregation of multidimensional time series of counts of events. The efficiencies provided by T-Cube support human users who benefit from very fast responses to queries and from dynamic visualizations of data at interactive speeds. Fast querying also enables large-scale mining of multidimensional categorical aggregates. Moreover, exhaustive searches for patterns in highly dimensional categorical data become computationally tractable. That minimizes the risk of missing something important by having to resort to selective surveillance, and it maximizes the chances of obtaining useful information right when and where it is needed.

Acknowledgments

This work was supported in part by the U.S. Department of Agriculture (award 1040770), Centers of Disease Control and Prevention (award R01-PH000028), National Science Foundation (grant IIS-0325581), and the International Development Research Centre of Canada (project 105130). Many thanks to Andrew Moore, Jeff Schneider, Daniel Neill, Josep Roure, Maheshkumar Sabhnani, Purnamrita Sarkar, John Ostlund, Lujie Chen,

Saswati Ray, Michael Baysek, and Anna Michalska for contributing information used in the text.

References

Auton Lab 2009. T-Cube Web Interface. http://www.autonlab.org/autonweb/19117.html (accessed August 14, 2009).

Burkom, H.S., Elbert, Y., Feldman, A., and Lin, J. 2004. The Role of Data Aggregation in Biosurveillance Detection Strategies with Applications from ESSENCE. *Morbidity and Mortality Weekly Report (Supplement)*, 53:67–73.

Dubrawski A., Baysek M., Mikus S., McDaniel C., Mowry B., Moyer L., et al. 2007a. Applying Outbreak Detection Algorithms to Prognostics. In *Proceedings of the 2007 AAAI Fall Symposium on Artificial Intelligence in Prognostics*, Arlington, VA, November 2007.

Dubrawski A., Ostlund J., Chen L., and Moore A. 2007b. Computationally Efficient Scoring of Activity using Demographics and Connectivity of Entities. Information Technology and Management (2010) 11:77–89.

Dubrawski A., Sabhnani M., Knight M., Baysek M., Neill D., Ray S., et al. 2009a. T-Cube Web Interface in Support of Real-Time Bio-surveillance Program. In *Proceedings of the 3rd IEEE/ACM International Conference on Information and Communication Technologies and Development ICTD2009*, Doha, Qatar, April 2009.

Dubrawski A., Sarkar P., and Chen L. 2009b. Tradeoffs between Agility and Reliability of Predictions in Dynamic Social Networks Used to Model Risk of Microbial Contamination of Food. In *Proceedings of the International Conference on Advances in Social Networks Analysis and Mining ASONAM 2009*, Athens, Greece, July 2009.

Food Safety and Inspection Service 2008. U.S. Department of Agriculture: Public Health Risk-Based Inspection System for Processing and Slaughter. Technical Report: http://www.fsis.usda.gov/OPPDE/NACMPI/Feb2008/ Processing_Slaughter_Tech_Rpt_041808.pdf (accessed August 14, 2009), and Appendix E—Data Analyses: http://www.fsis.usda.gov/OPPDE/NACMPI/Feb2008/Processing_Appendix_E_041808.pdf (accessed August 14, 2009), April 19, 2008.

Kulldorff, M. 1997. A Spatial Scan Statistic. *Communications in Statistics: Theory and Methods*. 26(6):1481–1496.

Kulldorff, M., Mostashari, F., Duczmal, L., Yih, K., Kleinman, K., and Platt, R. 2007. Multivariate Spatial Scan Statistics for Disease Surveillance. *Statistics in Medicine*. 26(8):1824–1833.

Moore, A., and Lee, M. 1998. Cached Sufficient Statistics for Efficient Machine Learning with Large Datasets. *Journal of Artificial Intelligence Research*, 8:67–91.

Naus, J., and Wallenstein, S. 2006. Temporal Surveillance Using Scan Statistics. *Statistics in Medicine*. 25:311–324.

Neill, D.B., and Cooper, G.F. 2009. A Multivariate Bayesian Scan Statistic for Early Event Detection and Characterization. *Machine Learning* (in press).

Neill, D.B., and Moore, A.W. 2004. A Fast Multi-resolution Method for Detection of Significant Spatial Disease Clusters. In *Advances in Neural Information Processing Systems 2004*. 16:651–658.

Page, E.S. 1954. Continuous Inspection Scheme. *Biometrika*. 41(1/2):100–115.

Ray S., Michalska A., Sabhnani M., et al. 2008. T-Cube Web Interface: A Tool for Immediate Visualization, Interactive Manipulation and Analysis of Large Sets of Multivariate Time Series. In *Proceedings of the AMIA Annual Symposium*, Washington, DC, 2008.

Roure J., Dubrawski A., and Schneider J. 2007. A Study into Detection of Bio-events in Multiple Streams of Surveillance Data. In D. Zeng et al. (Eds.): *BioSurveillance 2007, Lecture Notes in Computer Science* 4506:124–133.

Sabhnani M., Moore A., and Dubrawski A. 2007. T-Cube: A Data Structure for Fast Extraction of Time Series from Large Datasets. Technical Report CMU-ML-07-114, Carnegie Mellon University, 2007.

Sarkar P., Chen L., and Dubrawski A. 2008. Dynamic Network Model for Predicting Occurrences of Salmonella at Food Facilities, D. Zeng et al. (Eds.): *BioSecure 2008, Lecture Notes in Computer Science* 5354:6–63.

Sarkar P., and Moore A. 2005. Dynamic Social Network Analysis Using Latent Space Models. In *Proceedings of the 19th Annual Conference on Neural Information Processing Systems*, Vancouver, Canada, December 2005.

10

Introduction to China's Infectious Disease Surveillance System

Jin Shuigao and Ma Jiaqi

National Center for Public Health Surveillance and Information Services

Chinese Center for Disease Control and Prevention

Beijing, China

CONTENTS

10.1 The Evolution of China's Disease Surveillance System

To understand China's notifiable disease reporting process, it is necessary to introduce China's health administration system. This section provides a brief introduction to health care and public health administration system in China. Figure 10.1 illustrates the administrative infrastructure.

The column on the right-hand side of Figure 10.1 corresponds to China's administrative system beginning in 1949, when the People's Republic of China was established. At each governmental level, except that of the township, there is a health bureau. At each administrative level, except, again, at the level of township, there are also different levels of the Chinese Center for

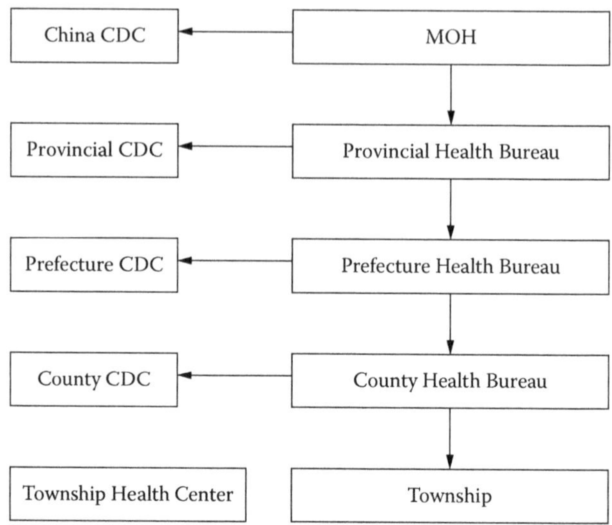

FIGURE 10.1
Infrastructure of the Chinese Health Administration System.

Disease Control and Prevention (CDC*), which serve in disease control and treatment. Also present are the many different levels of hospitals—provincial, prefecture, and county. However, unlike the CDCs, hospitals have a less tight relationship with the health bureau at each level and function independently of the CDCs in disease control and prevention. There are more than 3,500 CDCs, 19,852 hospitals, and 41,000 township/community health centers in the country (Ministry of Health China 2007).

10.1.1 The Notifiable Diseases in China

China's disease reporting system was developed in the mid-1950s, when notifiable diseases were required to be reported according to their severity into three categories (A, B, and C). Category A contains cholera and plague, those diseases considered the most severe among all infectious diseases, and cases are required to be reported as soon as possible. Following in severity, Category B contains 27 diseases with cases required to be reported within 6 hours after detection. Category C contains those diseases that are less severe but still require reporting to authorities.

The diseases in Categories B and C have changed slightly over the past 50 years according to epidemic situations. For example, in 1996, tuberculosis

* Before 2002, CDC units were known as anti-epidemic stations (EPS). Also, the Chinese Academy of Preventive Medicine (CAPM) was the former name of the Chinese Center for Disease Control and Prevention.

TABLE 10.1

Notifiable Diseases in the China Information System for Disease Control and Prevention (CISDCP)

Category	Diseases
A	Cholera, plague
B	Anthrax, bacillary, and amebic dysentery, brucellosis, dengue fever, diphtheria, gonorrhea, hemorrhagic fever with renal syndrome, high pathogenecity avian influenza, HIV/AIDS, Japanese encephalitis, leptospirosis, malaria, measles, meningococcal meningitis, neonatal tetanus, pertussis, poliomyelitis, rabies, SARS, scarlet fever, schistosomiasis, syphilis, tuberculosis, typhoid/paratyphoid fever, viral hepatitis
C	Acute hemorrhagic conjunctivitis, echinococcosis, epidemic typhus/endemic typhus, filariasis, infectious diarrhea, influenza, leprosy, kala-azar, mumps, rubella

was elevated to Category B status from Category C. Conversely, some diseases, such as forest encephalitis, which was removed from Category C in 1990, have been downgraded and no longer require reporting due to progress on the disease control front. Nonetheless, new emergent infectious diseases have been added to the list: HIV/AIDS in the 1990s, SARS in 2003, and highly pathogenic avian influenza (HPAI) in 2004. Tables 10.1 and 10.2 provide the current list and codes of notifiable diseases for China's disease surveillance system (Jin et al. 2006).

10.1.2 The Notifiable Disease Reporting Processes in China

China's disease surveillance system has gone through three stages of reporting over the past 50 years. During the first stage (from the mid-1950s to 1987), all hospitals were required to send a certification card with individual case information to the local, usually county level, antiepidemic station through the Chinese postal system. Data, aggregated by county and month, were then sent through the post from the lower level antiepidemic stations to the upper ones as illustrated in Figure 10.2.

In the second stage (1987–2003), information technology and Web-based applications were rapidly developed and broadly applied worldwide. The Chinese Academy of Preventive Medicine (former name of the Chinese Center for Disease Control and Prevention) was responsible for data aggregation at the national level and so developed a new system for data collection to allow data transfer between lower and upper administrative level. The postal system was no longer used for data transfer, and instead, was replaced by the computer and Internet, saving much time that was previously needed for data aggregation and transfer. With the new technology, detailed case-level data were still collected at the county level, summarized on a monthly basis, and sent upwards.

TABLE 10.2

Notifiable Diseases in the China Information System for Disease Control and Prevention (CISDCP)

Chinese code	Name in Chinese	English name	ICD-10	Grade
0100	鼠疫	Plague	A20.901	A
0200	霍乱	Cholera	A00.901	A
0300	肝炎	Viral hepatitis		B
0400	痢疾	Dysentery		B
0500	伤寒+副伤寒	Typhoid/paratyphoid fever		B
0600	艾滋病	HIV/AIDS	B24.01	B
0700	淋病	Gonorrhea	A54.901	B
0800	梅毒	Syphilis		B
0900	脊灰	Poliomyelitis	A80.901	B
1000	麻疹	Measles	B05.901	B
1100	百日咳	Whooping cough	A37.901	B
1200	白喉	Diphtheria	A36.901	B
1300	流脑	Meningococcal meningitis	A39.002+	B
1400	猩红热	Scarlet fever	A38.01	B
1500	出血热	Epidemic hemorrhagic fever, EHF	A98.502+	B
1600	狂犬病	Rabies	A82.901	B
1700	钩体病	Leptospirosis	A27.901	B
1800	布病	Brucellosis	A23.901	B
1900	炭疽	Anthrax	A22.901	B
2000	斑疹伤寒	Epidemic typhus, endemic typhus	A75.901	C
2100	乙脑	Epidemic encephalitis B	A83.001	B
2200	黑热病	Kala-azar	B55.001	C
2300	疟疾	Malaria	B54.02	B
2400	登革热	Dengue fever	A90.01	B
2500	新生儿破伤风	Neonatal tetanus	A33.01	B
2600	肺结核	Tuberculosis	A16.202	B
2700	传染性非典	SARS	U04.901	B
3100	血吸虫病	Schistosomiasis	B65.202	B
3200	丝虫病	Filariasis	B74.901	C
3300	包虫病	Echinococcosis	B67.901	C
3400	麻风病	Lepriasis	A30.901	C
3500	流行性感冒	Influenza	A49.201	C

TABLE 10.2 (CONTINUED)

Notifiable diseases in the China Information System for Disease Control and Prevention (CISDCP)

Chinese code	Name in Chinese	English name	ICD-10	Grade
3600	流行性腮腺炎	Mumps	B26.901	C
3700	风疹	Rubella	B06.901	C
3800	急性出血性结膜炎	Acute hemorrhagic conjunctivitis	H10.301	C
3900	其它感染性腹泻病	Infectious diarrhea	A04.903	C
9900	人禽流感	Avian influenza virus		B

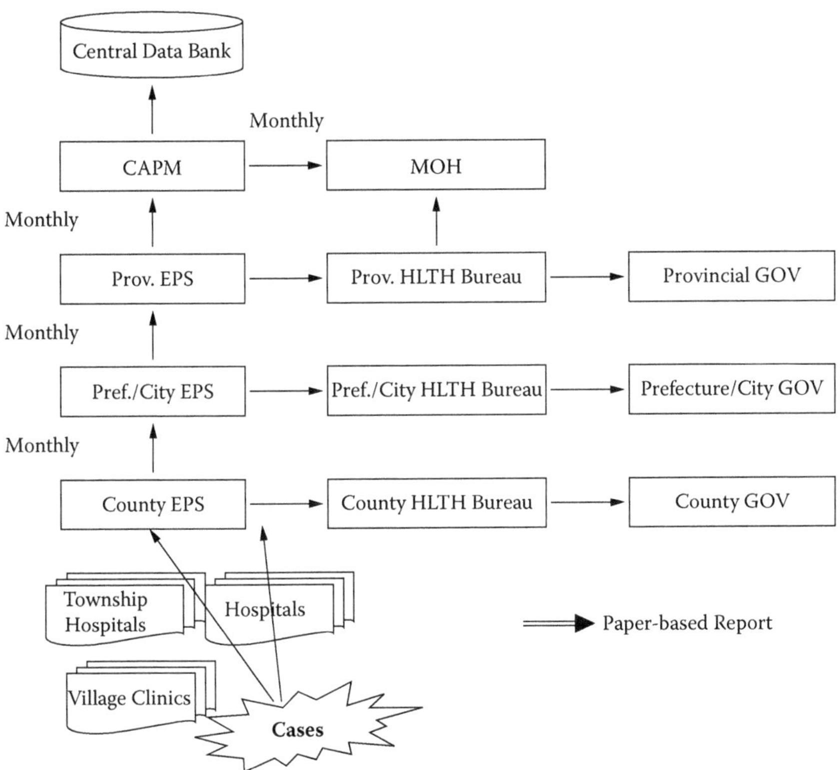

FIGURE 10.2
The Infectious Disease Reporting System in China (1950–1987).

During the third and current stage (2004–present), the SARS outbreak occurred in early 2003. This event stressed the disease surveillance system and exposed weaknesses with the prior disease reporting processes, particularly in data collection and transfer. The major problems identified were (Jin 2004)

1. Delays in disease reporting: Because the prior system had collected data on a monthly basis, it was difficult to effect early detection and warnings for infectious disease outbreaks.
2. Incomplete reports due to aggregate data: With data being first aggregated by county for reports to upper level CDCs (or EPSs), it was quite challenging to trace back outbreaks and investigate risk factors in clusters.
3. Lack of feedback and transparency: With no routine feedback mechanism from the upper to the lower levels, local authorities did not receive actionable information on disease activity in the region.

From the lessons learned from SARS, the Chinese government made the decision to enhance the public health system and place development of a new infectious disease surveillance system as one of its highest priorities.

10.2 System Development

The development of China's infectious disease surveillance system, the China Information System for Disease Control and Prevention (CISDCP), was led by China National Center for Disease Control and Prevention (CDC) in 2003 with nationwide support. This section summarizes its architecture and major features.

The main goals of the new surveillance system were as follows (Ma 2006, Wang 2004, Wang 2006):

1. To establish a five-level disease control and prevention network with a vertical top-down infrastructure (Figure 10.3) and to create a Regional Public Health Information Network (Figure 10.4).

   The five-level network consisted of levels extending from the centralized national level to the township. In the upper levels (national, provincial, and prefecture/city), an intranet was established, while on the bottom levels (county and township), PC stations were deployed.

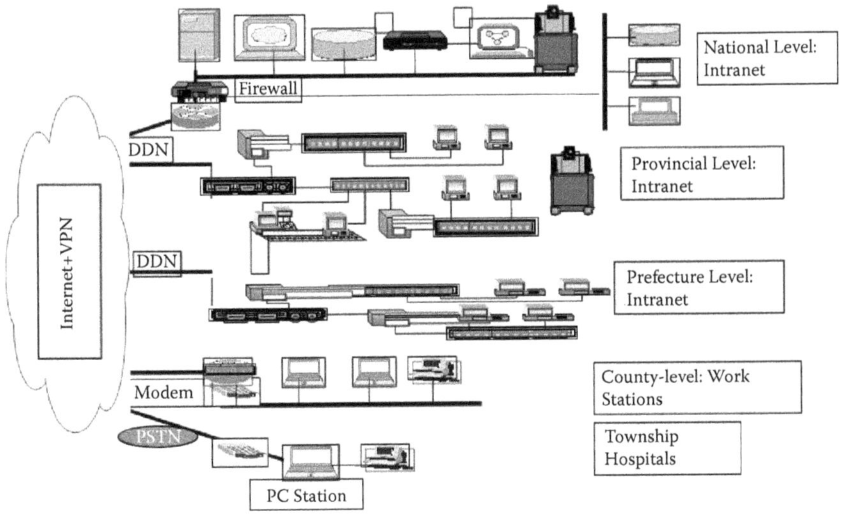

FIGURE 10.3
China's Public Health Information Network's infrastructure.

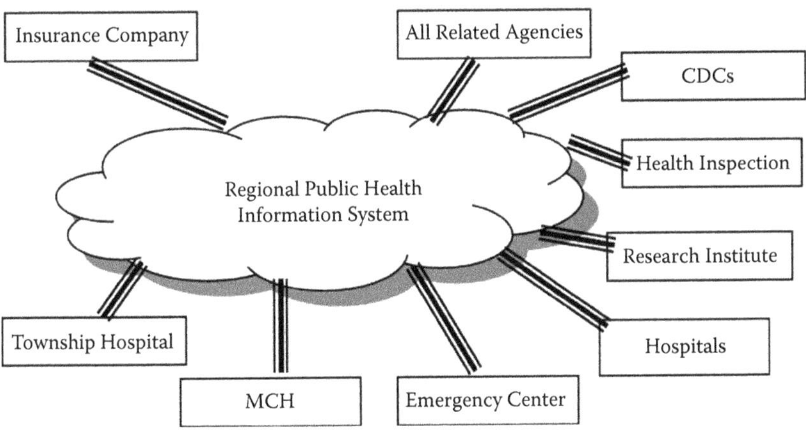

FIGURE 10.4
China's Regional Public Health Information Network's framework.

2. To establish platform ability with the major function of supporting notifiable infectious disease surveillance and public health emergency response wherein data from various information systems would be exchangeable.
3. To establish a system at the Chinese National Center for Disease Control and Prevention level that would cover all hospitals and health facilities, and contain a centralized data bank. Each individual case

of the 37 notifiable diseases and public health emergency events will be directly reported to this system immediately over the Internet.

4. To have the new surveillance system serve as the core of a Regional Public Health Information Network, and ensure all stakeholders share information so as to maximize the utilization of regional health data. Stakeholders included health administrative agencies, disease control, and preventive institutions, hospitals, insurance companies, and residents.

10.3 System Implementation and Its Progress and Impacts to Date

The China Information System for Disease Control and Prevention (CISDCP), China's infectious disease surveillance system, went live on January 1, 2004. Figure 10.5 illustrates the data flow (Ma 2006). The system integrated processes for the collection, auditing, analysis and reporting of data, and ran on a "case-based, real-time, online" basis. Cases diagnosed at hospitals were required to be reported and sent to the central data bank at the national CDC level at the time of detection via the Web. Local CDCs at each level perform audits of data before submission into the database for further analysis and interpretation. Only authorized users within the local health bureaus and CDCs have access to the data bank, based on roles and corresponding privileges.

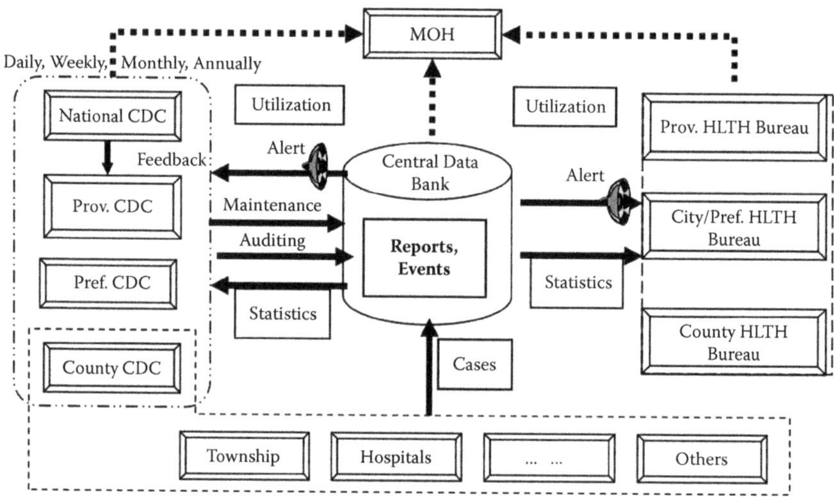

FIGURE 10.5
Data flow within China's Infectious Disease Surveillance System.

10.3.1 System Technical Architecture

The CISDCP system was developed using Java 2 Platform Enterprise Edition (J2EE) Web technology with a component model and relational database. This adoption allowed the system to receive and process information from various medical institutions via the Internet, virtual private networks, and ADSL connections. It also was possible for the system to be connected to other systems using standard data interface technology. This system also served as an information network platform for transmitting and accessing data through Web-service data exchange technologies. Disease surveillance and management processes, along with reporting and response protocols for public health emergency events, were customized according to workflow of the Chinese CDC. The system architecture is illustrated in Figure 10.6.

CISDCP also has built in a Web-based geographic information system (GIS) for the visualization of spatial information for epidemics and plotting of case clusters. An example of GIS drill-down maps that supported early warnings for an infectious disease outbreak in 2006 can be seen in Figure 10.7.

10.3.2 System Coverage and Utilization

The China Information System for Disease Control and Prevention supports all health administrative bureaus and CDCs across 31 provinces, 375 cities/prefectures, and 3,104 counties/districts. Users from about 18,700 hospitals (about 94% of the total of hospitals at the county level or above) and 41,000 township health centers (75%) access the system on daily basis. More

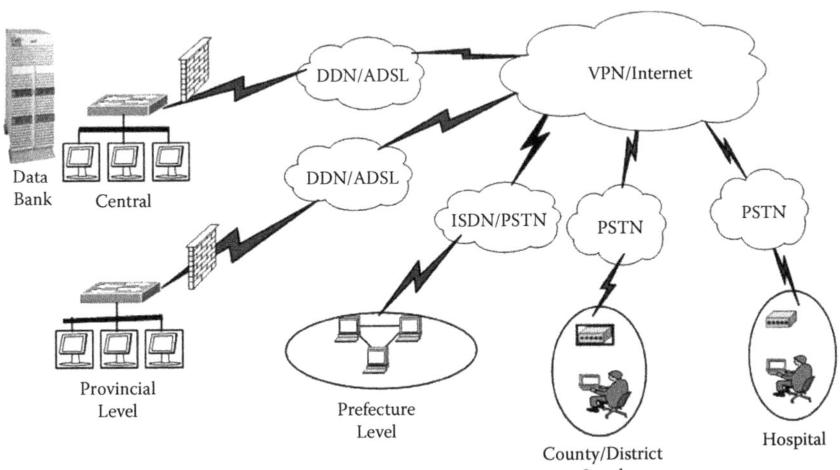

FIGURE 10.6
System architecture of China's Infectious Disease Surveillance System.

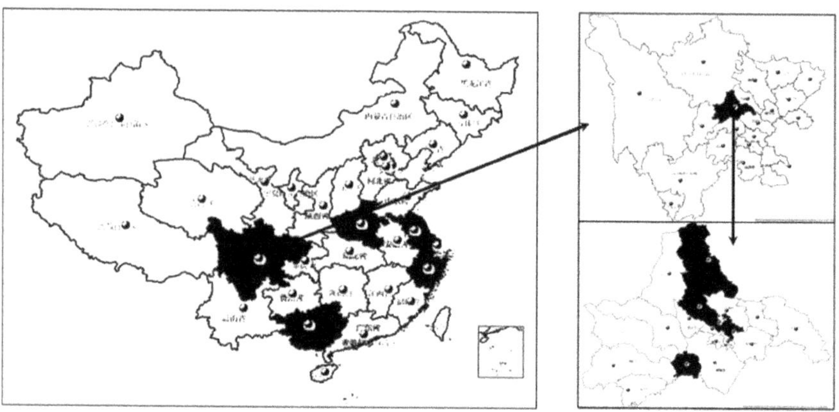

FIGURE 10.7
Example of GIS for Chinese Infectious Disease Surveillance.

than 50,000 entry points for reporting exist nationwide, which has greatly improved the timeliness and accuracy of reporting, facilitated disease-outbreak containment, and resulted in an overall improvement in infectious disease control and public health management. On average, there are 15,000 cases reported daily from hospitals and health centers across the country.

10.3.3 System Impact and Achievements

Since its deployment, the CISDCP Web-based disease surveillance system has played an unparalleled role in the discovery and containment of infectious diseases in a timely fashion. As a result, the system has done much to protect the lives and health of an entire population, and reduce the financial and human burden of infectious diseases on the Chinese society as a whole. The main achievements of the system are listed below (Wang 2004, 2007):

1. Since 2004, real-time, case-specific reports direct to the centralized data bank have taken the place of the previous system's reports of monthly aggregated data. The new system also boasts a 10-fold increase in overall reporting speed.
2. More cases have been able to be identified, and data reporting is more timely and complete. Because reports are sent to the central data bank directly, delays, such as those that happened during the 2003 SARS outbreak, in data transmission from the local to national level are avoided. In the first year of system use (2004), the total number of infectious disease cases increased by 33% compared to 2003. This pattern continued the following years, with an increase from 390 million cases reported in 2004 to 443 million reported in 2005. It has now reached a stable state. Missing reports

have also been greatly reduced with the real-time, Web-based reporting tool.
3. More accurate and timely reporting has led to the early detection and containment of outbreaks. This has not only protected the public from illness but also has mitigated other potential negative impacts (e.g., socioeconomic consequences) associated with infectious disease spread. The surveillance system maximizes the efficiency of outbreak response efforts by mobilizing response teams quickly and appropriately.
4. The implementation of CISDCP has improved the health care infrastructure in China, and also paved the way for technological networking infrastructure in local medical institutions. In addition, it has increased the computer proficiency of healthcare personnel nationwide.

10.3.4 Experience Obtained and Lessons Learned

Many lessons were learned with these experiences with respect to management and technology. These are summarized below:

1. Strong leadership and commitment from both the central as well as local government is key to ensure a surveillance system's success. Immediately after the SARS outbreak in 2003, the central Chinese government proposed a plan to strengthen the country's public health system; development of a public health information system was given utmost national priority. Movements towards this health goal were planned across all levels of the Chinese government. Moreover, what was also essential to success of CISDCP development was that both the central and local governmental treasury departments work together to provide the funds for system development.
2. The platform design and utilization of standards in the system was important to facilitate interoperability between CISDCP and other systems. Previously, reporting processes at each level only considered its own design and data standards, making data exchange between some levels extremely difficult if not impossible. Developers were successful in avoiding system isolation and the emergence of silos with CISDCP.
3. The national Chinese CDC was careful to orient the new system towards its aims for early detection of disease outbreaks and issuing early warnings of public health emergencies. Focus was put on requiring data collection of individual case data rather than county-based monthly aggregate data. Also, reports were changed to be transmitted via the Internet directly to the central data bank, located and managed in Beijing at the national level. This change in workflow was successful to save time, resources, and information loss due to upstream data transmission.

10.3.5 System Development Challenges

Challenges were met in the development of the CISDCP. The major ones experienced are summarized below:

1. Variation between geographic areas required system modifications/concessions. It is given that China is a very large country with great variation across regions in terms of economic development. It follows then, that it was neither easy nor possible to change the low level of information technology (IT) infrastructure that existed in some of the remote areas in time for system implementation. Also, recruitment and staff training presented a heavy burden in such areas. Consequently, 4% of the county-level hospitals and 25% of the township-level hospitals and clinics are still using phones to report disease case information to other institutions that have Internet access.
2. Lack of enough qualified personnel affected staffing for system implementation. Public health information systems depend on having reliable and trained personnel with multidisciplinary training in policy, administration, public health, technology, health informatics, and so on. Currently, in China, there are not enough individuals who fit this description to meet demands.
3. There has been difficulty in data-sharing with nonhealth institutions. Collaboration between public health agencies, hospitals, and clinics is very efficient within the healthcare system. However, information sharing and collaboration between health and nonhealth organizations and departments, such as China's national agriculture department, is not yet in coordinated. Animal and human health disease surveillance databases are not currently linked.
4. There are weak linkages with hospital information systems (HIS). While cases detected by hospitals are required to be reported to the CDC over the Internet, there is no direct linkage between hospital information systems and case reporting systems. Currently, hospitals manually enter disease case data into the surveillance system, which leads to duplicate efforts and a slight time delay in reporting.

10.4 The System's Future Directions

China's infectious disease surveillance system will continue to evolve and undergo improvement in the coming years. Future directions with respect to system expansion, data and information exchange, and the regional information network are discussed below:

1. Expansion of the CISDCP beyond infectious diseases to other diseases and health-related risk factors is necessary. Although CISDCP was initially developed for infectious disease control and prevention, it has served as a successful example for the centralized surveillance of disease in China. It is logical to leverage such valuable experiences and integrate other disease surveillance processes and systems into the common CISDCP platform.
2. Data utilization and organization for information sharing remains a major challenge. The technological developments of the information system for data collection, standardization, and data transfer and storage have been a great first step. However, data to support decision making are also critical. For this, efforts to share data not only between agencies within health system but also between those outside the health system will be necessary.
3. Information exchange between the CISDCP and the regional health information network (RHIN) and electronic health records (EHR) will be helpful. Interoperable electronic health records (EHR) is one of the major goals named in China's recent health reform plan. The next major goal for the national disease surveillance system is to have it directly link to the regional health information network and the interoperable EHRs to come. An EHR-based RHIN could make for hospital information systems and public health information systems to link more tightly, which will enable more timely information sharing and make syndromic surveillance possible.

10.5 Conclusions

China established CISDCP, its disease control and prevention information system, in 2004. This system encompasses all of China's health care facilities and public health institutes. It facilitates the collection, auditing, analysis, and reporting of disease data. Individual cases detected in hospitals are required to be sent immediately to the central data bank housed at the national Chinese Center for Disease Control and Prevention (CDC). Daily, weekly, monthly, and annual reports are generated and disseminated to stakeholders. CISDCP has made it possible for the early detection of infectious disease cases and outbreaks and for timely warnings of public emergencies for more effective response. The system is the largest real-time case reporting system in the world, and is run off of a common and flexible platform system architecture. This model has allowed the Chinese CDC to make a huge leap in disease control and public health management, and tremendously modernized China's disease surveillance capabilities.

References

Jin, S.G. 2004. Information collection and analysis of public health emergency. *Chinese Journal of Preventive Medicine.* 38(4):282–284.

Jin, S.G., Jiang, T., and Ma, J.Q. 2006. Introduction of China infectious disease surveillance system. *China Digital Medicine.* 1(1):20–22.

Ma, J.Q., et al. 2006, Web-based platform disease surveillance system in China. *Disease Surveillance.* 21(1):1–3.

Ministry of Health China. 2007. *China Health Statistical Yearbook* (2007). Peking Union Medical College Press, Beijing, China, 6–8.

Wang, L.D. 2004. Challenges and countermeasures in disease control and prevention in China. *International Medicine and Health Guidance News* (13):5–10.

Wang Longde, Y., Wang, Jin S.G., Wu, Z.Y., Chin, D., Koplan, J.P., et al. (2008). Emergency and control of infectious diseases in China. In Han Qide, Eds. *The Lancet: China and Global Health in 21st Century*—The Lancet Series. Beijing University Medical Press. Beijing, 17–27.

11

Biosurveillance and Public Health Practice: A Case Study of North Carolina's NC DETECT System

S. Cornelia Kaydos-Daniels, PhD, MSPH
RTI International
Research Triangle Park, NC

Lucia Rojas Smith DrPH, MPH
RTI International
Washington, DC

Amy I. Ising, MSIS
University of North Carolina
Chapel Hill, NC

Clifton Barnett, MSIS
University of North Carolina
Chapel Hill, NC

Tonya Farris, MPH
RTI International
Washington, DC

Anna E. Waller, ScD
University of North Carolina
Chapel Hill, NC

Scott Wetterhall, MD, MPH
RTI International
Atlanta GA

CONTENTS

11.1 Introduction

Biosurveillance systems were initially developed primarily to facilitate early detection for biological, chemical, radiological, or terrorist threats to public health (Lombardo, Burkom, and Pavlin 2004; Loonsk 2004). As these systems evolved, their application to a wide array of public health threats has become more routine (Ginsberg et al. 2008; Hope et al. 2008; Leonardi et al. 2006; Ma et al. 2006; Marx et al. 2003), and thus they have demonstrated their value and utility for strengthening public health preparedness.

North Carolina was an early adopter of biosurveillance technology, and here we describe the state's experience in developing and deploying its biosurveillance system, highlighting the challenges and successes that can inform similar efforts in other states.

11.1.1 The Establishment of NC DETECT

In 1999, the North Carolina Healthcare Information and Communications Alliance, Inc. (NCHICA), convened a group of emergency medicine clinicians and researchers, hospital administrators, and health informatics professionals to discuss how the use of routinely collected emergency department (ED) data could be captured and used to better understand and research the clinical aspects of emergency medicine. Not long after the group began meeting, the Centers for Disease Control and Prevention (CDC) became involved and added public health interests to the group.

One of the first tasks facing the group was to gather data from various EDs in a structured and systematic manner into a single database. An initial grant from CDC enabled the University of North Carolina–Chapel Hill (UNC-CH) to create a database, and pilot the concept that electronic data from disparate EDs could be collected and analyzed on a routine basis to inform public health. This CDC-funded project came to be known as the North Carolina Emergency Department Database (NCEDD) and included three hospitals.

After the events of September 11, 2001, and the anthrax cases that followed, the North Carolina Department of Health and Human Services, Division of Public Health (DPH) used a portion of its federally allocated funds from the CDC *Public Health Preparedness and Response for Bioterrorism Program* to continue the work of the NCEDD. The number of participating hospitals grew from 3 to 24, and data were collected daily from each ED. Although the sharing of patient data with public health entities was allowed under the Health Insurance Portability and Accountability Act, some hospital administrators were uneasy about possible liabilities. DPH therefore worked with the North Carolina Hospital Association (NCHA) to introduce legislation requiring hospitals in North Carolina to provide timely ED visit data for public health surveillance. In 2004, the North Carolina legislature authorized the establishment of the North Carolina Hospital Emergency Surveillance System (NCHESS) and directed the state's 24-hour acute care hospital-affiliated EDs (at that time, 112) to provide data to NCEDD for public health surveillance purposes, effective January 1, 2005.

In 2004, NCEDD became known as the North Carolina Disease Event Tracking and Epidemiologic Collection Tool (NC DETECT). Currently, NCHA supervises data collection from EDs. The DPH contracts with the UNC–CH Department of Emergency Medicine (DEM) to oversee the NC DETECT surveillance system and to manage the storage and analysis of the ED data. As of January 1, 2009, 98% (at that time, 110) of the 112 EDs covered by the mandate provide data at least daily to NC DETECT. The remaining EDs are in the process of joining the system (www.ncdetect.org).

Additionally, NC DETECT receives data from the Carolinas Poison Center (CPC) poison control hotline, which covers the entire state of North Carolina;

the statewide Pre-Hospital Medical Information System, which captures information on all ambulance runs; select urgent care centers in one metropolitan area; two veterinary data sources; and Veterans Administration (VA) hospitals in the state. This evaluation focuses on ED data.

11.1.2 NC DETECT Data Syndromes

At the time that we conducted this evaluation in 2007, NC DETECT classified ED visits into eight syndromes as presented in Table 11.1, based on presenting symptoms captured in chief complaints (CC), triage notes (TN), and initial body temperature measurements, when available. All syndrome definitions, except GI-All, require both a constitutional symptom (e.g., fever, body aches) and a syndrome-specific symptom or mention of the condition (e.g., sore throat, vomiting). Syndrome-specific symptoms relate specifically to the syndrome or organ of interest (e.g., shortness of breath for respiratory illness or vomiting for gastrointestinal illness). Constitutional symptoms are less specific, reflect generalized illness, and are not representative of any specific organ system or specific syndrome (e.g., fever or myalgias). In 2007, triage notes were available for approximately 30% of the ED visits reported to NC DETECT.

In addition to CC, TN, and initial temperature, other data elements collected by NC DETECT include date of birth; sex; city, state, county, and ZIP code of patient's residence; ED facility; first date and time of ED visit; systolic and diastolic blood pressure; mode of transport to ED; ED discharge diagnoses, coded cause of injury, ED disposition, and coded procedures. Records may be updated as additional electronic information becomes available; this is particularly necessary for ICD-9-CM-coded diagnoses, cause of injury, and procedures.

Not all ED visits reported to NC DETECT fit into a syndrome, and if an ED visit meets the criteria for more than one syndrome, it was binned into each of those syndromes. ED visits are not limited to syndromes associated with infectious diseases but could include any possible illness or injury. All ED visit data are available for analysis even if they did not fit into a syndrome.

TABLE 11.1

NC DETECT Syndromes and Sample Chief Complaints*

Syndrome	Sample chief complaints
Botulism-like	Vomiting, blurred vision, headache
Fever/rash	Fever, rash on body
Gastrointestinal—severe	Fever, vomiting
Gastrointestinal—all	Vomiting
Influenza-like illness	Fever, headache, cough, nausea, vomiting
Meningoencephalitis	Fever, stiffness in neck
Respiratory	Sweating, shortness of breath

**Current as of 2007.*

New syndromes could be developed or existing ones modified to cover the specifics of a public health outbreak or incident.

11.1.3 NC DETECT Data Collection, Processing, and Analysis

All data collected in NC DETECT are secondary data. They are collected in electronic data systems for other purposes and NC DETECT receives an extract of what is already being captured. The NCHA, through NCHESS, establishes the data feed from each participating hospital to a third-party data aggregator. The data aggregator then makes a file of the collected ED visit data available for download to NC DETECT twice a day. The UNC DEM performs extraction, translation, and loading of the data into the emergency department database in NC DETECT, monitors and addresses data quality issues, bins the visits into the various syndrome categories, analyzes the data using CDC algorithms from the Early Aberration Reporting System (EARS), and presents the data through a sophisticated Web portal to a variety of users around the state. The EARS algorithms are programmed to detect unusual clusters of illness based on syndrome, date, facility, and county of residence. If an unusual cluster is identified, it is highlighted with a "signal" to alert the appropriate NC DETECT users when they log in to the system.

The statewide CPC receives more than 120,000 calls each year, and data are sent to NC DETECT every hour. Calls include human exposures, animal exposures, and informational calls. Of the human exposure calls, 99% are assigned at least one clinical effect. Categories of the clinical effects include cardio, dermal, fever, gastro, hemorrhagic/hepatic, neuro, ocular, renal, and respiratory.

The UNC DEM produces reports of the analyses, which are available to authorized NC DETECT users via the Web portal. Users view alerts, the information for each "case" in an alert, and can investigate and notate alerts further. Epidemiologist users are also able to post comments for individual alerts, including results of further investigation, communications with colleagues, and determinations that no additional follow-up is required. The NC DETECT application also allows users to conduct their own queries and analyses unrelated to any specific alert.

11.1.4 NC DETECT Users

Users of NC DETECT data include hospital-based epidemiologists, local health departments, regional public health preparedness teams, and DPH as presented in Table 11.2. Users who perform investigations as part of their job functions generally have broader data access for their respective jurisdictions than other user roles. DPH users and hospital users are also able to access additional systems outside of NC DETECT to review medical charts of patients seen at select hospitals remotely.

TABLE 11.2

Type and Number of Users of NCDETECT

User Type	Number
North Carolina State College of Veterinary Medicine Laboratories (CVML)	1
DPH General Communicable Disease Control Branch (GCDC)	22
DPH Non-GCDC	11
Public Health Epidemiologist (PHE)	10
Hospital user (non-PHE)	26
Local Health Department (LHD)	30
Public Health Regional Surveillance Teams (PHRST)	20
Total	35

11.2 Methods

The RTI Evaluators worked with UNC DEM to identify key informants associated with NC DETECT (see Table 11.3). Once key informants were identified, a select number of informants were invited to participate in interviews.

The evaluators developed a general interview guide that included open-ended questions organized around the key domains of inquiry for the evaluation. The interview guide was customized for each key informant or group of informants to include the most relevant questions (end users, for example, were unlikely to be able to provide meaningful information about the costs of maintaining the system or the history of its establishment).

Interviews were conducted during the summer of 2007 by the evaluators in person when possible; otherwise, interviews were via telephone and were approximately 60 to 90 minutes in duration. Group interviews were conducted for users of similar types who worked in the same establishment; for example, several members of the NC DETECT program at UNC–CH were interviewed as a group. All interviews were recorded, with the interviewees' permission, to ensure the accuracy of the transcripts.

The evaluators created written transcripts from the interview recordings. They analyzed the transcripts qualitatively by applying a technique known as *content analysis*, which groups or categorizes large sections of text into smaller content categories based on explicit rules of coding (Stemler 2001). In this study, codes were established a priori, based on the themes and research questions of interest in N'Vivo, a software application used for qualitative data analysis. One analyst coded the entire transcript set while a second checked the coding for consistency and relevance.

TABLE 11.3
Key Informants

Key informant roles	Number interviewed
Hospital public health epidemiologist	4
Hospital infection control manager	2
County public health preparedness coordinator	1
PHRST personnel	1
State epidemiologists/section chiefs/directors	4
Hospital clinical applications analyst	1
NC DETECT staff	3
Other	2
Total	18

11.3. Findings

11.3.1 How Has Biosurveillance Been Used?

The utility of NC DETECT for early detection was limited, in the view of some informants, because some conditions and illnesses would never or rarely present themselves in a hospital setting or some outbreaks may be too small to detect. As one informant explained, "It does not pick up small things; it does not pick up single patients. Let's say I had one patient with botulism. They've got botulism surveillance now and I have been checking that, but I would probably be told by a physician that I have a botulism case, before I picked it up on NC DETECT."

Nonetheless, key informants voiced a clear consensus that NC DETECT was a valuable tool in the early investigational phase of an outbreak. For example, one hospital-based user reported that for certain syndromes, such as meningoencephalitis, she investigates all cases to confirm whether it is the first report of the disease. In the course of investigating signals in NC DETECT, this user further examines admissions data, laboratory data, and the ED logs to generate reports for other stakeholders. She therefore uses NC DETECT to initially identify possible outbreak and alert others, and then uses additional data sources to complete her investigations of signals.

Key informants have used NC DETECT most extensively for *situation awareness*. Several hospital-based users mentioned how NC DETECT has been helpful in monitoring disease trends. The winter of 2006–2007 was a particularly severe season for Norovirus in North Carolina (and across the United States). NC DETECT was used by these key informants to monitor Norovirus outbreaks in the community through the gastrointestinal syndrome.

One hospital-based epidemiologist uses NC DETECT for situation awareness in the hospital when there is a high level of influenza or other acute respiratory illness. This enhanced level of understanding about the outbreak within the hospital informs decisions about when to implement heightened measures to control infection. These would include prompting employees to be vaccinated, discouraging persons from visiting inpatients, erecting hygiene stations in the ED that contain respiratory masks for patients, hand sanitizers, and/or disposable bags for use during times when there is a high incidence of gastrointestinal illness.

At the time of the interview, the VA system was not part of the NC DETECT system, but the PHE there had access to NC DETECT, and could run reports for the region or state and manually compare VA data and trends with those of other EDs. The VA and other PHEs use NC DETECT data to validate disease trends that are happening in the community. As one user put it, "It gives you a little better view of different areas and it gives you a better overview of what North Carolina is seeing as a group. It is nice not to operate in a vacuum, which is what most of us [hospitals] did before this."

Situation awareness and early detection are also enhanced by the flexibility of the NC DETECT application. DPH uses local and national information on disease occurrences to create specialized syndromes; it is relatively easy for code to be written for new syndromes, or to alter existing syndromes to detect specific key words. For example, during a nationwide recall of a common brand of peanut butter because of salmonella contamination, a filter was put in place to separate out cases of gastrointestinal symptoms in which the persons reported eating peanut butter. The resulting investigation showed no additional cases in North Carolina of salmonella because of the contaminated peanut butter.

NC DETECT has also been used by DPH to respond to public health threats. During a heat wave in August 2007, DPH and the NC DETECT team created a filter for heat-related illnesses. DPH monitored the syndrome signals, and within days of the end of the heat wave had issued a press release about patients who sought emergency care at EDs for heat-related illness. Health warnings during previous heat waves had targeted children and the elderly; but the NC DETECT data revealed that those most likely to experience heat-related illness were adults who worked outside and were overwhelmingly male. This enhanced understanding of susceptible populations was used by DPH to more effectively target prevention messages and heat-related warnings.

Another example of the use of NC DETECT for situation awareness and response was an incident in 2006 in which a chemical storage facility exploded and burned in central North Carolina. DPH and the UNC DEM created a filter with key words to find patients reporting exposure to the fumes.

11.3.2 How Has Biosurveillance Been Integrated with Traditional Surveillance Activities?

NC DETECT complements traditional surveillance activities, including reporting. PHEs in the hospitals all reported that they check NC DETECT signals daily, as a part of their routine surveillance responsibilities. For these epidemiologists, the focus of their work is on what illnesses are circulating in the community and presenting at the ED. They use NC DETECT data from their hospitals, plus potentially other hospitals in the same system, and compare trends and signals with regional and state data. They use additional sources of data, including medical charts, laboratory data, and medical testing results to investigate signals further. As cases are investigated, users can add comments into the NC DETECT system that a signal has been investigated, and can report the outcome of the investigation.

Hospital-based users send weekly reports of their surveillance activities to local health departments, DPH, and hospital administrators. One PHE said that in addition to the above, she posts her reports on the hospital intranet, so anyone with hospital privileges can view the reports. She also sends reports directly to the director of the ED, as well as ED physicians and pediatricians. Sometimes the local health director (at the local health department) asks her to send her reports or notices to local physicians who are not connected to the hospital, so that they are also aware of community illnesses.

Regional state-based response teams use NC DETECT as part of their surveillance activities for the regions. They may not check the system as often as PHEs, but review signals daily when warranted by an ongoing disease outbreak. Because a region may include up to 25 counties, the epidemiologists review signals by county, and can view a line listing of each signal to inform them at which hospital the patient presented. Some counties may require more attention than others, depending on whether the local health department or a PHE also reviews cases for a county (or a large hospital with a large patient population from a single county).

State-based epidemiologists monitor the signals from NC DETECT daily. For approximately half of the hospitals on the NC DETECT system, DPH can directly access patient medical records to investigate signals. The epidemiologists add comments to signals in NC DETECT as they are investigated, and review comments other users have entered for signals. They validate trend data with other sources of disease data for the state, mainly reportable disease data.

NC DETECT is also used to supplement and complement other forms of public health surveillance of nonreportable illnesses and conditions. One hospital-based user described her efforts to facilitate local injury control activities with NC DETECT. She created special sets of queries to identify the number and type of injuries presenting to the ED. These data were subsequently used by a local nonprofit injury prevention program to secure grant funding and inform the planning of a new children's hospital. This innovative use of NC DETECT is especially noteworthy because it filled a gap in the public health surveillance system. The local health department lacked the resources to carry out injury prevention or surveillance, and the only available data on injuries were based on state and national estimates. In the view of this informant, the local data were much more compelling to potential funders and community injury stakeholders. As she explains, "[NC DETECT] has been used for a variety of things, from just the general advocacy level all the way up to programming … highlighting and justifying to the national organization … what [the local groups] are … working on."

11.3.3 What Has Been the Value Added of Biosurveillance to Traditional Surveillance?

NC DETECT has added value to traditional disease surveillance by enhancing sensitivity, timeliness, flexibility, case detection, and communication. Key informants reported additional uses for which NC DETECT could be adapted and used because of the amount of data generated.

11.3.3.1 Validity

The use of syndromes instead of diagnoses is more sensitive (thereby increasing case counts) and less specific than traditional disease surveillance. Biosurveillance allows for more immediate identification and investigation of possible outbreaks, but the enhanced sensitivity of the system also results in the greater probability of "false positive" signals. A user could see a spike in cases of gastrointestinal illness, only to discover upon further investigation that the cases were unrelated and possibly not even because of a foodborne pathogen. Multiple users could also be tracking the same cluster of cases. This presents an opportunity for scarce resources to be wasted. As one informant explained, "That's the biggest downfall, the false positive. I investigate a signal and find out that half of them are false positive."

11.3.3.2 Timeliness

NC DETECT makes use of data that are already being collected and entered into databases at EDs as patients are seen; thus, real-time data are downloaded every 12 hours. Those data are available to users for analysis and report generation immediately via the NC DETECT Web portal; UNC DEM also produces custom reports when requested.

Traditional surveillance of reportable diseases relies on clinicians and laboratories to complete reportable disease cards and mail, fax, or call in the information to the local health department. Because completing and mailing a card is additional work for physicians/laboratories, reporting rates are notoriously low. Traditional surveillance for reportable diseases is by definition passive and generally includes a final diagnosis. The time between when a patient first presents to the clinician or a specimen is received by a laboratory and a report is sent to the health department can be lengthy.

NC DETECT, in contrast, which is still a passive system, imposes no extra burden on the part of the hospitals in terms of reporting, but in the view of key informants is more timely and complete than traditional surveillance. As one DPH user explained, "This system is a trigger.... Users still follow up cases of interest, but they are alerted to the presence of these cases much earlier than with traditional surveillance, partially because they do not have to wait for a final diagnosis."

To address these potential problems, NC DETECT has a comment area that can be viewed by all users and where they can note what they have learned through their investigations. NC DETECT users reported that they make notes in the comment area and this saves them time. Also, as patients receive diagnoses within the hospital electronic information system, they are downloaded to NC DETECT, which then automatically updates the records. The strong consensus among the users was that NC DETECT was a net gain in terms of timeliness. Even though the majority of the aberrations they review are not true outbreaks, they do not view the time spent as excessive or consuming.

In other examples of NC DETECT's enhancement of timeliness, parents, upon learning about a mercury exposure from their children's school, called CPC inquiring about the effects of mercury. NC DETECT received data related to these calls in near real time that could then be monitored by DPH users. DPH saw the signal and promptly investigated it, and alerted the local health department.

The North Carolina coast frequently experiences hurricanes, and surveillance for hurricane-related injuries and ED visits is used for emergency planning and resource allocation. In the past, it has taken approximately 3 months for an epidemiologist to abstract ED charts for a week before and after a hurricane hits (to compare time periods). With NC DETECT, the same data can be (and have been) obtained in a matter of hours.

11.3.3.3 Flexibility

NC DETECT is mainly used for ongoing real-time surveillance of particular illness syndromes. New syndromes or filters can be requested at any time by NC DETECT users and added to the system by UNC DEM NC DETECT staff, which greatly enhances the system's flexibility. A new filter can be used to detect new cases at system EDs, and can also be used to retrospectively find cases. This feature has been used extensively by DPH users to enhance surveillance of specific illnesses and syndromes. Some examples have been previously mentioned, including the filters for heat-related illnesses and for gastrointestinal illness related to peanut butter consumption, and a chemical explosion.

Creating specific new filters would be more difficult if it were not for the inclusion of the "triage note" in the NC DETECT database. The triage note greatly increases the amount of information available to NC DETECT. For example, the chief complaint could be "diarrhea and vomiting," which classifies the case as gastrointestinal syndrome. If the triage note indicates "patient reports eating peanut butter of the same brand that was recalled," then the case would be added to the syndrome for that particular outbreak. The triage note improves the quality of the data users see, and improves their efficiency during investigations.

11.3.3.4 Case Detection

NC DETECT also enhances traditional systems of surveillance because cases of disease that may otherwise go unreported can be detected using the system. The user described earlier who follows up every case of meningoencephalitis in NC DETECT also noted that if the case is ultimately diagnosed as meningococcal meningitis, she reports it to DPH, knowing that it may not be reported through any other means. Alternatively, DPH can follow up on a single case detected in NC DETECT either directly through the medical record, or by placing a call to the local health department or hospital. A key advantage of a distributed system that allows multiple users to see the data is it reduces the potential for an important case or cluster to be missed. If a hospital user, for example, misses a case or cluster, then it could be identified by another user at the local health department or the DPH.

Triage notes are an important feature of the system's case detection capabilities. One outbreak of foodborne disease among young adults occurred during the winter holiday break. Using the triage notes area, epidemiologists were able to identify a cluster of cases in students from a university not in session at the time. The outbreak was investigated, and the likely cause was determined to be a food item at a sorority social function held just before the students left the university for their vacation. It is unlikely this outbreak would have been detected with a traditional surveillance system because the cases became geographically dispersed once they left campus and thus more difficult to identify.

11.3.3.5 Communication

Several users reported that NC DETECT has greatly improved communication within and among hospitals and public health authorities. Reports produced by NC DETECT data are prepared and sent to the local health departments, regional public health teams, DPH, hospital administrators, clinicians, and even to the community. The ability to view disease trends across the state has also helped hospital-based epidemiologists and infection control practitioners feel more informed and linked to other hospitals. One user also indicated that because of NC DETECT "we talk a lot more on how to deal with illness than we did before."

The findings also suggest that the electronic flow of information among users had not diminished personal communication but on the contrary had increased its intensity and depth. As one user explained, investigating signals requires "a lot of human contact" and communication flows related to NC DETECT enhance other interactions as well. As one user put it, "I think it has greatly improved our relationship with hospital communication. I have heard health directors say before, even if it is something that is not a flag that we call them about … , they are more likely to call us now about other things … even if they are not NC DETECT."

More specifically, key informants described how the Annotation Report feature of NC DETECT—where users can post general comments—streamlines communication about an investigation and reduces duplication of effort and following up signals of no significance. Users also thought the Annotation Reports enhanced the documentation of an investigation so the information exchanged is captured in an accessible and retrievable manner for current and future purposes.

The exchange of information among public health practitioners has also improved as a consequence of NC DETECT according to informants. Many local health departments do not have the resources to staff an epidemiologist, so regional epidemiologists use NC DETECT to keep local health officers informed about a potential or confirmed outbreak in their jurisdiction.

11.3.4 What Has Been the Value Added of Biosurveillance to Sentinel Influenza Surveillance?

Influenza is not a reportable disease in North Carolina, unless it results in death in a person under 18 years of age. As a result, surveillance for influenza has traditionally relied on the Sentinel Providers Network (SPN). This is a group of individual physicians who have agreed to tally cases of influenza-like illness (ILI) and diagnosed cases of influenza and report them to CDC weekly during the influenza season (see http://www.epi.state.nc.us/epi/gcdc/flu.html). There are multiple drawbacks to this system. First, not all physicians are sentinel providers, and representation may vary across the state. Second, the SPN is not active year-round, so outbreaks of influenza in the summer (for example) may not be detected at all. Third, testing to definitively diagnose influenza becomes less frequent as the flu season progresses and the strains circulating are well established.

ILI cases are reported to NC DETECT all year, and, like all other cases, are updated every 12 hours. The data from NC DETECT are therefore more timely than the SPN data and, additionally, will detect cases in the off-season.

Therefore, the raw numbers of cases of ILI are much higher for NC DETECT than the SPN. The NC DETECT data for ILI may present more severe cases of ILI and a different age or socioeconomic population than those represented in the SPN data. DPH uses NC DETECT data and SPN data to validate each other, and for the past two influenza seasons have found that the two surveillance systems correlate well in terms of timing and relative size of peaks (http://www.epi.state.nc.us/epi/gcdc/flu2006.html).

In the event of a pandemic, users predict the value of NC DETECT will be "huge," although opinions varied about what aspects of the pandemic would benefit most from NC DETECT. One user thought it would be most useful in informing decisions regarding where antivirals and response would be most needed, while others thought it would be most useful for early detection, particularly if pandemic influenza struck outside of the normal influenza season, when SPN was not active.

One user predicted that NC DETECT would be very useful during a pandemic because it would require no additional effort for the hospitals to enter data, whereas the SPN might break down if physicians were swamped with ill patients (or they themselves became ill). On the other hand, as another user noted, in a pandemic hospitals would be similarly overwhelmed and routine data entry might drop off or cease altogether. Also, patients may be presenting to off-site emergency wards with limited capabilities for reporting. Several users pointed out that during the peak of a true pandemic, providing care to ill persons would be paramount, and collecting and analyzing surveillance data could come later.

11.3.5 What Have Been the Challenges to Implementing Biosurveillance?

Key informants had several thoughts about barriers to the implementation of the system. One stakeholder who has been involved with NC DETECT since it was a pilot project in 1999 summed up the barriers as he perceived them:

> Policy is the number one [barrier]. Technology was the relatively easy part. We had to overcome policy concerns and liability concerns. And I would say the lesson learned there was to create safe harbors whenever possible for easing the concerns of providers in providing information. Number two impediment is priorities. The number of initiatives and projects before hospitals is enormous. So getting a high priority on this is an issue.

Other informants echoed these sentiments and emphasized the complexity and enormity of the task of building a statewide system, as well as securing the buy-in of key stakeholders:

> … It takes a lot of determination, commitment both from within the higher up in the agency … it is extremely complex in that way. When we

> captured data from 111 hospitals almost everyone had their own system; sometimes we were lucky enough to have the same vendor covering several hospitals and you can have a group approach, but in many cases it is hospital by hospital to build a system, monitor it, and come back to get it running again when there is a problem.

Depending on the compatibility between the hospital's computer network and software and that of NC DETECT, the ease of implementation varied widely. The average time between an initial test and a live date on the NCHESS ELERT system is approximately 251 days. Changes to the NC DETECT or the hospital's software can also cause technical problems that can add additional time to implementation. One informant reported that it took 6 weeks for his hospital to get his system working again after the ED implemented a change in the software used for tracking medical records.

The format of the triage notes has also posed a technical challenge for NC DETECT. The triage note is in free-text format, meaning that whatever the triage nurse posts can be downloaded into NC DETECT. It is common for nurses to include "negatives" in the triage note, for example, "patient reported no fever, no nausea, no dizziness," or more commonly to save time, "patient reports no fever, nausea, dizziness." In the first example, it is relatively easy to write a program to understand that the "no" meant the absence of dizziness but much more difficult in the second example. Despite the limitations of the triage notes, the fact that the majority of hospitals never or rarely enter triage notes was a problem in the view of some users. A few informants suggested having a more standardized approach to posting triage notes to address some of these concerns.

The cost of implementing and maintaining the system was viewed by some key informants as a barrier. Informants perceived the contract with UNC DEM as relatively expensive to support, but believe that the benefits of NC DETECT are clear and compelling enough to warrant its expense. DPH uses bioterrorism funds granted by CDC to support NC DETECT; however, the level of funding from that source is expected to decline over time.

11.3.6 What Factors Have Facilitated the Implementation of Biosurveillance?

There were a number of important factors that facilitated the development of NC DETECT. Foremost among these was the vision and commitment of public health leaders, hospital stakeholders, NCHICA, and policymakers to pass a law mandating the participation of hospitals with 24-hour EDs. Key informants agreed that without the law, building a statewide system would have been much more difficult.

A second facilitating factor pointed out by key informants was the high level of technical expertise of the UNC DEM. At the time the system was being developed, syndromic surveillance was still a novel concept, and the

UNC DEM decided to develop its own system based on emergent technology to meet the needs of the state and the many other users expected to use the system. Key informants indicated that the state was truly fortunate in having the technical capacity to address the complexity and scope of the effort.

The system was designed to be seamlessly integrated into the normal data flow of all participating EDs, and this was also an important factor that impacted its universal acceptance. There was no additional work required to enter or download data. Moreover, hospital users found the system easy to use and to incorporate into their daily routine. One informant described it thusly: "I think the real incentive is that NC DETECT has become part of the daily work flow in many hospitals today."

The costs to the hospitals for participating in NC DETECT were, by and large, minimal and limited to the time spent by IT staff at the onset to implement software, configure it, and work out technical issues. Hospitals were also given $5,000 as a nominal incentive. The minimal cost burden to the hospital was viewed by some informants as a factor that greatly facilitated their support. Hospitals, however, do continue to absorb costs required to maintain their data feeds to NC DETECT.

11.3.7 Recommendations for Improving NC DETECT

Although users unanimously were of the opinion that NC DETECT is a highly valuable system, there were some enhancements that were suggested. These are as below:

- Expand the sources of data. At present, NC DETECT data are currently limited to 24-hour EDs, the Poison Control Center, EMS, and some laboratories. Syndromes seen at these locations may not be representative of illnesses across the state, especially in terms of severity or patient population. Presumably persons without a regular doctor or with more severe disease present to EDs rather than their personal physician or even urgent care centers. Consequently, less severe illnesses may be missed by NC DETECT.
- DPH and NC DETECT informants recognized this opportunity, and were working to add to the system other sources of data such as urgent care centers, the four VA hospitals in the state, military hospitals, and pharmacies. Informants indicated that they would like to see private practices and school health clinics added to the system; however, this would require a uniform and widespread adoption of electronic medical records. One informant also saw the potential usefulness of data from wildlife stations and veterinary feeds. NC DETECT currently receives data from a wildlife center and the North Carolina College of Veterinary Medicine, but these have not been widely used.

- Expand the application of the NC DETECT data. Several users remarked that NC DETECT is not being used to its full advantage. The amount of data collected and analyzed is considered enormous, but the capacity to exploit its full potential remains limited by the user's lack of time and knowledge of the application. As one informant explained: "We just don't have enough resources, so we have data but probably not enough people to interpret this data, too." Informants also observed that NC DETECT had data related to asthma, mental health, injuries, and domestic violence that could inform surveillance and public health programs.
- Most users with whom we spoke only use the system to run preprogrammed reports; only one had taken advantage of the application's query function to produce customized analyses. However, even she noted that the number and complexity of the E-codes and sub-codes was the major stumbling block in carrying out her analyses.
- These comments suggest that enhancing the usability of NC DETECT will require (1) making time-saving modifications that allow current users to more fully exploit the capabilities of the system for outbreak detection and investigation; and (2) evolving the system to serve nontraditional users; in other words growing NC DETECT's "market share." A system that has utility for a wide range of uses among a diverse set of stakeholders is more likely to be sustainable and justifiable in terms of cost to benefits.
- Enhance the positive predictive value of the detection algorithms. Some informants thought the number of false alarms was unacceptably high and needed to be reduced.
- Establish guidelines for investigation of signals. Informants voiced a need in particular for consistent guidelines and protocols for investigating signals so an inordinate amount of time is not wasted on following up on "false alarms" or duplicating others' work. For example, one guideline could be that all users who investigate a signal document their findings in the comment areas.

11.4. Conclusions

NC DETECT has contributed to early detection, although its utility is limited at present. Informants cited examples of how NC DETECT has been used to detect cases of illness that may not have been identified otherwise (e.g., foodborne outbreak from a sorority house), but in most cases, NC DETECT is used to confirm or monitor an outbreak. There is, however, some indication that NC DETECT may improve the early detection of ILI by producing data that are comparable to and more timely than those produced by the sentinel surveillance system. The enhancements in timeliness, according to informants, would be critical in the event of pandemic influenza. The addition of other data, such as ambulatory care visits and pharmacy sales, could enhance system performance for early detection.

NC DETECT has demonstrated its greatest utility in terms of situation awareness and response. Situation awareness was enhanced through the use of filters that allowed DPH to conduct active surveillance for cases of salmonella related to tainted peanut butter, and respiratory distress because of chemical exposures from a chemical spill. Public health response was enhanced when NC DETECT data revealed that heat warnings were not reaching a vulnerable risk group of young adult males who work outdoors. The real-time nature of the data also allows investigations to proceed more quickly without having to wait for a final confirmatory diagnosis.

Key informants also cited enhanced communication between and among hospitals and public officials as another key value of NC DETECT that enhanced situation awareness and response. The frequency of communications had increased as well as the productivity of those interactions. Users reported how they could quickly exchange information about a suspect case(s), thereby avoiding duplication of effort or the alternative of missing a potentially important case altogether.

The evidence from the case study suggests that NC DETECT has become a core tool for public health epidemiologists, infection control officers, and other public health practitioners in North Carolina. Several key factors have aided the development and adoption of NC DETECT statewide and these include:

- The engagement and commitment of key stakeholder groups, in particular the state's hospital association and the DPH
- Passage of legislation mandating hospital participation
- The informatics capabilities of UNC to develop and support the system
- The relatively low burden to hospitals in terms of time, equipment, and manpower to participate in NC DETECT
- The application's perceived ease of use and low time burden for users

The key barriers to implementation and development of NC DETECT have been primarily of a technical nature, although the program has developed processes for identifying and addressing technical challenges and providing technical assistance to data providers and users. The moves to meet challenges going forward include:

- Continuing to improve the positive predictive value of the system and building applications that allow users to follow up and rule out "false alarms" quickly so daily workflow is not encumbered
- Developing strategies and tools that allow users to do more in less time
- Reaching out to new users who could mine the data for other public health purposes

NC DETECT has made important contributions and enhancements to North Carolina's public health surveillance system and can serve as a model for other states working to initiate and develop biosurveillance systems.

References

Ginsberg, M., J. Johnson, J. I. Tokars, C. Martin, R. English, G. Rainisch, et al. (2008). Monitoring health effects of wildfires using the BioSense system—San Diego County, October 2007. *MMWR* 57(27):741–47.

Hope, K., T. Merritt, K. Eastwood, K. Main, D. N. Durrheim, D. Muscatello, et al. (2008). The public health value of emergency department syndromic surveillance following a natural disaster. *Communicable Disease Intelligence* 32(1):92–94.

Leonardi, G. S., S. Hajat, R. S. Kovats, G. E. Smith, D. Cooper, and E. Gerard. (2006). Syndromic surveillance use to detect the early effects of heat-waves: An analysis of NHS direct data in England. *Soz Praventivmed* 51(4):194–201.

Lombardo, J. S., H. Burkom, and J. Pavlin. (2004). ESSENCE II and the framework for evaluating syndromic surveillance systems. *MMWR* 53(Supplement):159–65.

Loonsk, J. W. (2004). BioSense: A national initiative for early detection and quantification of public health emergencies. *MMWR* 53(Supplement):53–55.

Ma, H., J. I. Tokars, R. English, T. L. Smith, C. Bradley, L. Sokolow, et al. (2006). Surveillance of West Nile virus activity using BioSense laboratory test order data. *Advances in Disease Surveillance* 1(1):45. http://www.isdsjournal.org/article/view/224/167.

Marx, M. A., C. V. Rodriguez, J. Greenko, D. Das, R. Heffernan, A. M. Karpati, et al. (2005). Diarrheal illness detected through syndromic surveillance after a massive power outage: New York City, August 2003. *American Journal of Public Health* 96(30):547–53.

Stemler, S. (2001). An overview of content analysis. *Practical Assessment, Research and Evaluation,* 7(17). http://PAREonline.net/getvn.asp?v=7&n=17.

12

Aberration Detection in R Illustrated by Danish Mortality Monitoring

Michael Höhle
Ludwig-Maximilians-Universität München
Munich, Germany
and
Munich Center of Health Sciences
Munich, Germany

Anne Mazick
Statens Serum Institute
Copenhagen, Denmark

CONTENTS

KEYWORDS Disease outbreak, Monitoring, Surveillance, Change point detection

12.1 Introduction

The objective of biosurveillance in this chapter is the detection of emerging incidence clusters in time of a health-related event. Reviews on temporal surveillance can be found, for example, in Sonesson and Bock (2003), Bravata et al. (2004), Buckeridge et al. (2005), and Tennant et al. (2007). In recent years, a pleasant development has been a synthesis of surveillance methods with methods from statistical process control (see, for example, Woodall (2006) for a survey).

One important aspect to ensure a transfer of methodological developments into practice is the availability of appropriate software implementations and their documentation. With the present chapter, we want to introduce one such open-source software implementation into a public health context: the R package `surveillance`. In order to demonstrate functionality, we use Danish mortality data from the ongoing European monitoring of excess mortality for public health action (EuroMOMO) project (Anonymous, 2009).

The R system is a free software environment for statistical computing and graphics distributed under a GNU-style copyleft license and running under Unix, Windows, and Mac (R Development Core Team, 2009). Several documents and books provide an introduction, such as Dalgaard (2008), Venables et al. (2009), and Muenchen (2009). The add-on package `surveillance` offers functionality for the visualization, monitoring, and simulation of count data time series in R for public health surveillance and biosurveillance. It provides an implementation of different aberration detection algorithms for epidemiologists and an infrastructure for developers of new algorithms. The package is freely available under the GNU GPL license and obtainable from the Comprehensive R Archive Network (CRAN). To install the package from CRAN, the following call in R has to be performed once:

```
R> install.packages ("surveillance")
```

After installation, the package is loaded using:

```
R> library ("surveillance")
```

The focus in the present chapter is on using the aberration detection algorithms in the package for univariate count data time series, but the package also contains example outbreak data from the German SurvStat@RKI database (Robert Koch Institute, 2009) functionality for the simulation of outbreak data, and the comparison of algorithms. Höhle (2007) provides basic information about the package; further information can be found at the package homepage located at `http://surveillance.r-forge.r-project.org/`. The present text introduces a number of new developments in the package, for example, using the S4 `sts` class for gathering data and methods, and using likelihood ratio-based cumulative sum (CUSUM) algorithms.

At the time of this writing, only few other R packages exist aimed at helping epidemiologists in their outbreak detection and outbreak investigation. Retrospective cluster detection is available, for example, in the `DCluster` package (Gõmez-Rubio et al., 2005) and visualization of outbreak data can be performed by `epitools` (Aragon, 2008). Retrospective and—to some extent—prospective investigations of structural changes in time series can also be performed by the package `strucchange` (Zeileis et al., 2002), which, however, aims more at the econometrics community.

12.1.1 The EuroMOMO Project

The program European Monitoring of Excess Mortality for Public Health Action (EuroMOMO) is a 3-year project representing a network of 23 partners from 21 countries in the European region. The project is cofunded by the European Commission and coordinated by Statens Serum Institut Denmark (Mazick, 2007; Anonymous, 2009).

The aim of EuroMOMO is to develop and strengthen real-time monitoring of mortality across Europe; this will enhance the management of serious public health risks such as pandemic influenza, heat waves, and cold snaps. EuroMOMO's general objective is to develop and operate a routine public health system that monitors all-cause mortality in order to detect and measure—in a timely manner—excess number of deaths related to influenza and other known or emerging public health threats across European countries. Main actions include the creation of an inventory of existing mortality monitoring systems in Europe; the definition of minimal requirements for a mortality monitoring system; retrospective analysis of mortality data; identification of an optimal common analytical approach; and piloting of such a consensus system for mortality monitoring in several European countries.

Mortality monitoring is useful for early detection and monitoring of severe impacts of health threats and is as such an indicator-based surveillance system that provides important information within the framework of epidemic intelligence. The latter comprises the collection, collation, analysis, and assessment of information from different sources to rapidly identify and respond to known and unknown public health threats (Kaiser et al., 2006). Vital statistics are accessible for all European countries. However, often these data are not readily available in a timely manner during health crises or for imminent health threats. On the other hand, decision makers will request up-to-date mortality data in case of the threat of epidemics or emergence of new diseases (for example, pandemic influenza, AIDS, or SARS). As these threats are not restricted by borders, not only a national but also a common European approach to detect and estimate the magnitude of deaths is required. This is especially important as the methodology of monitoring mortality is complex, and there is a risk of European countries sharing incompatible information if different methodologies are used. However, in Europe, real-time monitoring of mortality is presently neither carried out uniformly nor in many European countries.

The main outcome of mortality monitoring is excess mortality, which can be defined as observed mortality in a given time period (e.g., a week) minus the expected mortality for that time period. Ongoing data analysis involving modeling the expected number of deaths for a given geographical unit and for different population groups is needed, and there are several candidate models available that have been tested or are in use in a few European countries (Conti et al., 2005, Gergonne et al., 2005, Josseran et al., 2006, Nogueira et al., 2005, and Simõn et al., 2005). However, in order to compare estimates of excess deaths, a common versatile statistical model is needed, and the key output of EuroMOMO is to provide a European consensus model for mortality monitoring that is applicable all over Europe and which is piloted and ready to implement.

The structure of this chapter is as follows: Section 12.2 provides an overview of the `surveillance` package, Section 12.3 constitutes the statistical framework of aberration detection, which is then considered in details for the Farrington method and the negative binomial CUSUM in Sections 12.4 and 12.5. After a description of the theory and syntax of invocation, Danish mortality data are used in each section to illustrate the methods. Section 12.6 concludes the chapter with a discussion.

12.2 Overview of the `surveillance` Package

The functionality in `surveillance` can be divided into two categories: prospective change-point (aka.aberration) detection algorithms for univariate time series of counts, and retrospective modeling of possibly multivariate times series of counts.

Classical public health aberration detection algorithms for univariate time series found in `surveillance` are, for example, the function `cdc` implementing the approach described (Stroup et al., 1989) and the function `farrington` (Farrington, 1996). More statistical process control–oriented approaches can be found as functions `cusum` (Rossi et al., 1999), `rogerson` (Rogerson and Yamada, 2004), and `glrnb` (Höhle and Paul, 2008).

Retrospective time-series modeling is available in `algo.hmm`, implementing the hidden Markov model approach in (Le Strat and Carrat, 1999) and `algo.hhh`, implementing the branching process approach (Held et al., 2005, Paul et al., 2008). Furthermore, `algo.twins` contains an implementation of the two-component endemic and epidemic approach described in (Held et al., 2006).

In what follows, focus will be on aberration detection methods. A prerequisite to their use is an understanding of the data structure and related access and visualization methods for the data.

12.2.1 Data Structure and Data Input

The S4 class `sts` (an abbreviation for "surveillance time series") provides a data structure for handling the multivariate time series of counts of the form $\{y_{it}; i=1,\ldots,m, t=1,\ldots,n\}$. Here, n denotes the length of the time series, and m denotes the number of entities being monitored, for example, geographical regions, hospitals, or age groups. A slot `observed` of `sts` contains an $n \times m$ matrix representing the y_{it} counts. The slot start denotes the origin of the time series given by a vector of length two containing the year and the epoch within that year. Furthermore, `freq` denotes the number of observations per year, for example, 365 for daily data, 52 for weekly data, and 12 for monthly data. An integer slot `epoch` denotes the time index $1 \leq t \leq n$ of each row in observed.

To import data into R and `surveillance`, one can use R's `read.table` or `read.csv` functions to read ASCII text or comma-separated value files. A different option is to use the package `foreign` to import SAS, SPSS, Stata or dBase files or the RODBC database interface to import from Microsoft Access/Excel or SQL databases. An `sts` object is then created from the resulting matrix of counts. We start the analysis of the Danish 1994–2008 mortality data by reading a CSV file (782 rows and 8 columns) containing the weekly number of all-cause mortality, and use this to create an sts object.

```
R> momo.ts <- read.csv ("mortality-dk.csv", header = TRUE,
check.names = FALSE)
R> dates <- as.Date ("1994-01-03") + 7 * 0:(nrow(momo.ts) - 1)
R> momo <- new("sts", epoch = as.numeric(dates), start = c(1994,
1), freq = 52, observed = momo.ts, epochAsDate = TRUE)
```

The eight columns correspond to the eight age groups <1, 1–4, 5–14, 15–44, 45–64, 65–74, 75–84, and ≥85 years as defined by the EuroMOMO project to be a relevant age stratification. Deaths are registered by the day of death. A special feature of the EuroMOMO data is that weeks are handled as defined by the ISO 8601 standard (Anonymous, 2004). This standard defines week-numbering for a year to start at the first Monday of week 01 and to end at the last Sunday before the new ISO year. Here, week 01 of a year is the week with the year's first Thursday in it. As a consequence, a year consists of either 52 or 53 full weeks. Usually, one operates in `surveillance` with a fixed number of epochs per period, for example, 52 weeks per year as given by the `freq` argument. But by specifically setting the `epoch` slot to a numeric representation of the corresponding Monday of each week and setting the `epochAsDate` attribute, we can use the `Date` class in R to easily handle this ISO week complication.

The resulting `sts` object `momo` can now be accessed and manipulated using standard matrix and data frame like access, `momo[1:10,"[0,1)"]` gives an sts object containing the first 10 weeks of the <1 age group and `dim(momo)` returns the dimension of the momo time series (that is, 782 × 8). Other operations are the aggregation of the time series over several epochs or entities by the `aggregate` function or linking the multivariate times series to geographical regions of an ESRI shapefile. Plot functions provide visualization of the multivariate time series in time, space, and space–time. In the subsequent analysis of the Danish mortality data, we focus on the country-aggregated time series stratified by age. Here, age stratification is used to differentiate between different mortality risk groups, and country level is used to ensure sufficiently large strata in a population of 5.5 millions. For larger EuroMOMO countries, a further stratification by geographical region might, however, be relevant. The following code illustrates various uses of the plot function for the momo object with corresponding output shown in Figures 12.1 and 12.2:

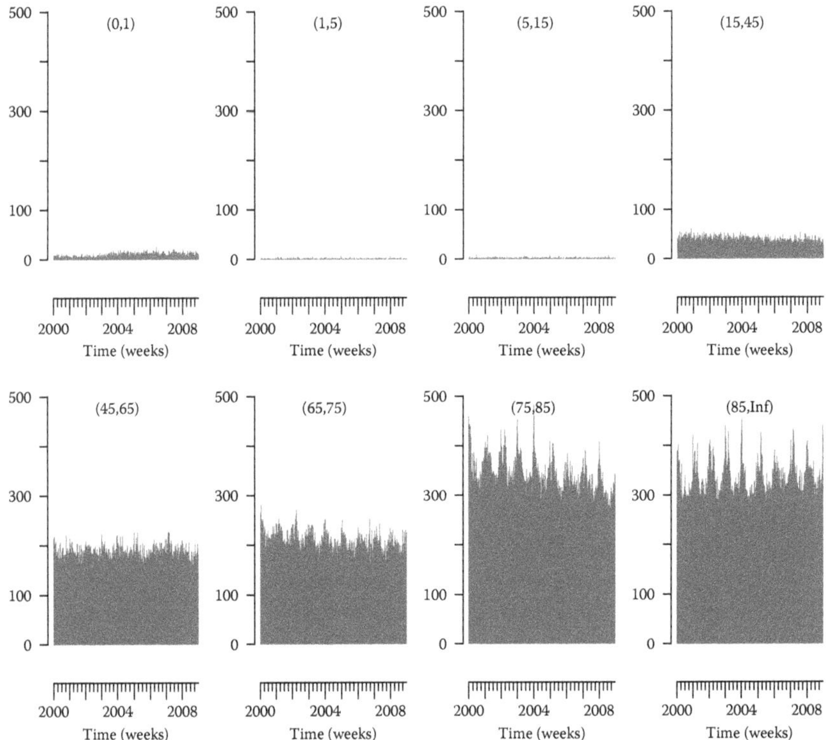

FIGURE 12.1
Weekly number of all-cause mortality in Denmark in the eight age groups during 2000–2008. Each axis tick denotes a quarter (3-month period), and the larger tick marks denote the 1st quarter of the year (starting with ISO week 01).

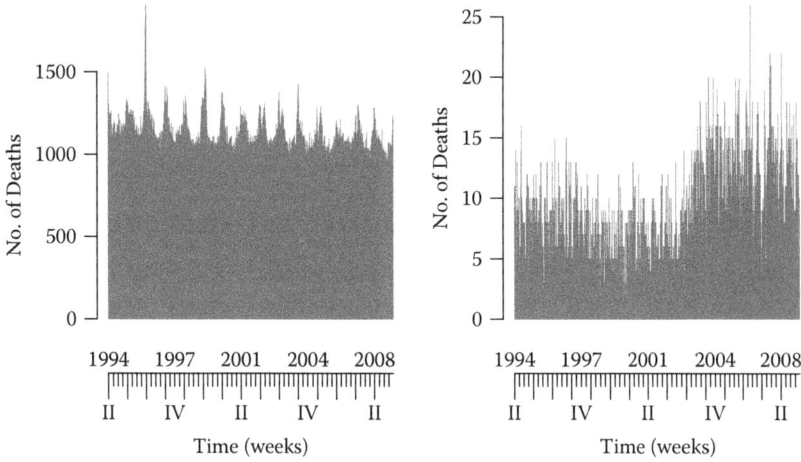

FIGURE 12.2
(Left) Weekly number of all-cause deaths in Denmark 1994–2008 aggregated over all age groups, and (right) the weekly data of the <1 age group. The increase of mortality in this group is due to a change in the gestational age defining a stillbirth, which was lowered from 28 weeks to 22 weeks in 2004.

```
R> plot(momo[year(momo) >= 2000, ], type = observed time |
unit)
R> plot(momo, ylab = "No. of deaths", type = observed time)
R> plot(momo[, "[0,1)"], ylab = "No. of deaths")
```

In the above lines, the type argument controls the view on the multivariate time series object. If no such argument is provided as in the third call, a default choice is used.

Figure 12.1 shows that monitoring of weekly mortality in Denmark requires handling both weekly time series containing small count numbers and series having large counts. For the four age groups in the top row of the figure, it will be important to take the count data nature into account, because a Gaussian approximation is expected to work poorly here. As a consequence, we will in our work focus on statistical modeling and aberration detection handling small counts. The methods should, however, be flexible enough to also handle time series with large counts as, for example, in the bottom row of Figure 12.1. An additional advantage of being able to handle small counts is that this also allows for further stratification of the data into, for example, geographical regions or gender. Furthermore, the time series can contain temporal trends, such as the downward trend for the 65–74 group or the mortality increase in the ≥85 group due to increasing longevity. Similar examples are the seasonal patterns for the 75–84 and ≥85 age groups, where an increased mortality during winter and spring is observed. In order to accommodate such nonstationarity, we want to investigate modeling and aberration detection approaches, taking such trend and seasonality into account.

12.3 Statistical Framework for Aberration Detection

Denote by $\{y_t, t = 1,2,\ldots\}$ the univariate time series to monitor. In this chapter, y_t will always be a discrete univariate random variable, but continuous and multivariate versions are just as conceivable. The aim of aberration detection is to on-line detect an important change in the process occurring at an unknown time t. This could, for example, be a change in the process parameters resulting in a change in level or variation of the process. Using terminology from statistical process control, the process can thus be in one of two states at each time point t: *in-control,* that is, $s < \tau$, or *out-of-control* (that is, $s \geq \tau$). The binary 0/1 indicator $x(t)$ will denote the true but unknown state of the process at time t, assuming that $x(t) = 1$ means out-of-control.

At time $s \geq 1$, where a decision about the state of $x(s)$ is to be made, the available process information is $\boldsymbol{y}_s = \{y_t; t \leq s\}$. A detection method is now a rule that predicts the unknown state of $x(s)$ based on $\boldsymbol{y}_s$. This is done by computing a summary $r(\boldsymbol{y}_s)$ based on $\boldsymbol{y}_s$, which is then compared to a threshold value g and, consequently,

$$\hat{x}(s) = I(r(\boldsymbol{y}_s) > g),$$

where $I(\times)$ is an indicator function, that is, the function returns 1 if $r(\boldsymbol{y}_s) > g$ and zero otherwise. The time of the first out-of-control alarm is then a random variable

$$T_A = \min\{s \geq 1 : r(\boldsymbol{y}_s) > g\}. \quad (12.1)$$

After the change to the out-of-control state at time τ, the decision rule should as quickly as possible sound an alarm. However, it might take a number of observations after τ before enough evidence has been collected to do so. Two important target variables for evaluating the performance of a detection method are the *in-control run-length* $T_A|\tau = \infty$, that is, the number of epochs before the first wrong alarm, and the *out-of-control run-length* $T_A|\tau = 1$, that is, the number of epochs to detect an already occurred change. Various summaries such as expectation or median can be computed of these run-length variables. Specifically, the expectation of the in-control run-length $\mathrm{E}(T_A|\tau = \infty)$—known as the *average in-control run-length* or $P(T_A \text{ Y } t_a|\tau = \infty)$—the probability to get a false alarm within the first t_a epochs of the monitoring—is often used as a criterion when evaluating the performance of a detection method. A more thorough discussion on such criteria can be found, for example, in Frisén (2003).

12.4 The Farrington Algorithm

The aim of the Farrington et al. (1996) algorithm was to develop a robust and fast method applicable for the routine monitoring of weekly reports on infections for many different pathogens at the former Communicable Disease Surveillance Centre (now Health Protection Agency) in the United Kingdom. For the current time point $t_0 = (t_0^{\text{week}}, t_0^{\text{year}})$, that is, week, t_0^{week}, in year, t_0^{year}; this is done by formulating a statistical algorithm for predicting the observed number of counts y_{t0}. This prediction is based on a subset of the historic data: Centered around the current week, t_0^{week}, for example, week 23, one includes w values to the left and right of that week together with the week itself, for example, week 21–25, if $w = 2$. This is done for each of the years $t_0^{\text{year}-1}, \ldots, t_0^{\text{year}-b}$. Thus, a total of $b \cdot (2w + 1)$ reference values are extracted. Now, an overdispersed Poisson generalized linear model (GLM) with log-link is fitted to the reference values. The GLM has the following mean structure:

$$E(y_t) = \mu_t, \quad \text{where } \log(\mu_t) = \alpha + \beta t, \tag{12.2}$$

and $\text{Var}(y_t) = \varphi\mu_t$ with α, β, and $\varphi>0$ being coefficients to estimate. See, for example, Fahrmeir and Tutz (2001) for further information about GLMs. One can show that an approximate $(1 - \alpha) \cdot 100\%$ prediction interval for y_{t0} based on this GLM has an upper limit,

$$u_{t_0} = \hat{\mu}_{t_0} + z_{1-\alpha/2} \cdot \sqrt{\text{Var}(y_{t_0} - \hat{\mu}_{t_0})} = \hat{\mu}_{t_0} \cdot \left(1 + z_{1-\alpha/2} \cdot \sqrt{\frac{\phi\hat{\mu}_{t_0} + \text{Var}(\hat{\mu}_{t_0})}{\hat{\mu}_{t_0}^2}}\right),$$

where $z_{1-\alpha/2}$ is the $1 - \alpha/2$ quantile of the standard normal distribution, while $\hat{\mu}_{t_0}, \hat{\phi}$ and $\text{Var}(\hat{\mu}_{t_0})$ can be obtained from the GLM output. If the observed value y_{t0} is greater than u_{t0}, then the time point t_0 is flagged as an outbreak, that is, in the notation of Section 12.3:

$$\hat{x}(t_0) = I\left(\frac{y_{t_0}}{u_{t_0}} > 1\right). \tag{12.3}$$

The Farrington algorithm contains a number of additional refinements for improving the prediction of y_{t0}, for example, by correcting for past outbreaks among the reference values, by testing the need of the trend component in Equation 12.2, and by a skewness correction of the predictive distribution for low count series. In order to keep the current presentation compact, we refer to Farrington et al. (1996) for further details on these refinements. In `surveillance`, the function `farrington` is used to run the algorithm:

```
R> phase2 <- which(epoch(momo) >= "2007-10-01")
R> s.far <- farrington (momo[, "[0,1)"], control = list(range
= phase2, alpha = 0.01, b = 5, w = 4, powertrans = "none"))
```

We start the monitoring in week 40 of 2007 (that is, October 1, 2007) and let `phase2` denote the index of all ISO weeks to monitor. The call to function farrington then performs aberration detection for these weeks in the <1 age group. Note that all aberration detection algorithms in `surveillance` follow the same structure: The first argument denotes an object of class `sts` containing the data, the second argument contains a list of algorithm-specific control options, and a vector `range` with the time points to monitor. Specifically, the above code uses $\alpha = 0.01$ to form the upper limit of the predictive distribution, and $b = 5$ and $w = 4$ to generate the reference values. Figure 12.3 shows the results of the monitoring. In order to obtain the above-described procedure without any additional transformation, the argument `powertrans`="none" is used. Other options are "2/3", which provides a skewness correction, which is preferable in low count scenario. Similarly, "1/2" provides the variance stabilizing square-root transformation.

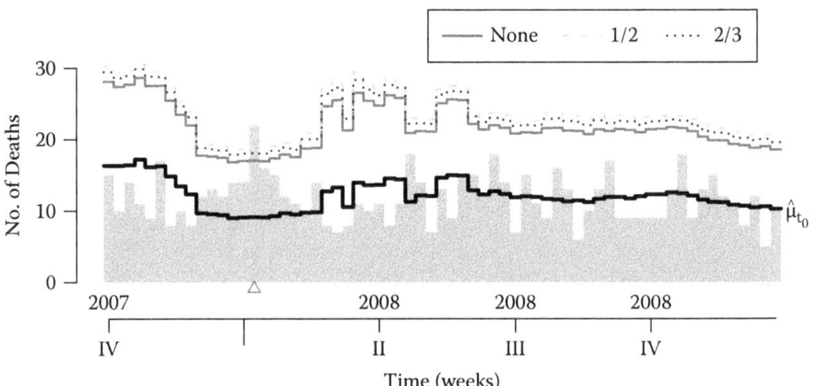

FIGURE 12.3
Aberration detection for the <1 age group using the Farrington et al. (1996) method. The upper three lines show the upper prediction limit as calculated using each of the three possible power transformations. The lower solid line denotes the expected model predicted number of cases for each time point t_0. Triangles indicate an alarm.

```
R> plot(s.far, ylab = "No. of deaths", xlab = "time (weeks)",
main = "")
```

The figure is interpreted as follows: Starting in ISO week 40 of 2007, we use only values from the past to construct a prediction interval for the observed number of counts for week 40. When comparing the actually observed number 15 with the upper limit $u_{t_0} = 28.1$, we have no reason to believe in an excess number of deaths and hence no alarm is generated. The upper limit would have been 30.3 or 29.4 cases for the two other transformations. The same procedure is now repeated for ISO week 41, etc. In week 02 of 2008, the observed number of counts exceeds the threshold of the "none" line for the first time, and hence an alarm is generated for that week. No further alarms are generated during the 65 weeks of surveillance. Once an alarm is sounded, the alarm must be verified and the public health significance investigated. In this instance, investigation of available epidemic intelligence did not reveal any specific explanation for the mortality peak that would indicate a significant public health event.

Note also the prospective behavior of the detection: At each time point, we are only allowed to look back in time, never ahead in time. Thus, detection mimics the arrival of new data each week, which would be the case in practical applications. Choosing a specific value for α is particularly dependent on the application and mode of operation. A value of, for example, $\alpha = 0.01$ means that for a particular week the probability of observing a value $y_{t_0} > u_{t_0}$ by pure chance under the estimated model is $\alpha/2 = 0.5\%$. If these probabilities are assumed independent for the individual weeks, the probability of observing a false alarm during the 65 epochs of the monitoring is thus $1-(1-0.005)^{65} = 0.28$. In Section 12.1, the actual run-length distribution of the algorithm is studied in further detail.

A call to an aberration detection algorithm fills the `alarm` slot of the `sts` object. This is an $n' \times m$ matrix of Booleans stating for each time point (aka. `epoch`) and series whether the time point was classified as aberration. Here, n' corresponds to the number of elements in the `range` argument of the call. Furthermore, the `upper-bound` slot contains an $n' \times m$ matrix of values corresponding to the minimum number of cases each week that would have resulted in an alarm. Finally, the slot `control` contains the list of control arguments that was used to invoke the aberration detection algorithm.

For the EuroMOMO project, an important aspect besides the detection of aberrations is the quantification of excess mortality. A first measure of this excess could be based on the predictive distribution. For example, Figure 12.3 shows the predicted expected number $\hat{\mu}_t$ of cases in-control, allowing for a definition of excess as, for example, $y_t - \hat{\mu}_t$. By computing confidence intervals for $\hat{\mu}_t$, one would also be able to assess the uncertainty of such an excess. As a further tool in this direction, Figure 12.4 shows the quantiles of the predictive distribution. The Farrington procedure sounds an alarm once the $1-\alpha/2$ quantile is exceeded.

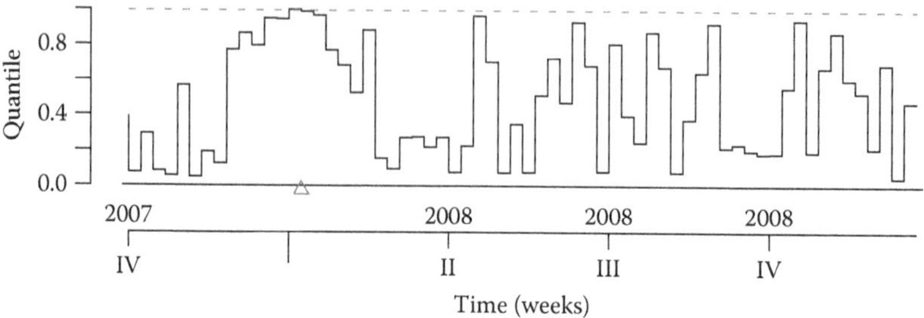

FIGURE 12.4
Quantiles of the predictive distribution. The dashed line indicates the $1-\alpha/2 = 0.995$ quantile used for the surveillance in Figure 12.3. Triangles indicate the alarms.

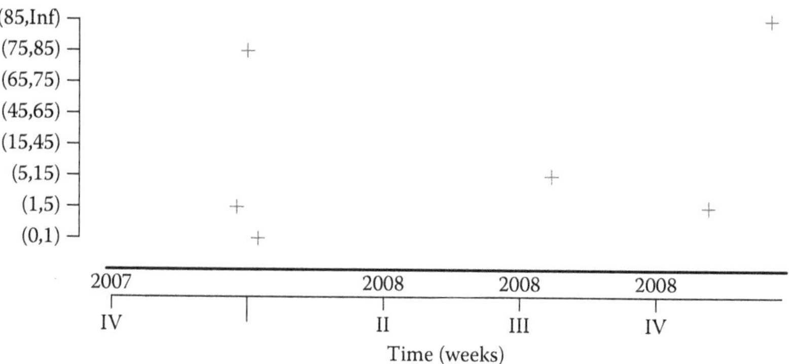

FIGURE 12.5
Overview of aberration detection for all eight age group time series using the Farrington algorithm with $\alpha = 0.01$.

One way to simultaneously monitor all eight age groups is to monitor each time series separately using, for example, the Farrington procedure. This is done by the following code:

```
R> s.far.all <- farrington(momo, control = list(range =
phase2, alpha = 0.01, b = 5, w = 4))
```

A plot of the alarms for each time series provides a graphical overview as shown in Figure 12.5. Monitoring each series independently as done above ignores possible correlations of the time series. Furthermore, if one wanted to keep the number of false alarms at the same level as for the surveillance of a single series, one could, however, have used an α, being one-eighth of what was used for the single time series case previously.

```
R> plot(s.far.all, type = alarm time, xlab = "time (weeks)")
```

In Figure 12.5, we observe no specific patterns of the alarms across age strata, except for single week alarms around the turn of the year 2007/2008 in age groups <1, 1–4 and 75–84. Note that the 2007/2008 season in Denmark did not exhibit any heavy influenza activity. Furthermore, the current surveillance does correct for any population demographics using the linear trend in Equation 12.2. It might, however, be worth investigating an additional adjustment for population size in the eight age strata as these are expected to change over the years.

As a further remark, in the notation of Section 12.3 the Farrington algorithm does not utilize all available information at decision time s = t_0, that is, $r_{\text{Farr}}(\boldsymbol{y}_s) = r_{\text{Farr}}(\boldsymbol{y}'_s)$ with $\boldsymbol{y}'_s \subset \boldsymbol{y}_s$. The effects of seasonality are handled robustly by using only "similar" weeks as reference values and hence no explicit seasonal model is needed. Such an approach is, however, suboptimal, if it is possible to adequately model the seasonal behavior as, for example, it is done in Section 12.5.

Even though more than a single y_s is used to compute $r(\boldsymbol{y}_s)$ in the Farrington algorithm, the decision in Equation 12.3 occurs by only comparing the current observation with the upper limit of the predictive distribution. Hence, no accumulation of evidence against the in-control situation occurs. In the next section, we reconsider this task from a statistical process control viewpoint and describe an approach taking accumulation into account.

12.5 Negative Binomial CUSUM

Reconsidering Equation 12.1 more from the viewpoint of statistical process control, the simplest class of detectors is the Shewhart detector, which for $r(\boldsymbol{y}_s)$ only utilizes information about the last time point, for example, by comparing the single y_s value to a fixed threshold value. In a parametric detection setup one assumes a known probability mass function (PMF) $f(\cdot;\theta)$ for y_s, which is parametrized by a parameter vector θ. If the parameter vector θ is assumed to be known in the in-control and out-of-control state, an optimal change-point detection can be achieved based on the partial likelihood ratio (Frisén, 2003). Let $L(s,t)$ with $s \geq t$ be the partial likelihood ratio between the out-of-control and in-control models at time s, given that τ = t. Assuming independence between the elements of ys when conditioning on the parameter θ, one obtains

$$L(s,t) = \frac{f(\boldsymbol{y}_s \mid \tau = t)}{f(\boldsymbol{y}_s \mid \tau > s)} = \frac{\prod_{i=1}^{t-1} f(y_i;\theta_0) \prod_{i=t}^{s} f(y_i;\theta_1)}{\prod_{i=1}^{s} f(y_i;\theta_0)} = \prod_{i=t}^{s} \frac{f(y_i;\theta_1)}{f(y_i;\theta_0)}.$$

For the Shewhart detector, optimal detection can be achieved by $r(s) = L(s,s)$. This detector is good at detecting large process shifts quickly, but if the shift is small but sustained, accumulating deviations over time is necessary in order to detect the change. The likelihood ratio based cumulative sum originally proposed by Page (1954) is one method to deal with accumulation and is advantageous for detecting sustained shifts. It uses

$$r(s) = \max\{1 \le t \le s : L(s,t)\}.$$

When the y_t are independent and identically distributed discrete random variables, such count data CUSUM detectors are well investigated (see, for example, Hawkins and Olwell (1998)). However, biosurveillance data often exhibit seasonal variations and time trends that violate the assumption of an identical distribution. As in Höhle et al. (2009), let

$$r(s) = \max_{1 \le t \le s}\left[\sum_{i=t}^{s} \log\left\{\frac{f(y_i;\theta_1)}{f(y_i;\theta_0)}\right\}\right], \tag{12.4}$$

where we have used the log-likelihood ratio (LLR) instead of the likelihood ratio. Let θ_0 denote the in-control and θ_1 the out-of-control parameters. If θ_0 and θ_1 are known, Equation 12.4 can be written in recursive form as follows:

$$r_0 = 0 \quad \text{and} \quad r_s = \max\left(0, r_{s-1} + \log\left\{\frac{f(y_s;\theta_1)}{f(y_s;\theta_0)}\right\}\right), \quad \text{for } s \ge 1. \tag{12.5}$$

One sees that for time points with LLR>0, that is, evidence against in-control, the LLR contributions are added up. On the other hand, no credit in the direction of the in-control is given because r_s cannot get below zero.

In practical applications, the in-control and out-of-control parameters are, however, hardly ever known beforehand. A typical procedure in this case is to use historical phase 1 data for the estimation of θ_0 with the assumption that these data originate from the in-control state. This estimate is then used as plug-in value in the above LLR. Simultaneously, the out-of-control parameter θ_1 is specified as a known function of θ_0, for example, as a known multiplicative increase in the mean. Developing appropriate count data time series models together with statistical inference for the estimation of θ_0 and θ_1 in a statistical process control framework is thus an important aspect of performing biosurveillance.

As we suspect the number of persons in the eight age groups to shift toward older age during the years, we want to take the population size of the eight age strata into account in our monitoring. We do so by using data from Statistics Denmark (2009) on the number of individuals on January 1, 1994–2008, in each of the eight age groups.

```
R> population(momo) <- as.matrix(read.csv("population-dk.csv",
check.names = FALSE))
```

We will in the following use a generalized log-link negative binomial model for the in-control situation of a specific age group, that is, $y_t \sim \text{NegBin}(\mu_{0,t}, \alpha)$ with

$$\log(\mu_{0,t}) = \beta_0 + \beta_1 \cdot t + c(t) + \beta_2 \cdot \text{pop}_t, \tag{12.6}$$

where $c(t)$ is a cyclic function with period 52 or 53, depending on the number of ISO weeks in the year of t, e.g., $c(0) = c(52)$ for years with 52 ISO weeks. Such behavior can, e.g., be obtained by sinusoidals (Serfling, 1963) or using cyclic splines (Wood, 2006). Furthermore, pop_t denotes the population size in the respective age group at time t. In the above negative binomial model $E(yt) = \mu_{0,t}$ and $\text{Var}(y_t) = \mu_{0,t} + \alpha \cdot \mu_{0,t}^2$, that is, α is a dispersion parameter, which we will assume to be constant over time. Thus, with $\alpha>0$, we are able to handle possible overdispersion of the count data time series. For $\alpha \to 0$, the negative binomial distribution tends to the Poisson distribution.

The out-of-control model for the mean is now assumed to be $\mu_{1,t} = \kappa \cdot \mu_{0,t}$ which on the log-link scale corresponds to a level shift in the intercept from β_0 to $\beta_0+\log(\kappa)$. The following R code estimates such a negative binomial GLM from the phase 1 data of the 75–84 age group using the `glm.nb` function (Venables and Ripley, 2002).

```
R> phase1 <- which(year(momo) == 2002 epochInYear(momo) ==
40):(phase2[1] - 1)
R> momo.df <- as.data.frame(momo)
R> m <- glm.nb('observed.[75,85)' 1 + epoch + sin(2 * pi *
epochInPeriod) + cos(2 * pi * epochInPeriod) + 'population.
[75,85)', data = momo.df[phase1,])
R> mu0 <- predict(m, newdata = momo.df[phase2, ], type =
"response")
```

Here, `phase1` contains the index of all time epochs in the phase 1 sample used to estimate the in-control parameters. A 5-year period has been used above. Then the function `as.data.frame` is applied to convert the `sts` object to the necessary `data.frame` used by `glm.nb`. For simplicity, a single harmonic is used for $c(t)$ consisting of one sine and one cosine term. The parameter estimates for the other terms are $\hat{\beta}_0 = 10.49$, $\hat{\beta}_1 = -9.54 \cdot 10^{-5}$, $\hat{\beta}_2 = -1.24 \cdot 10^{-5}$ and $\hat{\alpha} = 1.97 \cdot 10^{-3}$. In practical application, one should perform a model selection process to decide on covariates and an appropriate number of harmonics to include. For example, such a selection for the above model would reveal pop_t as being nonsignificant, whereas a total of three superimposed harmonics could be justified. For illustration we, however, proceed with the above

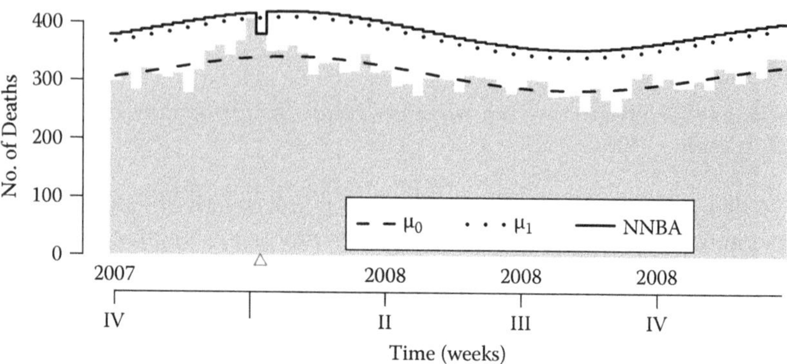

FIGURE 12.6
Aberration detection for the 75–84 age group series using a time-varying negative binomial CUSUM. Shown are the time-varying in-control and out-of-control means and the number needed before an alarm (NNBA). Triangles indicate alarms.

model and use `predict` to obtain the expected value $\mu_{0,t}$ during phase 2. Figure 12.6 illustrates the $\mu_{0,t}$ predictions based on this GLM model.

If, for example, one wanted to optimally detect a 20% increase in the mean, one would have $\kappa = 1.2$. Again, the choice of κ depends very much on the specific application and mode of operation. Together with the threshold g, the value of κ determines the distribution of the run-length as further investigated in Section 12.1. The resulting $\mu_{1,t}$ is shown in Figure 12.6. Also shown is the number needed before alarm (NNBA) at each time s. This number is obtained by reversing Equation 12.5 with known threshold g, that is, given r_{s-1} find the minimum y_s such that $r_s > g$.

```
R> kappa < - 1.2
R> s.nb < - glrnb(momo[, "[75,85)"], control = list(range =
phase2, alpha = 1/m$theta,mu0 = mu0, c.ARL = 4.75, theta =
log(kappa), ret= "cases"))
```

The above code extracts the dispersion parameter α from the `glm.nb` fit; note the slightly different parametrization of the dispersion parameter here. For the threshold g (in `glrnb` denoted `c.ARL`), we use the value of 4.75. This threshold value determines the distribution of the run-length T_A as investigated in detail in Section 12.1; specifically, we show that $g \approx 4.75$ results in $P(T_A \leq 65 | \tau = \infty) \approx 0.1$. The results from this call are illustrated in Figure 12.6. For week 02 in 2008, an alarm is generated. Notice that the number of cases in the previous week is not enough to sound an alarm itself, but helps to lower the NNBA in the following week, where it is just about exceeded. No further alarms are generated. The alarm is an example of excess mortality peaks in the elderly that occur regularly during winter around the change of the year and at the time of influenza epidemics.

12.5.1 Run-Length Properties

As mentioned previously, the behavior of the CUSUM depends very much on the choice of the threshold g. In order to guide the choice of g, we will look at the run-length distribution of $T_A|\tau = \infty$ under the fitted negative binomial model. Prediction of $\mu_{0,t}$ requires knowledge of all involved covariates during the monitoring period, e.g., in model (6), this would be the population size. For the monitored period of 65 weeks (2007-W40 – 2008-W52), these values are available, but if monitoring exceeded this period, we would have needed to predict covariate values as well before being able to compute $\mu_{0,t}$. Hence, it is practically more feasible to look at $P(T_A \le t_A|\ \tau = \infty)$ for a small t_A than to estimate, for example, $E(T_A|\tau = \infty)$ as here many more time points might be needed if the expectation is large. Furthermore, the distribution of T_A is also often skewed, which makes the expectation a bad summary of the central tendency.

Specifically, we want to choose g such that $P(T_A \le 65|\tau = \infty)$ is below some acceptable value, for example, 10%. In other words, the probability of a false alarm within the 65 weeks of our $\mu_{0,t}$ versus $\mu_{1,t}$ monitoring should be below 10%. To compute the probability under the selected model, two approaches exist: direct Monte Carlo estimation or a Markov chain approximation.

In the first approach, we use Monte Carlo estimation of $P(T_A \le 65|\tau = \infty)$. For each realization j, a time series of length 65 is simulated from the estimated negative binomial model with mean $\mu_{0,t}$, t=1, … , 65, and dispersion parameter α. Then the negative binomial CUSUM is applied to this time series and one checks if $T_A^j \le 65$. The probability of interest using k such realizations can then be estimated as $\sum_{j=1}^{k} I(T_A^j \le 65)/k$, where $I(\cdot)$ is the indicator function. Code-wise this can be done for k = 1000 for a grid of g's as follows.

```
R> simone.TAleq65 <- function(sts, g) {
observed(sts)[phase2,]<-rnbinom(length(mu0), mu = mu0, size =
mtheta)
one <-glrnb(sts, control = modifyList(control(s.nb),
list(c.ARL = g)))
return(any(alarms(one)))
}
R> g.grid <-seq(1.8, by = 0.5)
R> pMC <-sapply(g.grid, function(g) {
mean(replicate(1000,simone)))
})
```

Figure 12.7 shows the result. We note that $g \approx 4.75$ ensures that the false-alarm probability within the monitoring period drops below the desired level of 10%. If one is interested in $P(T_A \le 65|\tau = 1)$ instead, $\mu_{1,t}$ has to be used as argument mu in `rnbinom`.

A different option to compute this false-alarm probability for a likelihood ratio-based CUSUM is to use a Markov chain approximation to determine the PMF of the run-length variable. This approach implemented in

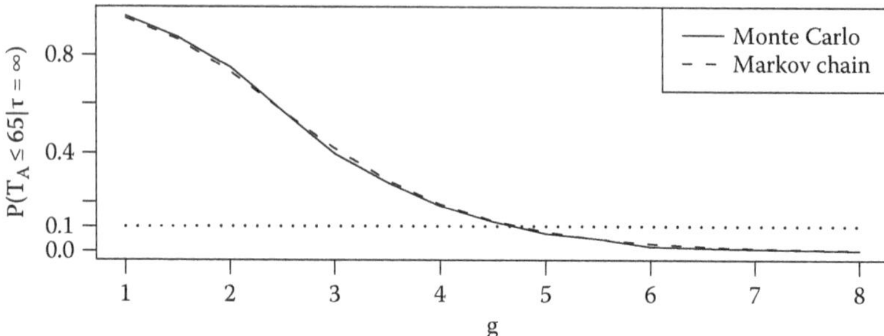

FIGURE 12.7
$P(T_A \leq 65 | \tau = \infty)$ as a function of the threshold g computed using both Monte Carlo simulation and a Markov chain approximation. A dotted line shows the desired value 0.10.

`surveillance` is a generalization of the work in Bissell (1984) to time varying count data CUSUMs.

```
R> dY <- function(y, mu, log = FALSE, alpha, ...)
dnbinom(y, mu = mu, size = 1/alpha, log = log)
R> pMarkovChain <- sapply(g.grid, function(g){
TA <-LRCUSUM.runlength(mu = t(mu0), mu0 = t(mu0), mu1 = kappa*
t(mu0), c.ARL = g, dfun = dY, n = rep(600, length(mu0)),
alpha = 1/mtheta)
return(tail(TAcdf, n = 1))
})
```

Here, `dY` is a function specifying the one-parameter PMF used in the likelihood ratio detector; in our case, this is the negative binomial PMF $f(y_t;\mu_t,\alpha)$. The above invocation of the function `LRCUSUM.runlength` derives the distribution of T_A when the value of μ_t is equal to $\mu_{0,t}$ (that is, in-control) for given specifications of in-control mean, out-of-control mean, and dispersion parameter. The function computes the loglikelihood ratio between all possible realizations of *yt*. However, to make computations feasible, an upper limit n is used at each time point, after which for $y_t > n$ the probability of y_t to occur under μ_t is negligible. Figure 12.7 shows the result and the close agreement with the Monte Carlo estimation. The Markov chain approximation is considerably faster though.

Returning to the monitoring of the <1 age group from Section 12.4, we would like to compare the Farrington algorithm with the negative binomial CUSUM. To do so, we use the in-control model $NegBin(\mu_{0,t},\alpha)$ for the CUSUM, with $\mu_{0,t}$ as in Figure 12.3 and α estimated by a similar GLM as in Section 5. The out-of-control mean is again given as $\mu_{1,t} = 1.2, \mu_{0,t}$. The threshold g should be chosen such that the two algorithms are as comparable as possible with respect to. for example, $P(T_A \leq 65 | \tau = \infty)$. A Monte Carlo estimation as just described is performed to determine this probability for the Farrington algorithm. The model used for this simulation is the above in-control negative binomial model.

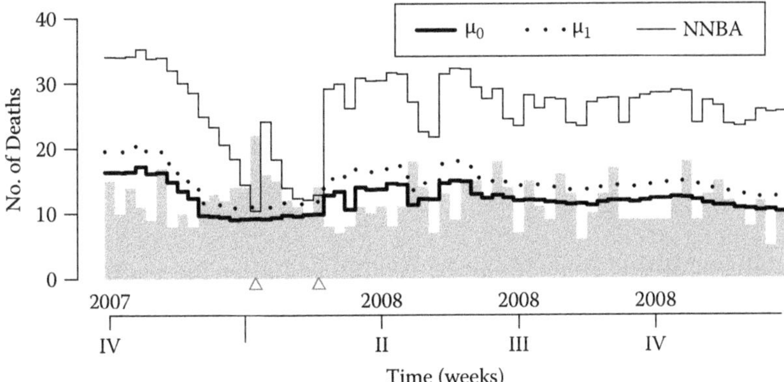

FIGURE 12.8
Negative binomial CUSUM for the <1 group. The interpretation of the lines shown is as in Figure 12.6.

Based on 1000 realizations of $I(T_A \le 65 | \tau = \infty)$, the probability is estimated to be 0.57, which is surprisingly high compared to the rough estimate of 0.28 in Section 12.4. However, the two numbers are not completely comparable as the simulation uses a negative binomial model and observations are not independent. If the above Monte Carlo estimated false-alarm probability of the Farrington algorithm should be near 10%, we would have to choose a much smaller α. Instead, we use the Markov chain approximation to determine that a threshold of $g \approx 2.2$ gives a similar probability for the negative binomial CUSUM. Figure 12.8 contains the result of the CUSUM monitoring with this threshold.

The CUSUM behaves slightly different than the Farrington algorithm in Figure 12.3. In the last weeks of 2007, an increased number of cases above the baseline is accumulated leading to a steady decrease of NNBA. In week 01, the threshold is nearly reached, but as for the Farrington procedure, an alarm is first generated for week 02 in 2008. However, the sustained excess above baseline leads to a further alarm in week 08, which was not detected by the Farrington algorithm, as here, the excess alone in that week is not enough to get beyond the threshold.

12.6 Conclusions

In this chapter, we have given an introduction to the capabilities of the open-source R package `surveillance` for epidemiological biosurveillance. Further advantages of choosing R to conduct such analyses exist: R produces high-quality graphics in a variety of formats, including TIFF, PNG, EPS, and PDF which, combined with Sweave or odfWeave Leisch (2002),

Max Kuhn, and Steve Weaston (2009), allows for automatic report generation using LaTeX/OpenOffice in literate programming fashion. Also HTML pages containing text, graphics, and tables of the results can automatically be generated from R using, for example, the package `R2HTML` (Lecoutre (2003) or `hwriter` Pau (2009)). Altogether, using the command

```
R> demo(biosurvbook)
```

the analyses of this chapter can be reproduced after the package has been loaded.

We introduced the time-varying negative binomial CUSUM as an alternative to the Farrington aberration detection method, as it is better embedded within the framework of statistical process control. A shortcoming of the suggested GLM modeling to determine in-control and out-of-control values is that any uncertainty of the estimation was ignored when plugging in the estimators for $\mu_{0,t}$ and $\mu_{1,t}$ into the CUSUM. Furthermore, no auto-correlation between observations was taken into account—neither in the GLM model nor in the likelihood ratio-based CUSUM. However, if trend and seasonality are adequately modeled, little auto-correlation is expected to remain as, for example, shown in the simulation study by Farrington et al. (1996). If auto-correlation is a concern, different modeling strategies can be applied: generalized estimating equations (used for mortality modeling in, for example, Fouillet et al. (2008); integer auto-regressive models (Freeland and McCabe 2004, Held et al. 2005, Wei 2007), or pairwise likelihood models (Varin and Vidoni (2006)). An auto-regressive approach is, for example, implemented in the function `glrnb` by using the control argument `change = "epi"` (see Höhle and Paul, 2008 for details on the methodology). The same reference also discusses how to estimate the out-of-control state κ at each time point using generalized likelihood ratio CUSUMs instead of a fixed prior specification. An alternative to the independence assuming likelihood ratio-based CUSUM is the Shiryaev-Roberts detector, which also works for auto-correlated observations (see for example Frisén (2003) for details). As an example, the spatio-temporal cluster detection of Assunção and Correa (2009)—implemented as function `stcd in surveillance`—uses this detector. Further package developments are the extension to categorical time series, for example, the monitoring of binomial and multinomial data.

With respect to the Danish mortality monitoring, the presented analyses illustrated the potential of using `surveillance` and R for this task since they provide methods for the visualization, modeling, and aberration detection. A big advantage of the regression-based models in the CUSUM detection is their flexibility for extending them with additional covariates as illustrated by population size. Such covariates could for example, be the number of influenza-like illness cases or temperature. A limitation of the current methods is that mortality reporting is governed by a delay between the day of death and the reporting to health authorities. Quantification and handling of such reporting delay is thus a precondition for valuable prospective monitoring. Approaches exist for dealing with such reporting delay (see, e.g., Heisterkamp et al. 2006), but these are currently not available for routine use in `surveillance` and have also not methodologically been adapted to the CUSUM context. Finally, the open-source and copyleft approach of the R system and `surveillance` is well suited for the EuroMOMO project aim of obtaining a mortality monitoring system operating in many different countries.

Acknowledgments

We thank Christiane Dargatz for proofreading the manuscript. The EuroMOMO project has received funding from the European Union in the framework of the Public Health Programme. However, the responsibility for the content lies solely with the authors, and the European Union is not responsible for any use that may be made of the information.

References

Anonymous (2004). Data elements and interchange formats—Information interchange—Representation of dates and times, Jan 12, ISO 8601:2004(E), The International Organization for Standardization.

Anonymous (2009). European monitoring of excess mortality for public health action, Project homepage: http://www.euromomo.eu/, last access: June 9, 2009.

Assunçáo, R. and T. Correa (2009). Surveillance to detect emerging space-time clusters. *Computational Statistics and Data Analysis 53*(*8*), 2817–2830.

Bissell, A. F. (1984). The performance of control charts and cusums under linear trend. *Applied Statistics 33*(2), 145–151.

Bravata, D. M., K. M. McDonald, W. M. Smith, C. Rydzak, H. Szeto, D. L. Buckeridge, C. Haberland, and D. K. Owens (2004). Systematic review: surveillance systems for early detection of bioterrorism-related diseases. *Annals of Internal Medicine 140*(*11*), 910–922.

Buckeridge, D. L., H. Burkom, M. Campbell, W. R. Hogan, and A. W. Moore (2005). Algorithms for rapid outbreak detection: a research synthesis. *Journal of Biomedical Informatics 38*(2), 99–113.

Conti, S., P. Meli, G. Minelli, R. Solimini, V. Toccaceli, M. Vichi, C. Beltrano, and L. Perini (2005). Epidemiologic study of mortality during the Summer 2003 heat wave in Italy. *Environmental Research 98*(*3*), 390–399.

Dalgaard, P. (2008). *Introductory Statistics with R 2008*, 2nd ed., Springer.

Fahrmeir, L. and G. Tutz (2001). *Multivariate Statistical Modelling Based on Generalized Linear Models*, 2nd ed., Springer.

Farrington, C. P, N. J. Andrews, A. D. Beale, and M. A. Catchpole (1996). A statistical algorithm for the early detection of outbreaks of infectious Disease, *Journal of the Royal Statistical Society, Series A 159*, 547–563.

Fouillet, A., G. Rey, V. Wagner, K. Laaidi, P. Empereur-Bissonnet, A. Le Tertre, P. Frayssinet, P. Bessemoulin, F. Laurent, P. De Crouy-Chanel, E. Jougla, and D. Hémon (2008). Has the impact of heat waves on mortality changed in France since the European heat wave of summer 2003? A study of the 2006 heat wave. *International Journal of Epidemiology 37*, 309–317.

Freeland, R. K. and B. P. M. McCabe (2004). Analysis of low count time series data by Poisson autoregression. *Journal of Time Series Analysis 25(5)*, 701–722.

Frisén, M. (2003). Statistical surveillance: optimality and methods. *International Statistical Review 71*(2), 403–434.

Frisén, M. (1992). Evaluations of methods for statistical surveillance. *Statistics in Medicine 11*, 1489–1502.

Gõmez-Rubio V., J. Ferrándiz-Ferragud, and A. López-Quílez (2005). Detecting clusters of disease with R. *Journal of Geographical Systems*, *7*(2), 189–206.

Gergonne, B., R. Pebody, N. Andrews, W. Bird, M. Gibbs, and C. Griffiths (2005). Mortality early warning system based on weekly death registrations in England, *Oral presentation 154*, Annual Conference, Warwick, U.K., September 12–14, 2005, Abstracts: oral presentations and posters. London: Health Protection Agency, 107.

Hawkins, D. M. and D. H. Olwell (1998). *Cumulative Sum Charts and Charting for Quality Improvement*. Statistics for Engineering and Physical Science, Springer.

Heisterkamp, S. H., A. L. M. Dekkers, and J. C. M. Heijne (2006). Automated detection of infectious disease outbreaks: hierarchical time series models. *Statistics in Medcine 25*, 4179–4196.

Höhle, M. (2007). Surveillance: An R package for the monitoring of infectious diseases. *Computational Statistics 22 (4)*, 571–582.

Held, L., M. Hofmann, M. Höhle, and V. Schmid (2006). A two component model for counts of infectious diseases. *Biostatistics 7*, 422–437.

Held, L., M. Höhle, and M. Hofmann (2005). A statistical framework for the analysis of multivariate infectious disease surveillance data. *Statistical Modelling 5*, 187–199.

Höhle, M. and M. Paul (2008). Count data regression charts for the monitoring of surveillance time series. *Computational Statistics and Data Analysis 52*(9), 4357–4368.

Höhle, M., M. Paul, and L. Held (2009). Statistical approaches to the surveillance of infectious diseases for veterinary public health. *Preventive Veterinary Medicine, 91*(1), 2–10.

Josseran, L., J. Nicolau, N. Caillère, P. Astagneau, and G. Brücker (2006). Syndromic surveillance based on emergency department activity and crude mortality: two examples. *Eurosurveillance 11*(*12*), 01 Dec, pii=668.

Kaiser, R., D. Ćoulombier, M. Baldari, D. Morgan, and C. Paquet (2006). What is epidemic intelligence, and how is it being improved in Europe? *Eurosurveillance 11*(*5*), 02 Feb, pii=2892.

Kuhn, Max and Steve Weaston (2009). odfWeave: Sweave processing of Open Document Format (ODF) files. R package version 0.7.10.

Lecoutre, E. (2003). The R2HTML Package *R News 3(3)*, 33–36.

Leisch, F. (2002). Sweave: Dynamic generation of statistical reports using literate data analysis. In W. Härdle and B. Rönz, eds., *Compstat 2002—Proceedings in Computational Statistics*, 575–580.

Le Strat, Y. and F. Carrat (1999). Monitoring Epidemiologic surveillance data using hidden Markov models. *Statistics in Medicine 18*, 3463–3478.

Mazick, A. (2007). Monitoring excess mortality for public health action: potential for a future European network. *Eurosurveillance 121*, pii=3107.

Muenchen, R. A. (2009). *R for SAS and SPSS Users*, Springer.

Nogueira, P. J., J. M. Falcão, M. T. Contreiras, E. Paixão, J. Brandão, and I. Batista (2005). Mortality in Portugal associated with the heat wave of August 2003: Early estimation of effect, using a rapid method *Eurosurveillance 10(7)*, July 01, pii=553.

Page, E. S. (1954). Wong, W.-K., A. Moore, G. Cooper, and M. Wagner (2003). Control charts for the mean of a normal population. *Journal of the Royal Statistical Society, Series B*, 16(1), 131–135.

Pau, G. (2009). `hwriter`: HTML Writer—Outputs R objects in HTML format, R package version 1.1, http://www.ebi.ac.uk/gpau/hwriter/.

Paul, M., L. Held, and A. M. Toschke (2008). Multivariate modelling of infectious disease surveillance data, *Statistics in Medicine*, pp. 6250–6267.

R Development Core Team (2009). *R: A Language and Environment for Statistical Computing*, R Foundation for Statistical Computing, Vienna, Austria, `http://www.R-project.org`.

Robert Koch Institute (2009). SurvStat@RKI, `http://www3.rki.de/SurvStat`, Last access: June 9, 2009.

Rogerson, P. A. and I. Yamada (2004). Approaches to syndromic surveillance when data consist of small regional counts. *Morbidity and Mortality Weekly Report 53*, 79–85.

Rossi, G., L. Lampugnani, and M. Marchi (1999). An approximate CUSUM procedure for surveillance of health events. *Statistics in Medicine 18*, 2111–2122.

Serfling, R. E. (1963). Methods for current statistical analysis of excess pneumonia-influenza deaths. *Public Health Reports* (78), 494–506.

Simín F., G. Lopez-Abente, E. Ballester, and F. Martínez (2005). Mortality in Spain during the heat waves of summer 2003. *Eurosurveillance*, July 01, *10(7)*, pii=555.

Sonesson C. and D. Bock (2003). A review and discussion of prospective statistical surveillance in public health. *Journal of the Royal Statistical Society*, Series A, *166(1)*, 5–12.

Statistics Denmark (2009). StatBank Denmark, Available from `http://statbank.dk`, Date of query: June 6, 2009.

Stroup, D. F., G. D. Williamson, J. L. Herndon, and J. M. Karon (1989). Detection of aberrations in the occurrence of notifiable diseases surveillance data. *Statistics in Medicine 8*, 323–329.

Tennant, R., M. A. Mohammed, J. J. Coleman, and U. Martin (2007). Monitoring patients using control charts: a systematic review. *International Journal of Quality in Health Care 19(4)*, 187–194.

Tomas, A. (2008). epitools: Epidemiology Tools, R package version 0.5-2.

Varin C. and P. Vidoni (2006). Pairwise likelihood inference for ordinal categorical time series. *Computational Statistics and Data Analysis* 51, 2365–2373.

Venables, W. N. and B. D. Ripley (2002). *Modern Applied Statistics with S*, 4th ed., Springer.

Venables, W. N. and D. M. Smith, and the R Development Core Team (2009). An Introduction to R, 2.9.0, The R Project for Statistical Computing, Available from http://cran.r-project.org/manuals.html.

Wei, C. H. (2007). Controlling correlated processes of Poisson counts. *Quality and Reliability Engineering International 23*, 741–754.

Wood, S. (2006). *Generalized Additive Models: An Introduction with R*, Chapman & Hall/CRC.

Woodall W. H. (2006). The use of control charts in health-care and public-health surveillance. *Journal of Quality Technology*, *38*(2), 89–104.

Zeileis A. and F. Leisch, K. Hornik, and C. Kleiber (2002). `strucchange`: An R package for testing for structural change in linear regression models. *Journal of Statistical Software 7*(2), 1–38.

13

User Requirements toward a Real-Time Biosurveillance Program

Nuwan Waidyanatha
LIRNEasia
Kunming, China

Suma Prashant
Department of Electrical Engineering
Indian Institute of Technology–Madras
Chennai, India

CONTENTS

13.1 Introduction

Health officials in India and Sri Lanka do not receive health information in a timely manner in order to prevent diseases from reaching epidemic states. This was the case with chikungunya viral fever (Epidemiology Unit Sri Lanka 2007), a communicable disease that did not require the Epidemiology Unit to be "notified." The current surveillance system does not provide the much-needed "real-time" information flow and analysis to determine that scattered cases are becoming a collective event needing reporting. The lack of real-time disease detection can be overcome with reliable and robust ICTs and intelligent software (Ganapathy and Ravindra 2008; Mechael 2006; Sabhnani et al. 2005; Wagner et al. 2008).

The RTBP pilot promises to strengthen existing disease surveillance and notification communication systems, reduce latencies in detecting and communicating disease information, and set a standard interoperable protocol for disease information communication with national and international health-related organizations in the region (Wagner et al. 2008).

Other initiatives of similar nature use mobile phones (or m-Health programs) for disease surveillance. Three such programs are Cell-Life, Episurveyor (Kinkade and Verclas 2008), and e-MICI (DeRenzi et al. 2008), all developed for monitoring epidemiological information. However, these applications are geared toward collecting data on specific, known diseases: HIV/AIDS, tuberculosis, malaria, child illnesses, etc. Moreover, they run on high-end mobile phones or PDAs. The RTBP developed a system that can survey all patient cases (disease and syndrome) in accordance with the World Health Organization's policy of disease surveillance systems for monitoring all diseases (World Health Organization [WHO] Regional Office of Asia 2004).

RTBP is being strengthened around the ICT-based surveillance and notification system. Pilot implementation in the two nations is a research project aimed at evaluating a wider scale deployment in India and Sri Lanka with the possibility of extending the RTBP to the region. The RTBP is made possible through a research grant from the International Development Research Centre of Canada.

In this chapter, the reader will be introduced to the present disease surveillance and notification or control systems practiced in Sri Lanka and Tamil Nadu. Thereafter, the top-down, bottom-up approach used to develop the user requirements and the outcome of the process will be described, along with a preview of future work ahead.

13.2 Sri Lanka Disease Surveillance and Notification System

Sri Lanka is an island off the southern tip of India with a multiethnic population close to 21 million. The geography of the tropical country ranges from a coastal belt to highlands, with a demarcation of wet zones, arid zones, and dry zones; the average temperature varies between 15° and 40°C. There are two main seasons, dry and rainy, where southeast and northwest monsoons hammer the island with heavy rains during the months of April–June and November–January, respectively, with intermediary showers in-between the monsoons. Exported labor, tourism, textiles, tea, and spices are the major source of foreign income. The country is an agricultural society.

13.2.1 National Epidemiology Unit Organizational Structure

History of disease surveillance in Sri Lanka dates back to the late 19th century. The *Quarantine and Prevention of Disease Ordinance* was introduced in 1890 to implement the notification system on communicable disease in the country. Figure 13.1 shows the institutional hierarchy.

The Director General, Provincial Director, and Regional Director of Health Services engage in the policy and decision making processes. The main responsibility of the Chief Epidemiologist is the analysis of surveillance data. The Regional Epidemiologist overseas the regional level decision making and mediation of surveillance information. The Medical Officer of Health plays a key role in surveillance and notification by reporting to the higher levels and launching the actions prescribed by higher levels. The Public Health Inspector assists in the investigation, reporting, and assisting in the preventive and curative measures in the field. *Suwadana Centre Volunteers are* part of the Comprehensive Community Health Program of the Sarvodaya movement, which facilitate primary health care in the villages, and work alongside the Medical Officer of Health and Public Health Inspector in their area.

13.2.2 Disease Surveillance and Notification Processes

The Quarantine and Prevention of Disease Surveillance Ordinance in Sri Lanka states that all medical practitioners or persons professing to treat

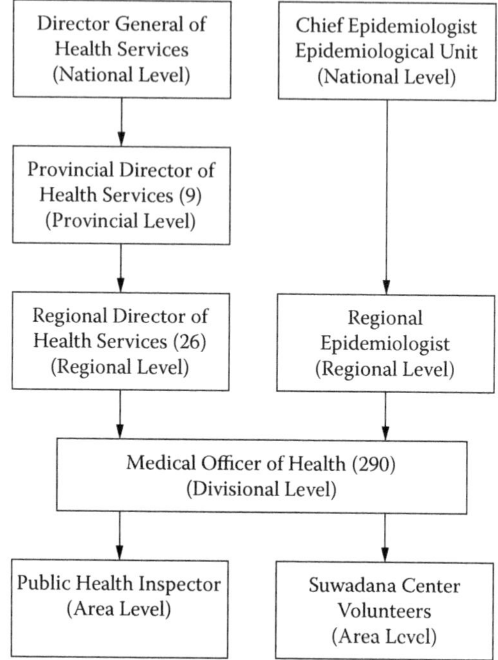

FIGURE 13.1
Organizational structure of the Sri Lanka Government Healthcare Officials (integer in parenthesis is the number of each entity in the country).

diseases and attending to patients (in government and private medical institutions, the intern house officers, grade medical officers, other medical officers and consultants, general practitioners, and family physicians) suspecting any "notifiable" disease type marked as Group A, Group B, and SARS, should report the case to the relevant public health authorities (Epidemiology Unit of Sri Lanka 2005). *Group A* diseases (cholera, plague, or yellow fever) should be reported to the Director General of Health Services, Deputy Director General of Public Health Services, Epidemiologist, Regional Epidemiologist, and Divisional Director of Health Services/Medical Officer of Health, using form I (H-544) communicated via telephone, fax, or telegram. *Group B* diseases (acute flaccid paralysis [or poliomyelitis], enteric fever, tetanus, chicken pox, food poisoning, typhus fever, dengue fever [or dengue hemorrhagic fever], human rabies, whooping cough, diphtheria, leptospirosis, tuberculosis, dysentery, malaria, viral hepatitis, encephalitis, measles, mumps, rubella (or congenial rubella syndrome), meningitis, simple fever continued over 7 days, or any other disease occurring in epidemic proportion) should be reported to either the divisional Director of Health Services or medical officer of health or both using form I (H-544) via the postal service.

Severe acute respiratory syndrome (SARS) is reported to the Director General of Health Services, Deputy Director General Public Health Services, Director Quarantine, Air Port Health Officer, Port Health Officer, Epidemiologist, Regional Epidemiologist, Divisional Director of Health Services, and Medical Officer of Health using form I (H-544) by telephone, fax, or telegram.

Tuberculosis is reported to the Director of the National Program for Tuberculosis, Tuberculosis Control, and Chest Diseases using form II (H-816). The disease should be reported immediately at the time of first suspicion without waiting for laboratory test results or confirmatory tests. Making the notification at the earliest possible time is of paramount importance, thus enabling the field public health staff to start the necessary preventive and control measures immediately.

The notification card (Notification of a Communicable Disease H-544) should be filled with special emphasis on writing the patient's residential address (where it is suspected the patient contacted the disease) so that the range Public Health Inspector can trace the residence easily. The notification card should be addressed and sent via the postal service to the medical officer of health in the area where the patient is residing in.

A medical officer notifying a suspected case should complete a *Notification of a Communicable Disease Form* H-544). All such cases notified are entered in the *Ward Notification Register.* All wards should have a Ward Notification Register. Correct patient's name and address, age and sex of the patient, disease suspected, date of notification, to whom the case is referred to, and special remarks are included in these ward notification registers.

The completed notifications should be sent to the director/medical superintendent/district medical officer of the institution daily where data are entered in an Institutional Notification Register and mailed to the Medical Officer of Health of the relevant area. Figure 13.2 depicts Sri Lanka's process of disease notification and reporting.

The Medical Officer of Health on receipt of the notification will enter the data in the Notification Register of the health office and forward it to the relevant Public Health Inspector (PHI) in the ward of which the patient is a resident and presumably contracted the disease. The notification register contains the following data in a table format: serial number, patient's name, address, age, sex, disease, date of notification, notified by whom, date notification card received, Public Health Inspector area, date notification card was sent to the Public Health Inspector, date notification card received from the Public Health Inspector, and further remarks.

On receipt of H-544 the Public Health Inspector enters the data in her letter to the ward register and then visits the patient's household. During her visit, she carries out a basic public health investigation of the reported case in order to confirm or refute the disease. Upon her findings, she continues the investigation in the community to find any additional cases and take the necessary measures to stop disease spread in the community, including relevant health education. Then the public health inspector completes form

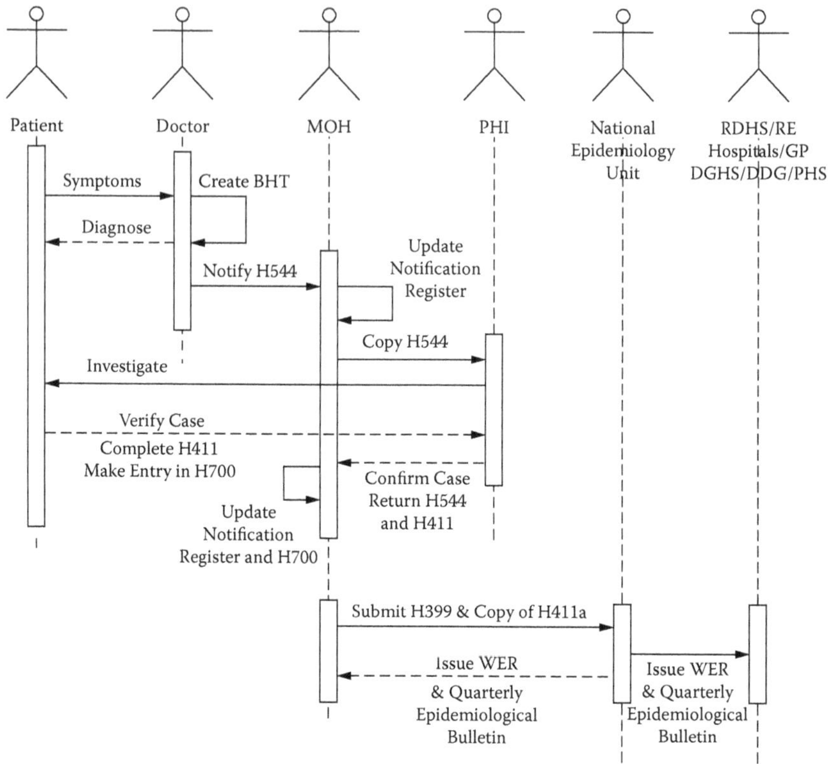

FIGURE 13.2
Sri Lanka system's sequence of disease notification and reporting.

H-411 (*Communicable Disease Report Part 1*) and enters data in her outward register. The data of all confirmed cases are also entered in the *Infectious Diseases Register* (H-700) at the Public Health Inspector Office. The public health inspector will then return the completed H-411 and H-544 to the medical officer of health.

At the latter's office, on receiving the H-544 and H-411 forms from the public health inspector, the Medical Officer of Health updates the notification register and then enters data of confirmed cases in the Infectious Diseases Register (H-700). For each confirmed case the form H-411a is completed using the data on the form H-411 sent by the Public Health Inspector.

Every week the medical officer of health completes the *Weekly Return of Communicable Disease* (WRCD–H-399) based on notifications in the Infectious Diseases Register. The H-399 and H-411 forms for the particular week are sent to the Epidemiological Unit in Colombo with copy to the regional epidemiologist. A third copy is retained in the Medical Officer of Health Office for future reference. This is the most important activity of the Medical Officer of Health in the notification system for which she is personally responsible. The officer has to fill in the Weekly Return of Communicable Disease (WRCD–H-399) and post it on Saturday each week (Epidemiology Unit of Sri Lanka 2005).

The Medical Officer of Health and Divisional Director of Health Services are also responsible for updating the maps and charts in the office according to the instructions given in the Divisional Circular Publication 110 of November 1, 1973 (Epidemiology Unit of Sri Lanka 2005).

For selected diseases that are under special surveillance, the Medical Officer of Health has to complete the special investigation forms and send same to the Epidemiology Unit. Every week the Epidemiology Unit prepares a consolidated summary of all Weekly Return of Communicable Disease (WRCD–H-399). This Weekly Epidemiological Report is sent to all health institutions in the country, including the Medical Officer of Health offices, thus completing the data flow cycle. Weekly Epidemiological Report (WER) contains the consolidated data on notifications by district, from all 290 reporting Medical Officer of Health areas in the country. You may also find a copy at: http://www.epid.gov.lk/wer.htm.

13.2.3 Sarvodaya Comprehensive Community Health Services

Besides the government's point of care health facilities, Sarvodaya, Sri Lanka's largest nongovernmental organization (NGO), has launched a campaign to develop primary health care facilities throughout Sri Lanka. There are more than 420 Suwadana Centers that are functioning on the island, 53 of which are in the Kurunegala District (where the RTBP pilot is carried out). The centers are run by trained volunteers known as the Suwadana Centre Volunteers (Novartis Foundation for Sustainable Development 2005).

Suwadana Centre offers a focal point for health education on an ongoing basis, monitoring the health status of the community (community surveillance), liaisoning with government health services, offering first-aid and treatment of minor ailments, organizing youth participation in health promotion, serving as a focal point for community disaster preparedness and management, and organizing periodic health clinics for specific target groups, pre- and postmaternal care, and small-scale laboratory tests.

The RTBP pilot utilizes the Suwadana Centre Volunteers in gathering data from the government and private health facilities in their jurisdiction. Periodically, the Suwadana Centre volunteers visit the hospital and clinics in their area to record and submit health data through mobile phones and software applications.

13.3 State of Tamil Nadu Disease Control System

India is the seventh largest country by geographical area, the second most populous country, and the most populous democracy in the world. India has a coastline of 7,517 kilometers and is bounded by the Indian Ocean on the south, the Arabian Sea on the west, and the Bay of Bengal on the east. India comprises 28 states and seven Union Territories and is bordered by Pakistan to the west; People's Republic of China (PRC), Nepal, and Bhutan to the north; and Bangladesh and Myanmar to the east. The economic reforms since 1991 have transformed it into one of the fastest-growing economies; however, it still suffers from high levels of poverty, illiteracy, and malnutrition. The World Bank has suggested that the most important priorities for India are public sector reform, infrastructure, agricultural, and rural development and HIV/AIDS.

13.3.1 Health Department Organizational Structure

The state of Tamil Nadu has an area of 130,058 sq. km. and a population of 62.41 million. There are 30 districts, 385 blocks, and 16,317 villages. The state has population density of 479 per sq. km. (the national average is 312). The population of the state continues to grow at a much faster rate (11.72% in the last decade) than the national rate (21.54%; Ministry of Statistics and Implementation Programme 2005).

The *National Surveillance Program for Communicable Diseases* was initiated in 1998 as a pilot project under the National Institute for Communicable Diseases,* which is the body that supervises the districts and analyzes the data for outbreaks in India. The National Institute for Communicable Diseases was established in 1963 to expand and reorganize the activities of the Malaria Institute of India (MII), which has remained in existence (now under a different name) since its inception in 1909. The reorganized institute was established to develop a national center for teaching and research in various disciplines of epidemiology and control of communicable diseases. The institute was envisaged to act as a center par excellence for providing multidisciplinary and integrated expertise in the control of communicable diseases. The institute was also entrusted with the task of developing reliable rapid economic epidemiologic tools that could be effectively applied in the field for the control of communicable diseases. The experience from the pilot is subsequently being expanded to build the Integrated Disease Surveillance Program for India. Figure 13.3 depicts the organizational structure of India's government health care officials.

The National Surveillance Program for Communicable Diseases has been launched to strengthen the disease surveillance system so that early warning signals are recognized and appropriate timely follow-up action is initiated. The main objective of the program is capacity building at district and state levels. "The World Health Organization is in the process of computerizing the surveillance system in the states of Tamil Nadu and Maharashtra. Computers have been provided to the districts and the relevant staff trained in computer

* A full description of the NIDC objectives are discussed at http://nicd.org/NICDObjectives.asp.

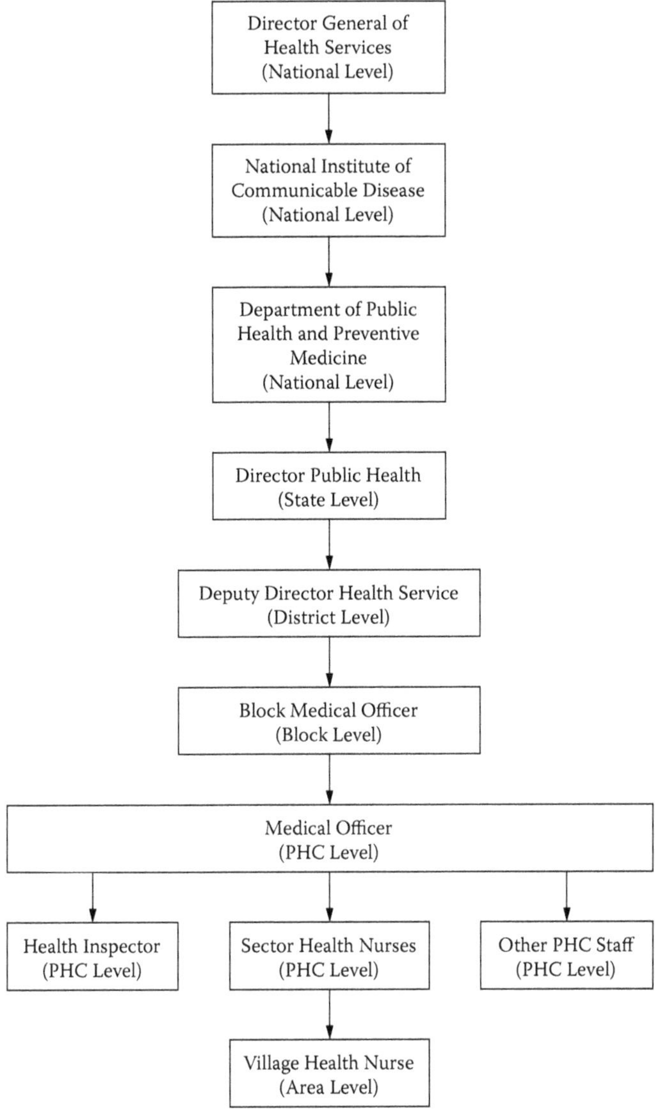

FIGURE 13.3
Organizational structure of the Indian Government Healthcare Officials.

applications vis-à-vis surveillance. This will result in faster transmission of information in both directions and prompt action in the management of outbreaks."*

* WHO instigated initiatives can be found at http://www.whoindia.org/EN/Section3/Section108.htm.

The *Department of Public Health and Preventive Medicine* implements various national and state health programs. This department also plans and implements measures to prevent the occurrence of communicable diseases, thereby reducing the burden of morbidity mortality and disability in the state. The provisions of primary health care, which includes maternity and child health services, require immunization of children against vaccine-preventable diseases, control of communicable diseases, control of malaria, filarial, Japanese encephalitis, elimination of leprosy, iodine deficiency disorder control program, prevention of food adulteration, health checkup of school children, health education of the community, collection of vital statistics under a birth and death registration system, environmental sanitation, prevention and control of waterborne diseases like acute diarrhea diseases, typhoid, dysentery prevention, and control of sexually transmitted diseases, including HIV/AIDS. The *Deputy Director of Health Services* does the ground work and takes immediate action if necessary, but always keeps the National Institute for Communicable Diseases updated on the statistics with periodic reports, seeking help whenever necessary.

The *Block Medical Officer* is a lead medical officer who can be consulted at several Primary Health Centre facilities. This medical officer oversees the other Primary Health Centre medical offices, if any. A *medical officer* is in each Primary Health Centre and is a medical doctor. The *Health Inspector* (HI) is part of the Deputy Director of Health Services' team that assists the Village Health Nurse in various activities such as conducting school health camps. The *Sector Health Nurse* reports to the Deputy Director of Health Services and is in charge of consolidating all Village Health Nurse and Primary Health Centre statistics from the health records for the Deputy Director of Health Services office. The *Village Health Nurse* reports to the Sector Health Nurse. Any suspicion of a disease with a high level of priority is immediately brought to the attention of the Primary Health Centre. The HI verifies it after analyzing the complaint.

13.3.2 Primary Health Centre Health Data Communication Processes

The various reports are Family Welfare, Morbidity (currently done online), Acute Direct Diseases, Fever, Immunization Report (by phone), Deliveries, Minor Surgeries, and Institution. Almost all of them are done paper and by fax except for Morbidity, which was recently launched online (Narain and Lal 2007).

If a cluster of common symptoms is observed, the Primary Health Centre notifies its Health Inspector and Village Health Nurse who in turn conduct a survey in the concerned villages. A communicable disease is verified by a Government Village Health Nurse. The Sector Health Nurse informs the Deputy Director of Health Services designated to the respective area. The Deputy Director of Health Services communicates the case to the Director

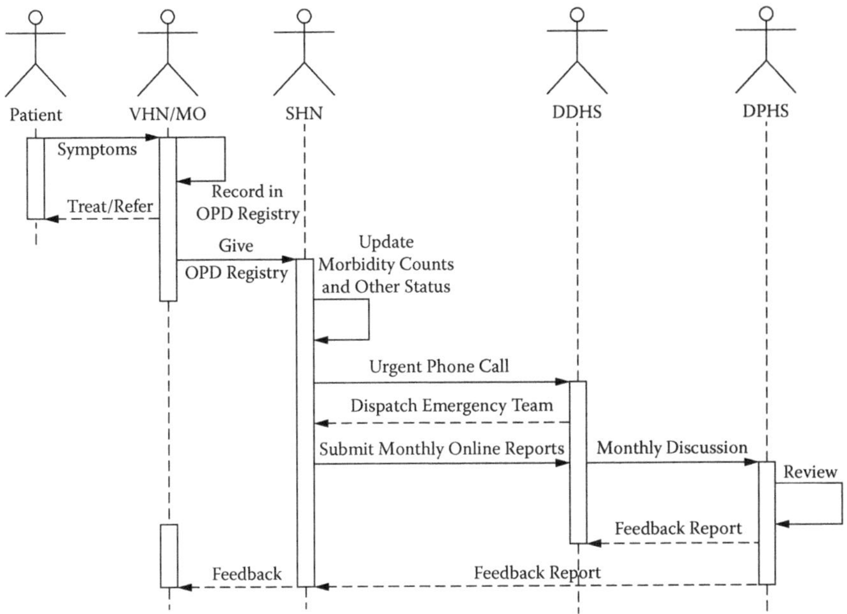

FIGURE 13.4
General State level notification process.

of Public Health Services designated to the state of Tamil Nadu. The information is then entered into a computerized database, which is shared with the National Institute for Communicable Diseases. Figure 13.4 illustrates the flow of information up- and downstream.

Primary Health Centre *Morbidity Report* entry input attributes contain the name of the Primary Health Centre. A drop-down list offers these selections: Primary Health Centre name, Report Date, Date object to select the date, Primary Health Centre OP Abstract—counts for Primary Health Centre outpatients by Male, Female for Adults, Children, and Total.

Public Health Centre outpatient morbidity counts are reported for a list of 50 diseases. Disease groups and list, for which morbidity counts are stratified by gender, age group, and total counts, are reported. This list belongs to the same Primary Health Centre morbidity form.

Here is the list of disease and the categorization for which morbidity counts are reported: *Respiratory System:* bronchial asthma, COPD, allergic bronchitis, LRI, including pneumonia, URI, tuberculosis, and other respiratory disease; *Cardiovascular system:* congenital heart disease, rheumatic heart disease, hypertension, ischemia, including LI, other diseases related to cardiovascular; *pyrexia-related diseases:* PUO, viral fever, typhoid fever, measles, chicken pox, malaria, others; *connective tissue disorder:* osteoarthritis, rheumatoid arthritis, other connective tissue disorders; *pregnancy-*

related disorders: pregnancy-induced hypertension, gestation diabetes mellitus, malnutrition, anemia, other related disorders; *skin:* eczema, tine infection, scabies, leprosy, other related skin diseases; *insect/animal bites:* dog bite, scorpion bite, snake bite; other insect and animal bites; *gastro-intestinal system:* acute diarrheal disease, abdominal colic, jaundice, worm infection, amoebiasis, acid peptic disease, food poisoning, apthus ulcer, other related GIT system; *genitourinary system:* urinary tract infection, menstrual disorder, RTI, malignancy, other related diseases including nephritic disease; *neurological disorder:* epilepsy, CVA, meningitis, other neurological disorders; *ENT:* sinusitis, ASOM CSOM middle ear infections, hearing defects, foreign body in ear, foreign body in nose, others; *ENT:* dental carries, dental fluorosis, other dental problems, gingivitis; *ophthalmic:* refractive errors, conjunctivitis, foreign body in eye, stye, other related diseases; *nutritional disorder:* anemia, Vitamin A deficiency, Vitamin B deficiency, malnutrition, other vitamin deficiencies; *endocrine system:* Diabetes mellitus, goiter, others; *all other causes:* accidents and injuries, burns, surgical-related diseases.

13.4. Top-Down, Bottom-Up Approach for Requirements Analysis

This section outlines the methodology applied to gather, verify, and document the set of User Requirement Specifications (commonly referred to as the URS or business study in software engineering principals). Figure 13.5 summarizes the processes involved in initiating and completing the user requirement specifications by taking up a top-down bottom-up approach (Gadomski et al. 1998). In order to optimize resources, one should complete the producing of the user requirement specifications in a single cycle. However, if necessary, repeat the cycle as many times until the user requirement specifications is stable.

The methodology is analogous to applying the axiomatic framework for designing systems and reducing system complexities; where the framework comprises customer, functional, design, and process domains for which customer attributes, functional requirements, design parameters, and process variables, respectively, are defined. The framework is a zigzag scheme, first starting with the set of functional requirements and constraints that adhere to the customer attributes; second, deriving the set of design parameters; and third, identifying the relevant process variable. Thereafter, we sequentially working backwards from the set of process variables to the design parameters and functional requirements to adjust them to reduce system complexities (Suh 2005).

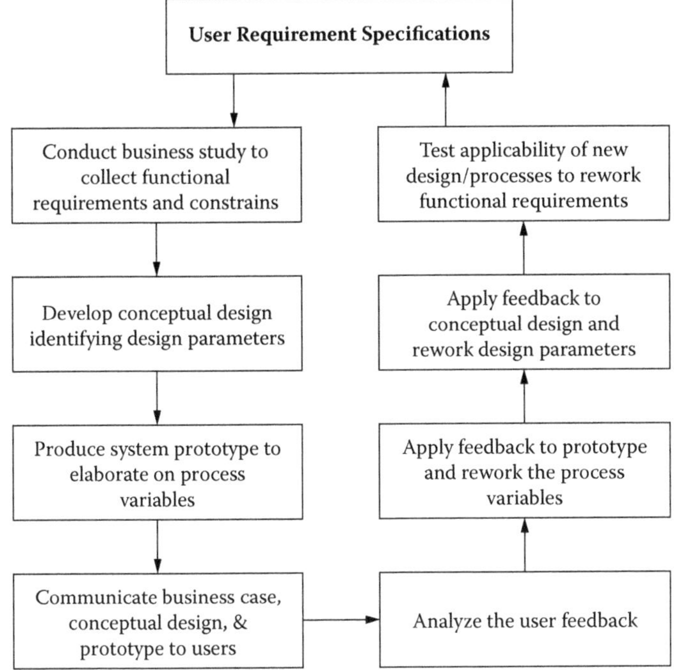

FIGURE 13.5
Top-down bottom-up work flow for developing set of user requirement specifications.

13.4.1 Business Study

Two teams, one in Sri Lanka and the other in Tamil Nadu, engaged in this process where team members were a mix of health domain professionals and technology professionals. The Indian team comprised members from the National Centre for Biological Sciences and the Indian Institute of Technology–Chennai's Rural Technology and Business Incubator. The team in Sri Lanka comprised members from Sarvodaya Shramadana Society, Post Graduate Institute of Medicine, and LIRNE*asia*.

Each team discussed the RTBP with the national-, state-, and district-level health officials. At the same time, they learned of the present disease surveillance and notification systems that are functioning. Through this consultation process the teams developed a set of reference content (notes). The document, known as the Preliminary Business Study, was communicated to all the project partners.

13.4.2 Conceptual Design

Each partner was provided with an agenda to define the conceptual design for their technology and process contributions. A partner planning meeting

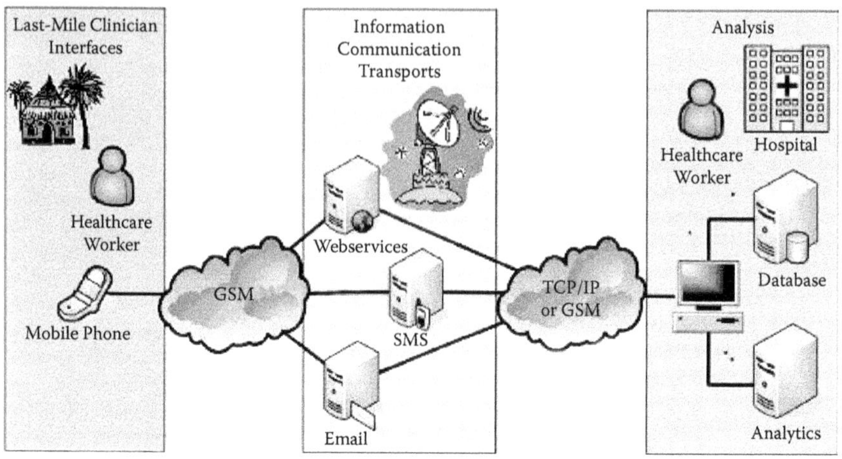

FIGURE 13.6
ICT system Architecture.

took place at the Indian Institute of Technology. The goal of the meeting was to communicate the project objectives as well as the lessons learned from the business study to the partners and give them opportunity to understand them well. The meeting also gave partners the opportunity to discuss their roles and responsibilities for addressing deliverables and reiterating the requirements. Figure 13.6 illustrates the ICT system's architecture.

13.4.3 Communicating with the Users

Once the prototypes were ready to be presented, the RTBP organized two separate meetings with health care workers, in Tamil Nadu and Sri Lanka, who were assisting with the RTBP research.

13.4.3.1 Sri Lanka Health Worker Meeting

The meeting was held at the Medical Officer of Health office auditorium in the town of Kuliyapitiya, Kurunegala District. The meeting was attended by the following: four Medical Officers of Health from Wariyapola, Kuliyapitiya, Pannala, and Udubedewa, overseeing the four Medical Officers of Health divisions in Kurunegala District, where the RTBP is being pilot-tested and 16 Suwadana Volunteers from the same Medical Officer of Health divisions attached to 16 Suwadana Centers (i.e., Comprehensive Community Healthcare Program Centers); four Sarvodaya Divisional Coordinators, supervising the selected RTBP villages, and the Kurunegala District Coordinator; resource persons including the Director Sarvodaya Shanthi Sena and Executive Director Sarvodaya from the Sarvodaya Head Office in Moratuwa; and technology partner representatives from the Post Graduate Institute of Medicine, Lanka Software Foundation, and Rural Technology and Business Incubator, and LIRNE*asia*.

The objective of the meeting was to bring together the Medical Officer of Health, Community Healthcare Workers, and other experts to discuss the RTBP research objectives; demonstrate the concept of using ICT for disease surveillance and notification through a community-based approach; provide an opportunity for participants to give feedback on the research design, specific objectives, and hypothesis; agree on the tasks, deliverables, and timeline; and conduct a survey through a questionnaire to understand the disease surveillance, notification-competency levels, and technology readiness of the Community Healthcare Workers.

13.4.3.2 Tami Nadu Health Worker Meeting

Indian Institute of Technology–Madras's Rural Technology and Business Incubator organized a workshop with the Village Health Nurses and Sector Health Nurses in Thirukoshtiyur Primary Health Centre in the Block of Thirupathur in Sivaganga district to get feedback on the first template of the mobile application developed for collecting patient case information. Thirupathur block has 24 Village Health Nurses, 23 of them participating in the workshop and giving active feedback on the mobile applications. The objectives of the workshop were to orient the Village Health Nurses on the RTBP project, to demonstrate the mobile application to the Village Health Nurses, to administer technology readiness and sample space assessment questionnaire, and to get their feedback and comments. The research assistants visited rural facilities to observe their daily activities, as well as consult with other health workers.

13.5 Deduced Set of User Requirements

User requirements derived in this section follow from the close analysis of the current disease surveillance and notification systems in both Sri Lanka and Tamil Nadu, discussed in the previous sections, as well as the consultations with the health workers and health officials in both countries. The main weaknesses deduced from the business analysis were:

1. The existing system thrives on a set of known diseases, labeled as "communicable" and/or "notifiable" diseases and not on detecting emerging diseases or other adverse health events.
2. The time taken in delivering the vital health information both upstream and downstream through paper, phone, and fax-based

systems up and down the health system organizational structure is greater than 10 days, normally about 30 days.

Therefore, the needs for user requirements are to

1. Design a system to detect all adverse events (including communicable diseases); thus, collect all patient health information for analysis in a timely manner (WHO Regional Office of Asia 2004).
2. Design a system that can directly communicate health information from the first point of healthcare to the key decision makers at central levels with provision for the same information to be accessed by all actors at the in-between stages in the health organizational structure to execute the required protocols.

First, we introduce the key actors, their roles, and the functionality required for the purpose of data collection, analysis, and reporting. Secondly we introduce the minimal set of attributes required to attain the system requirements for collection of health data, analysis, and reporting.

13.5.1 Functions, Actors, and Roles of RTBP

In general, the users are the healthcare workers, government or nongovernmental (or even private). Although the names (titles) assigned to the healthcare workers for the purpose of disease surveillance and notification is different between Sri Lanka and Tamil Nadu, the roles and responsibilities are quite similar. Table 13.1 describes the set of functions, actors (participants), and their roles and responsibilities, and similarities of the participants in the two countries. The columns labeled "Expected" under both Sri Lankan and Indian participants are the healthcare workers entrusted to carry out the prescribed function (protocols) and would be the resource person expected to carry out the respective functions, namely, the government health officials. The column labeled "Actual" indicates the resource person who will be actually carrying out the respective function for the purpose of the pilot project. Thus, when developing the system the designers kept in mind the broader perspective and audience that would use the system.

There are anticipated problems that may require more than technology. In Sri Lanka, Suwadana Centre Volunteers will be taking on the role of data entry operators for the purpose of the study. However, the Suwadana Centre Volunteers don't have the same level of training as the certified health workers (such as Public Health Inspectors or nurses). Health workers, besides Medical Officers, undergo 3–4 years of training in relevant healthcare matters associated with their work. Although all forms carry all three local languages, the Sri Lankan healthcare system functions in English. The Suwadana Centre Volunteers will not have the same level of English language competency as the health workers.

TABLE 13.1

RTBP ICT System Functions, Actors, and Roles and Responsibilities

Function	Sri Lankan actors		Indian actors		Roles and responsibilities
	Expected	**Actual**	**Expected**	**Actual**	
Data collection and submission	Public Health Inspector	Suwadana Centre Volunteer	Village Health Nurse, Sector Health Nurse	Village Health Nurse, Sector Health Nurse	Gather disease, symptoms, signs, gender, and age group records with respect to in- and outpatient visitations from the healthcare providers (hospitals, clinics, general practitioners, community health centers, etc.) in their jurisdiction; submit digitized data directly to a central relational database
Analysis	Medical Officer of Health, Regional Epidemiologist, Chief Epidemiologist	Medical Officer of Health	National Institute for Communicable Diseases, Deputy Director of Health Services	Deputy Director of Health Services	Periodically examine data stored in the central database for a given time period with the use of software tools to manually detect adverse events. Set the parameter thresholds and criteria for machine learning algorithms to auto-detect adverse events in the data
Decision making	Medical Officer of Health, Regional Epidemiologist, Chief Epidemiologist	Medical Officer of Health	Block Medical Officer, Deputy Director of Health Services, Director of Public Health Services, National Institute for Communicable Diseases	Deputy Director of Health Services Epidemiology Unit	When an adverse event (such as a possible disease outbreak or unusually increase of similar cases) is detected through the analysis process, the designated decision makers must decide whether or not the event is of significance to be communicated downstream to the designated healthcare workers in the vulnerable geographical areas

(Continued)

TABLE 13.1 (CONTINUED)

RTBP ICT System Functions, Actors, and Roles and Responsibilities

	Sri Lankan actors		Indian actors		
Function	**Expected**	**Actual**	**Expected**	**Actual**	**Roles and responsibilities**
Publishing or issuing of reports and alerts	Regional Epidemiologist, Chief Epidemiologist	Medical Officer of Health	National Institute for Communicable Diseases, Director, Public Health Services, Deputy Director Health Services	Deputy Director of Health Services–Epidemiology Unit	There are three types of reports: low, high, and urgent priority reports or alerts. *Low* and *high* priority reports are generated and disseminated on a weekly (or periodic) basis identifying substantially significant events (e.g., Weekly Epidemiological Report in Sri Lanka). Recipient: healthcare workers are not expected to take immediate action but closely monitor those diseases if they are of relevance. *Urgent* priority alerts are issued as and when a disease outbreak is detected and the health care workers in the vulnerable areas must be notified to take immediate action
Subscribing to receive reports alerts	Medical Officer of Health, Regional Director Health Services, Regional Epidemiologist, Hospitals, General Practitioners, Public Health Inspectors	Suwadana Centre Volunteers, Public Health Inspectors, and Medical Officer of Health	Village Health Nurses, Sector Health Nurses, Health Inspector, Deputy Director, Health Services, Block Medical Officer	Village Health Nurse, Sector Health Nurse, Health Inspector, Block Medical Officer	Subscribers can choose to receive either Urgent, High, or Low priority alerts. Based on the individual's responsibilities and the priority level of the alert the recipients will choose the course of action to be taken. If it is a low priority alert they may choose to be vigilant and observe and if it is a high priority alert the individual may choose to apply intervention and prevention actions to safeguard their respective communities

Village Health Nurses and Sector Health Nurses are to be entrusted in submitting the disease and syndrome data. However, Village Health Nurses and Sector Health Nurses are informed only if the Primary Health Centre detects a cluster of common symptoms. Ideally, we would want the Village Health Nurses and Sector Health Nurses to submit all symptoms. How they are to receive or extract information pertaining to all the symptoms reported by patients is a question.

Health officials: Medical Officer of Health staff in Sri Lanka and Deputy Director of Health Services office staff in Tamil Nadu will be conducting the automated and manual analysis of the data. It is doubtful that they will have the same level of advanced statistical analysis knowledge to detect adverse events that are not quite obvious, which usually an astute physician or epidemiologist has.

13.5.2 Optimal Set of Inputs, Outputs, and Functionality of ICT System

The partners or teams designing and developing the necessary standards, software, and protocols are expected to use the tables following as a guide for developing precise specifications, which will be documented in the *software requirement specifications*. It is evident that the designers and developers will need to expand on this and introduce more attributes and relationships to build working solutions.

13.5.2.1 Gathering of Disease and Syndrome Data

In Sri Lanka, the Suwadana Centre Volunteers, and in Tamil Nadu, Primary Health Centre staff (like the Sector Health Nurse) and Village Health Nurse will be providing a minimal set of information, through mobile phones, for the purpose of analysis and detection of adverse health events. The necessary and sufficient set of attributes is listed in Table 13.2. These health workers will visit the healthcare providers, periodically, or use other means to retrieve in- and outpatient data from the registries to digitize and send to the central database. They should be able to record the relevant data in a digital form at a rate of 15 seconds per record. Each of the health facilities in Tamil Nadu and Sri Lanka cater to a minimum of 100 patients on average per day. These patients visit the facilities between the hours of 8 a.m. until 1 p.m. in the afternoon. Hence, a medical officer will spend approximately 2–3 minutes with each patient. Given the time constraint, the data entry cannot take more than 10% of the patient care time, that is, 12–18 seconds, which sets the design benchmark for data entry at 15 seconds on average.

13.5.2.2 Relational Database for Storing Gathered Data

The relational database must, at least, possess the attributes defined in Table 13.3. The relational data structure (i.e., schema) will contain more

TABLE 13.2

Attributes of Visitation Data Digitized and Submitted by Health Workers

Attribute	Description	Example
Sender ID	Single value: A unique identifier to associate the data with the healthcare worker digitizing and submitting the data	Health system assigned unique identifier: name + National ID Number, National ID Number, or employee identification number
Provider or location	Single value: Healthcare provider: hospital, clinic, general practitioner, community healthcare enter, etc., where the data will be collected. This element will help identify location (or source) of the health record. It is anticipated that the patient will be from the nearby area. It is possible that a patient from outside of the area may visit the provider	Provider name: Kurunegala Base Hospital; provider type: hospital; provider town/village: Kurunegala; Provider name: Sevanipatti-PHC; provider type: Primary Health Centre; provider town/village: Sevanipatti; Provider name: Asiri Community; Healthcare Centre; provider type: clinic; provider town/village: Pannala
Disease	Single value: Disease name (diagnoses) based on the patient's symptoms and signs	Dengue, cholera, malaria
Symptoms	Multiple values: The complaints made by the patient to the doctor. The same diagnosis for two different patients may not always accompany the same symptoms	Fever, joint aches, vomit blood, rash (dengue), fever, joint ache (dengue), bloody stools (diarrhea)
Signs	Multiple values: The observations made by the practitioner (doctor) at the time of investigating the case	Swelling, rash, enlarged retinal, discoloration of tongue
Gender	Single value: Patient's sex; unknown can be used as a default value	Male, female, or unknown
Age group	Single value: Age category; it's at the discretion of the implementers as to how they wish to define the age categories	Adult/child, 0–10, 11–20, … , 91–100, infant (0–1), childs (2– 2), teenager (13–19), youth (20–25), adult (26–50), elder (50–100)
No. of cases	Single value: In a particular reporting period, more than one patient may share the same diagnosis, symptoms, and signs and be of the same gender and age group. In the event an aggregate can be reported instead of having to repeat the record	Default value = 1 General value = any "natural" number: 1, 2, 3, 4 ...
Case date	Single value: The date the patients or the cases were recorded by the provider (i.e., visitation date or admitted date)	August 8, 2009 August 1, 2009

TABLE 13.3

Information Stored in the Database

Attribute	Description	Example
Provider	Same as in Table 13.2	Provider name: Kurnegala Base Hospital, provider type: Hospital, provider town/village: Kurunegala Provider name: Sevanipatti-PHC, provider type: Primary Health Centre; provider town/village: Sevanipatti Provider name: Asiri Community Healthcare Centre, provider type: clinic; provider town/village: Pannala
Disease	Same as in Table 13.2; can be null. The database will try to resolve (suggest) a diagnosis based on the received symptoms	Dengue, cholera, malaria
Symptoms	Same as in Table 13.2; cannot be null	Fever, joint aches, vomit blood, rash (dengue), fever, joint ache (dengue), bloody stools (diarrhea)
Signs	Same as in Table 13.2; can be null	Swelling, rash, enlarged retina, discoloration of tongue
Gender	Same as in Table 13.2. If the input value is NULL, then will default to "Unknown"	Male, female, or unknown
Age group	Same as in Table 13.2; cannot be null	Adult/child, 0–10, 11–20, … , 91–100, infant (0–1), child (2–12), teenager (13–19), youth (20–25), adult (26–50), elder (50–100)
No. of cases	Same as in Table 13.2; can be null, if null, then will default to 1	Default value = 1 General value = any "natural" number: 1, 2, 3, 4 ...
Date	Same as in Table 13.2; can be null	01/08/09 01-Aug-09
ICD-10	Single value: International Code for Diseases version 10; the database will resolve the value based on the relationship of the codes associated with the diagnosis (disease). The healthcare workers will not be required to submit this data but the internal processes will fill in the voids.	A01.0 Typhoid fever A90–Dengue fever B01–Varicella (chickenpox) None; some diseases are not classified. So "none" should be a valid option
Long./lat.	Two values: GIS longitude and latitude will be resolved by the database by looking up the values from the preregistered GIS location information assigned to the provider's village/town or other location identifier.	Long. = 8.1414 Lat. = 3.4123
Other	Multiple values: other attributes the user can set or processes the user can execute to detect adverse events	Weather information

attributes than described in Table 13.2, especially with an emphasis on preserving data integrity. The data gathered (health records of patient disease and syndrome) by the healthcare workers from the provider will be stored in this database. The same data will be used in the event detection analysis.

13.5.2.3 Analysis for Detection of Events

Periodically, daily, every other day, or weekly, health officials will analyze the data for a given time frame to monitor and detect any emerging health threats. They may also execute other detection algorithms or processes for detection of possible adverse events. The users (detection and monitoring staff, namely, health officials) will need to filter the dataset through various combinations of selected parameters identified in Table 13.4.

13.5.2.4 Alerting and Reporting of Emerging Disease Outbreaks

Table 13.5 states the requirements for the production of weekly disease surveillance reports such as the Weekly Epidemiological Report and issuing alerts of potential threats such as emerging disease outbreaks. The health official issuing the alert will extract a summary of the weekly report (e.g., Weekly Epidemiological Report) and send the report to the healthcare workers each week, via e-mail, for example. In the event of detecting a significant health threat, the resources associated with detection and monitoring (e.g., Chief Epidemiologist) will notify the decision makers (e.g., Medical Officer of Health or Regional Epidemiologist) of the potential threat. Thereafter, the decision maker will decide the priority level and authorize the detection and monitoring staff to issue a bulletin (alert) to those health officials in the vulnerable areas. The weekly reports are regarded as low- or high-priority bulletins (reports) and the immediate notifications (alerts) are regarded as urgent-priority bulletins (Dias et al. 2007, Anderson et al. 2007).

13.6. Conclusions

The Tamil Nadu morbidity report's granularity of information is more so than the Sri Lankan weekly epidemiological report. Doctors in both countries use charts and admission or outpatient registries where a large portion of patients' data can be collected. Pervasive mobile technology can easily be leveraged in Asia (Zainudeen and De Silva 2007, Zenith 2008), while the expensive detection- and decision-assisting software (Sabhnani et al. 2005) must be located centrally; both mobile and server technologies must be easily scalable. The ICT system's success is highly dependent on the availability of data. It is uncertain at this point as to whether even the data available can be retrieved without political intervention/disruption or societal objection.

TABLE 13.4

Analysis Done by Health Officials (Epidemiologists) of the Collected Data Sets

Attributes	Description	Examples
Period	Two values: Start and end date of the series of data to be analyzed. Neither value can be null. Some logic will be used to suggest the start and dates for a period	October 11, 2006 to October 10, 2007 March 1, 2008 to March 31, 2008
Disease	Multiple values: Same as in Tables 13.2 and 13.3; user should have the option of selecting a single disease for analysis or a collection of diseases to analyze the data set, or by disease type	Cholera Mosquito-borne diseases: dengue, malaria Child diseases: typhoid, rubella, jaundice
Symptoms	Multiple values: Same as in Table 13.2 and 13.3; user should have the option of selecting a single symptom or a collection of symptoms to analyze the data	Cough Fever + cough Fever + joint ache + rash
Gender	Multiple values: Same as in Table 13.2 and 13.3; user should have the option of selecting Male or Female, Unknown, or a subset of the genders such as Male and Unknown to analyze the data set	Male Male, Unknown Male, Female, Unknown
Age group	Multiple values: Same as in Table 13.2 and 13.3; user should have the option of selecting one or a range of age groups	Child All (Child & Adult) Age: 10–25
Provider	Multiple values: Same as in Table 13.2 and 13.3; user should have the option of selecting one or a collection of providers.	Kurunegala base hospital Kurunegala base hospital + Kuliyapitiya hospital, + Pannala Peripheral Unit
Area	Multiple values: User should have the option of selecting a polygon (i.e., GIS area). The location will be subdivided as country, region, state, province, district, division, area, town/village	Pannala MOH Division Kurunegala District Sivaganga District Tamil Nadu State

13.7 Future Work

At the time of this writing this chapter, April 2009, the project had completed more than 85% of the implementation stage. A set of software requirement specifications were developed by the project's technology partners, and the individual software components were developed. The next steps involve

TABLE 13.5

Weekly Reports and Urgent Alerts Issued by Health Officials to Relevant Healthcare Workers

Attributes	Description	Examples
Headline	Single value: A headline describing one or more significant events; perhaps restricted to less than 100 characters	"Rains increase mosquito-borne diseases" "Chikungunya appears in North Central province" "Unusual fever-like disease emerging among children"
Priority	Single value: Indicating the urgency, severity, and certainty of the emerging disease with priority levels: *high*—healthcare worker should access alternate resources to learn more about the emerging disease and be vigilant, perhaps inform community, *low*—healthcare worker should be vigilant but does not need to take any action, or *urgent*—if message is intended for the healthcare worker (i.e., affects area healthcare worker is in), then take immediate intervention and prevention actions	Low High Urgent
Area	Multiple values: To identify the geographical areas the significant of the event	Western and central provinces Sivaganga, Colombo, Kurunegala districts Pannala, Wariyapola divisions Kuliyapitiya, Nathandiya, Pannala, towns, Sri Lanka
Description	Single value: Table of, at most, top five diseases and their counts or the most significant urgent priority adverse event and a description of the incident	Dengue (23), malaria (15), flu (145), chikungunya (12) "Be advised, 12 cases of chikungunya identified in Sivaganga district, rapidly spreading, take immediate action"
Resources	Multiple values: HTTP link to Web site with full report for users to access to obtain further information and instructions	http://www.epid.gov.lk/WER/ http://www.sahana.lk/DS/GIS/ WER General: +9198555123123 Deputy Director Health Services: +914455599889988
Effective	Single value: Date and time period the alert is effective for	From: 2009-05-24T13:30:00+05:30 To: 2009-05-29T16:30:00+05:30 ** +05:30 is the UTC offset for Sri Lanka and India.

integrating the software components, and introducing the standard operational procedures to the healthcare workers, as well as training them to operate the ICT system, and initial testing of the end-to-end system before initiating the evaluation period. Starting in June 2009 the RTBP would begin to collect data through the field-level healthcare workers, apply the analytic algorithms for detection of adverse events, and issue health alerts on events of interest. These actions would be monitored to measure the reliability and effectiveness of the system, as well as to collect evidence for policy makers to make a decision on the wider-scale deployment of this RTBP pilot.

Acknowledgments

The authors wish to acknowledge the International Development Research Centre of Canada for the research grant that makes it possible for the RTBP to be pilot tested in India and Sri Lanka.

Pubuduni Weerakoon and P. V. Ariyawansa were key resources from the Sarvodaya Shramadana Movement who engaged with the District of Kurunegala Medical Officer of Health in gathering information pertaining to the Sri Lanka disease surveillance system. Authors wish to thank Dr. Vinya Ariyartne (Executive Director, Sarvodaya) for liaising with the Ministry of Health in Sri Lanka to obtain necessary approvals for piloting the project in the District of Kurunegala. Dr. Roshan Hewapathirana of the Sri Lanka Post Graduate Institute of Medicine is to be thanked for his contribution in supplying literature with respect to the national disease surveillance and notification system of Sri Lanka.

The Indian Institute of Technology–Madras's Rural Technology and Business Incubator wishes to thank the following members for their respective contribution in gathering information included in this chapter; Field Coordinator N. Janakiraman and Geetha G., and for field supervision and workshop implementation, Dr. M. Ganesan. We extend our gratitude to the State of Tamil Nadu Health Department for their cooperation. Authors wish to thank Dr. K. Vijayraghavan (Director, National Centre for Biological Sciences in Bangalore, India) for introducing the project to the Tamil Nadu Health Department and obtaining approval for piloting.

References

Anderson, A., Gow, G., and Waidyanatha, N. (2007). Community based hazard warnings in rural Sri Lanka: Performance of alerting and notification in a last-mile message relay, *Proceedings IEEE 1st International WRECOM2007 Conference and Exhibition*, Rome, Italy.

DeRenzi, D., Lesh, N., Parikh., T., Sims, C., Mitchell., M., Chemba, M., et al. (2008). e-IMCI: Improving pediatric healthcare in low income countries. *Proceedings of the ACM CHI 2008 Conference on Human Factors in Computing Systems*, Florence, Italy. pp. 753–762.

Dias, D., Purasinghe, H., and Waidyanatha, N. (2007). Challenges of optimizing common alerting protocol for SMS based GSM devices in a last-mile hazard warning system in Sri Lanka, *Proceedings 19th Meeting Wireless World Research Forum, Chennai,* India. http://www.lirneasia.net/wpcontent/uploads/2007/11/challenges-of-optimizing-cap-on-smsovergsm-in-sri-lanka.pdf.

Epidemiology Unit Sri Lanka. (2007). Investigation of the Outbreak of Chikungunya 2006–2007. http://www.epid.gov.lk/pdf/chikungunya/OBOFCHIGYA.pdf.

Epidemiology Unit Sri Lanka. (2003). Strategic framework for health development in Sri Lanka. Ministry of Health, Nutrition, and Welfare. http://www.health.gov.lk/strategic_framework_for_health_d-DECEMBER%202006.htm. (Consulted December 2006).

Epidemiology Unit Sri Lanka. (2005). The Sri Lanka Epidemiological disease surveillance and notification handbook. http://www.epid.gov.lk/pdf/Final-Book.pdf.

Gadomski, A. M., Balducelli, C., Bologna, S., and DiCostanzo, G. (1998). Integrated parallel top-down and bottom-up approach to the development of agent-based intelligent DSS's for emergency management, in *Proceedings of The International Emergency Management Society's Fifth Annual Conference (TIEMS 98)*, May 19–22, Washington, DC.

Ganapathy, K. and Ravindra, A. (2008). mHealth: A Potential Tool for Healthcare Delivery in India. Making the e-Health Connection, Bellagio, Italy. http://www.comminit.com/en/node/277163.

Garg, S., Sundar, D., and Garg, I. (2005). M-Governance: A mobile computing framework for integrated disease surveillance in India. *Proceeding of the EURO mGOV 2005, from e-government to m-government,* Brighton, U.K. pp. 200–209.

Kinkade, H. and Verclas, K. (2008). Wireless Technology for Social Change: Trends in mobile phones by NGOs. Access to Communication Publication Series Volume 2. http://mobileactive.org/files/MobilizingSocialChange_full.pdf.

LIRNEasia Projects Page. (2008). Evaluating a Real-Time Biosurveillance Program: A Pilot Project, http://lirneasia.net/projects/2008-2010/evaluating-a-real-time-biosurveillance-program/.

Mechael, P. (2006). Exploring health-related uses of mobile phones: an Egyptian case study. Thesis submitted for the degree of PhD. London School of Hygiene and Tropical Medicine. http://www.medetel.lu/download/2006/parallel_sessions/abstract/0406/Mechael.doc.

Ministry of Statistics and Programme Implementation. (2005). Results at a Glance, Economic Census 2005, Chapter II. http://www.mospi.gov.in/chapter2.pdf.

Narain, J. P. and Lal, S. (2007). Implementing the revised international health regulations in India, *The National Medical Journal of India*, 20(50), pp. 221–224.

Novartis Foundation for Sustainable Development. (2005). Comprehensive Community Health Program in Sri Lanka: Project Description. http://www.novartisfoundation.org/platform/apps/Publication/getfmfile.asp?id=614&el=2346&se=1071197488&doc=129&dse=3.

Ohlbach, H., Schulz, K., and Weigel, F. (2005). Geospatial reasoning: Basic concepts and theory. Reasoning on the web. A1-D2 (REWERSE). Web link—http://rewerse.net/deliverables/m12/a1-d2.pdf. (Consulted March 2005).

Sabhnani, M., Neill, D., Moore, A., Dubrawski, A., and Wong, W. (2005). Efficient analytics for effective monitoring of biomedical security. *Proceedings of the International Conference on Information and Automation*, Colombo, Sri Lanka.

Suh, N. (2005). *Complexity: Theory and Applications*, 2nd ed., MIT Pappalardo series in Mechanical Engineering, Oxford University Press.

Vital Wave Consulting (2009). mHealth for Development: The Opportunity of Mobile Technology for Healthcare in the Developing World. Washington, D.C. and Berkshire, U.K.: UN Foundation-Vodafone Foundation Partnership.

Wagner, M., Dato, V., Alleswede, M., Aryel, R., and Fapohunda, A. (2008). Nation's current capacity for the early detection of Public Health Threats including Bioterrorism. Agency for Health Research and Quality. http://www.gaptheproject.eu/related-publications/Early%20Detection%20of%20PH%20Threats%20US.pdf/at_download/file.

Waidyanatha, N. (2008). Real-Time biosurveillance program: project partner meeting report, Chennai, India. http://lirneasia.net/wp-content/uploads/2008/08/rtbp-partner-meeting-report-v1.pdf. (Consulted August 2008).

World Health Organization. (2008). Chronical Kidney Disease of Unknown Aetiology (CKDu): A new threat to Health. http://www.whosrilanka.org/LinkFiles/WHO_Sri_Lanka_Home_Page_HL_Dec08_Insert_CKDu.pdf. (Consulted December 2008).

World Health Organization—Regional Office of South Asia. (2004). Comprehensive assessment of national surveillance system in Sri Lanka, Joint assessment report, SEA-HSD-269. (Consulted March 2003).

Zainudeen, A. and De Silva, H. (2007). Beyond Universal Access. CPRsouth: Research for improving ICT governance in the Asia-Pacific, Manila, Philippines. http://www.cprsouth.org/sites/default/files/Ayesha_Zainudeen.pdf.

Zenith. (2007). Sri Lanka mobile phone growth peaking: report. Lanka Business Online http://www.lankabusinessonline.com/fullstory.php?newsID=1205243831&no_view=1&SEARCH_TERM=5. (Consulted February 2007).

14

Using Common Alerting Protocol to Support a Real-Time Biosurveillance Program in Sri Lanka and India

Gordon A. Gow
University of Alberta
Edmonton, Canada

Nuwan Waidyanatha
LIRNEasia
Colombo, Sri Lanka

CONTENTS

14.1 Introduction

The Real-Time Biosurveillance Program (RTBP) is a multipartner research initiative to study the potential for new Information and Communication Technologies (ICTs) to improve early detection and notification of disease outbreaks in Sri Lanka and India. Experts in the field of biosurveillance and health informatics have argued that improvements in disease detection and notification can be achieved by introducing more efficient means of gathering, analyzing, and reporting on data from multiple locations (Wagner 2006). New information and communication technologies (ICTs) are regarded as a central means to achieve these efficiency gains. The primary research objective of the Real-Time Biosurveillance Program (RTBP) is to examine these claims more closely by producing evidence to indicate in what ways and to what extent the introduction of new ICTs might achieve efficiency gains when integrated with existing disease surveillance and detection systems.*

One important area of study is in the use of new ICTs to issue real-time alerts and notifications to local health officials. The RTBP research design includes the development of a test-bed using Common Alerting Protocol

* Conceptually, it may be important to distinguish between the terms biosurveillance and disease surveillance. For instance, Wagner (2006, p. 4) makes the point that "[t]he terms disease surveillance and public health surveillance connote disease surveillance practiced by governmental public health. Biosurveillance allows us to broaden the scope of our discussion to include many other organizations that monitor for disease, such as hospitals, agribusinesses, and zoos [emphasis in original]." Wagner also notes that the terms disease surveillance and public health surveillance may connote programs that focus on noninfectious diseases. Finally, Wagner suggests that, whereas public health surveillance may tend to focus primarily on disease outbreak detection, a central concern in biosurveillance is "disease outbreak characterization (e.g., determining the organism, source, route of transmission, spatial distribution, and number of affected individuals)."

(CAP) to support health alerting and data interchange. Under the current systems in Sri Lanka and India, patient data from regional and community health centers is gathered using paper-based forms and procedures. These forms are then sent to regional health officials where data analysis is carried out by qualified staff to identify potential disease outbreaks. Notifications are then issued from the regional health administrations to local authorities, again using paper-based reporting methods.

The RTBP testbed substitutes each of these existing procedures with ICT-based components. Patient data will be gathered using software application implemented on handheld electronic devices and transmitted to a central server using a wireless data link. Data will be drawn from the central server and analysis will be carried out using advanced software developed by the Carnegie Mellon University Auton Lab. Results are made available to regional and local health officials as electronic notifications accessible through a variety of devices, including mobile phones.

In addition to the test-bed component, the RTBP initiative is also examining interoperability issues associated with national and international health-related organizations in the region of Sri Lanka and southern India. It is anticipated that implementation of the alerting and notification component will provide important evidence regarding the opportunities and challenges associated with interjurisdictional alerting and notification for e-health systems in the region.

The RTBP Alerting and Notification Guide is based on the U.S. Center for Disease Control and Prevention's Public Health Information Network (PHIN) Communication and Alerting Guide (PCA). The PCA Guide has been identified as useful model on which to base the RTBP Guide because it addresses the problem of interjurisdictional alerting, provides a comprehensive set of alerting attributes identified through extensive consultation with public health experts, and expresses these attributes using Common Alerting Protocol (CAP) and Emergency Data Exchange Language (EDXL). RTBP will incorporate both CAP and EDXL as data interchange standards for use in the test bed in order to serve the primary objective of the project, and also to take into account other objectives related to system growth and regional interoperability.

14.2 The Role of Information Technology Standards in Health Alerting

The role of information technology standards is now recognized as an important element in the field of biosurveillance (Hogan and Wagner 2006). Generally speaking, the primary objective of any standard is to foster interoperability among the components parts within a complex system. According to CDC-PHIN, "[a] degree of standardization of alert format helps to ensure that public health organizations can communicate effectively within their jurisdictions and with other jurisdictions, especially during emergencies" (p. 9). From a health policy standpoint, a standards-based approach also has the potential to promote regional data sharing by ensuring a minimum degree of technical interoperability between platforms, thereby reducing transaction costs associated with system interconnection and data interchange.

Moreover, with a growing diversity of end-user devices being deployed at the community-level (e.g., mobile phones and other wireless devices), it is important that alerting and notification programs be guided by an approach based on the principle of extensibility in general (Botterell and Addams-Moring 2007). This principle essentially describes a design methodology that facilitates the integration of new devices and additional functionality into the system over time. This could include the ability to support a range of new end-user devices not anticipated at the initial stages of the project, the ability to introduce advanced distribution methods (e.g., precision geo-targeting and routing of messages), or the ability to support cross-jurisdictional and cascade alerting and notification as future enhancements to the system.

Within the context of a real-time biosurveillance system, it is especially important that the myriad components are capable of working together in a relatively seamless operation that extends from detection to alerting and notification. Information technology standards play a role at various architectural layers to support this objective, ensuring, for example, end-to-end interoperability of both hardware and software elements. In conjunction with software layer, it is important to consider the need for a standard to support data interchange between software applications. More specifically, a paramount consideration when issuing health alerts within the RTBP initiative has been to ensure that the system is extensible to the extent that it can support data interchange across a variety of end-user devices with quite different levels of capabilities, ranging from a standard HTML Web browser to the more constrained features of a JAVA-based application on a wireless device or Short Message Service (SMS) on a mobile phone.

A standardized alert format based on Common Alerting Protocol (CAP) v1.1, combined with Emergency Data Exchange Language (EDXL) Distribution Element, provides the basis for an extensible notification system well-suited to this objective (U.S. Centers for Disease Control and Prevention [CDC] 2008). The CAP/EDXL combination can support automated creation and distribution of alert messages to a wide range of end-user (last-mile) systems and devices, including mobile phones. Moreover, a standardized format using these protocols supports other activities related to biosurveillance projects, including data archiving and analysis of results for multi-agency situation awareness (MA-SA) activities as well as research (Organization for the Advancement of Structured Information Standards [OASIS] 2005).

In sum, there are three primary objectives served by providing a standardized format for issuing health alerts within the RTBP initiative:

1. Provide guidance for software development and ensure interoperability and extensibility across platforms and devices.
2. Provide a reference document for research-related activities related to health alerting and notification, including the identification and examination of various policy and procedural considerations related to health alerting within the scope of the project.
3. Provide a reference document to support future project expansion to include interjurisdictional/regional health alerting and cascade alerting.

In the following sections, we describe the steps taken toward an implementation of Common Alerting Protocol (CAP) for the Real-Time Biosurveillance Program (RTBP) initiative. The RTBP implementation is an adaptation based on pioneering work done by the U.S. Centers for Disease Control Public Health Information Network (CDC-PHIN) and contained in August 2008 in its PHIN Communication and Alerting Guide (hereafter referred to as "PHIN-PCA Guide"). The aim here is to demonstrate an instantiation of CAP as derived from the PHIN-PCA Guide, highlighting a number of specific issues and considerations associated with health alerting for a biosurveillance project in a developing country.

14.3 RTBP Alerting and Notification Subsystems

The RTBP alerting and notification functionality consists of four interconnected subsystems (see Figure 14.1):

- Message creation and validation
- Message distribution
- Message delivery
- Message acknowledgment

14.3.1 Message Creation and Validation

Message creation can be done manually or be automated through middleware linked to the detection/decision component. A software interface and associated application(s) to support manual message creation will need to be implemented for the RTBP. The foundation for such an application is currently available with the open source Sahana Disaster Management System Messaging Module (Sahana 2008). At present, the Messaging Module provides a set of generic menus and inputs based on Common Alerting Protocol v1.1.

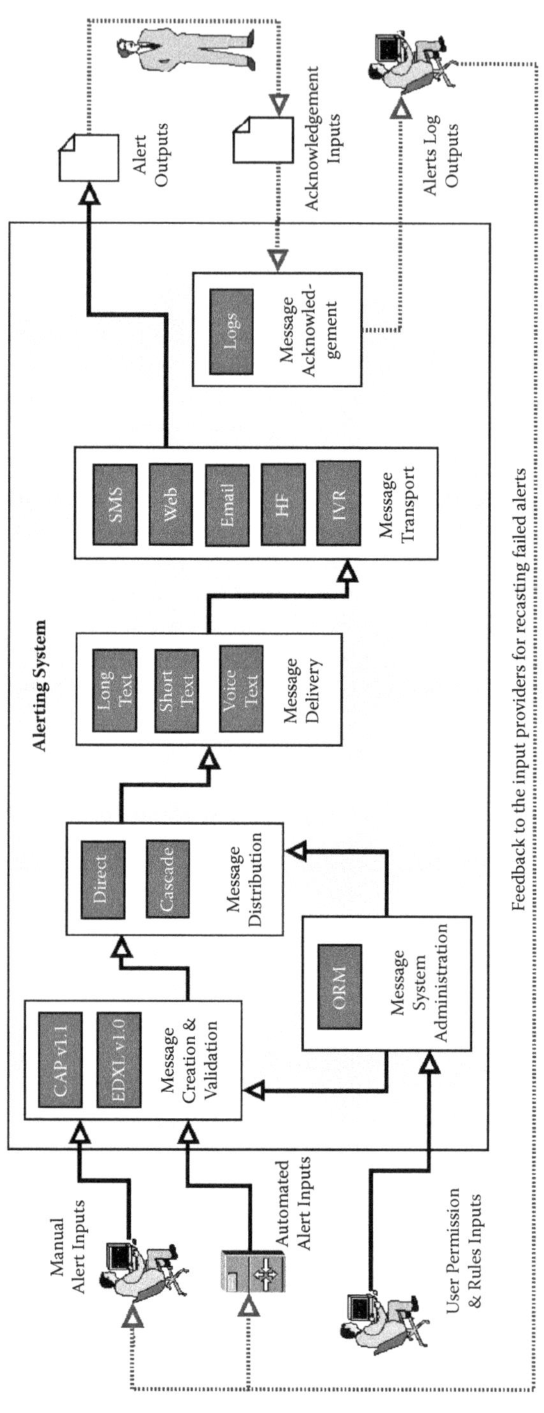

FIGURE 14.1
RTBP alert and notification system showing its various subsystems.

A degree of customization of the module will be necessary for it to conform to RTBP alerting and notification attributes and vocabulary described in this chapter.

As a system grows in size and scope, message creation and validation will also require administrative functionality that takes into consideration security provisions such as user access control and originator rights management. This will require a registry of usernames, passwords, and issuer rights profiles (set of privileges and rules) linked to the system's user interface.

14.3.2 Message Distribution

Once an alert or notification has been created, it must then be distributed to designated recipients. The PHIN-PCA Guide describes two primary methods for message distribution: direct alerting and cascade alerting.

1. *Direct alerting* is the normal process in which an alerting system delivers an alert to a human recipient. This is the normal mode of alerting when the recipient works within the organization or its jurisdiction. However, direct alerting can also be used to accomplish cross-jurisdictional alerting: an alerting system in one jurisdiction can send messages to recipients within another jurisdiction.
2. *Cascade alerting* is a process in which an alert is sent as a system-to-system message from one jurisdiction to another; the receiving system then distributes the alert to the appropriate recipients within the receiving jurisdiction. The message contains the alert along with parameters describing how and to whom the message should be delivered. Cascade alerting is the preferred method for sending cross-jurisdictional alerts. However, it requires greater technical sophistication to implement.

For the purpose of the RTBP testbed, direct alerting will be the primary focus initially. However, considerations for cascade alerting should be included in design and development efforts with a view to possibly test its implementation during a later stage in the project. Cascade alerting will likely have more relevance as cross-jurisdictional considerations come into play, and, as such, it may become an important consideration as the project evolves.

14.3.3 Message Delivery

Messages must reach their destination through an appropriate receiving device, be it a mobile phone, desktop PC, or other means. The contents of the CAP XML message must be rendered into a human readable form while taking into account the limits of bandwidth, processor capabilities, and message display constraints inherent to any particular device. Receiving devises contain a software application to carry out this function.

Message delivery options can be categorized into three types based on PHIN PCA designations:

- Long text—content rendered in a form appropriate for e-mail, fax, or Web presentation
- Short text—content rendered in a form appropriate for SMS and pagers
- Voice text—content rendered in a form appropriate for voice delivery or automated voice delivery by telephone

At present, the RTBP makes provisions for message delivery as long and short text. Sahana Messaging Module currently has an e-mail and SMS push function, but it will be adapted to include a Web-posting function compliant with CAP and EDXL.

14.3.4 Message Acknowledgment

In some cases, it may be advisable or desirable to include a back-channel for message acknowledgment from recipients. This would require a communication link back to the message delivery system to collect acknowledgment receipts and present these as a report.

14.4 Common Alerting Protocol (CAP)

Common Alerting Protocol or CAP is a nonproprietary digital message format that uses XML to standardize the content of alerts across all types of hazards and communication systems. Development of CAP was undertaken by a group of emergency managers and public safety professionals working together through the Partnership for Public Warning under the dual objectives to improve interoperability of alerting systems while offering an information architecture that would also support and advance best practices in public alerting.

The CAP format is designed to contain a broad range of information—the alert message, the specific hazard event, and the appropriate responses. Effective warning systems need to reach everyone who is at risk, wherever they are and whenever the event occurs. Yet, they must not alarm people unnecessarily. Systems must be easy to use, reliable, and secure. An effective warning message delivered by such a system must be accurate, specific, and action-oriented. Warning messages must also be understandable in terms of languages and special needs, with attention to the prior knowledge and experience of the receivers. It is also critical that times, places, and instructions are easily understood (CAP Cookbook 2009).

In 2004, CAP was reviewed and adopted by the Organization for the Advancement of Structured Information Standards (OASIS). The latest version of CAP (v1.1) was adopted in 2005. It has since been recognized and put into use by numerous public and private organizations involved in alerting activities, including the International Telecommunications Union and the U.S. Centers for Disease Control Public Health Information Network (CDC-PHIN). Adoption of CAP is expected to continue to grow in the coming years, as a variety of organizations seek ways to leverage digital platforms and distribution methods for alerts.

14.4.1 CAP Basic Message Structure

A CAP message is an XML document with a structured arrangement of information elements. Each CAP message contains an <alert> block, which may contain one or more <info> blocks, each of which may contain one or more <area> and <resource> elements. Taken together, these elements establish the basic structure of a CAP message. Figure 14.2 shows the basic CAP message structure adopted for the HazInfo Project in Sri Lanka (Evaluating Last-Mile Hazard Information Dissemination [HazInfo] 2007), using three <info> blocks per message to provide multilingual alerting in English (en), Tamil (ta), and Sinhalese (si) for various natural hazards, including tsunamis.

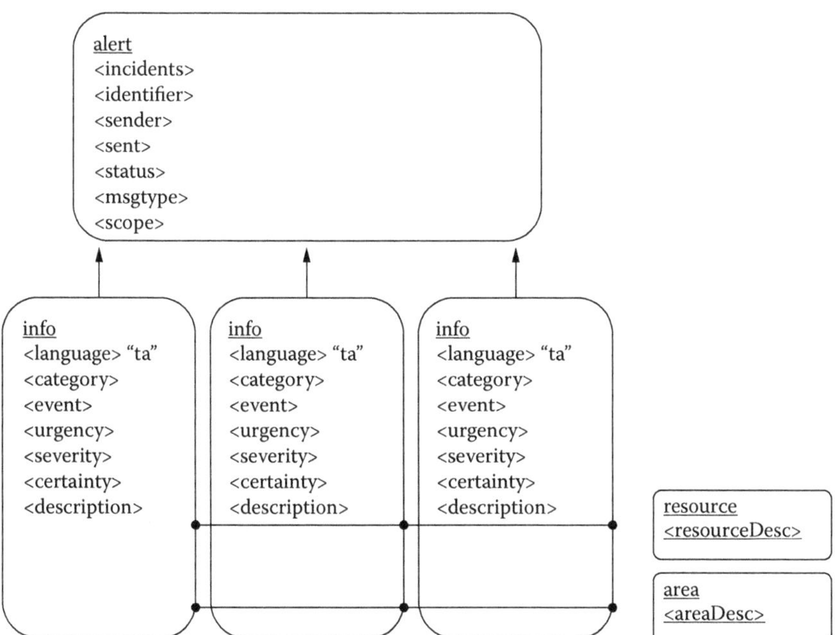

FIGURE 14.2
CAP message structure showing multiple "info" blocks used to provide multilingual alerting.

The contents of an alert message are contained in a set of prescribed sub-elements contained in the <alert> and <info> blocks. Some of these elements are required by CAP v1.1; others are optional or contingent on other factors. For example, the <alert> element must contain a set of prescribed sub-elements containing content that identifies the sender of the message, the type of message, and the time and date (time/date stamp) for the message.

14.4.2 CAP Profile Document

Whereas the CAP standard establishes the basic architecture of an alerting message through its prescribed elements and sub-elements, many of the actual values and usage conventions must be user-defined. As such, any implementation of CAP requires some further specification in terms of how various sub-elements (e.g., message ID) will be populated by an alerting system during message creation. Such specification may lead to the creation of a CAP profile document (see, for example, Common Alerting Protocol Canadian Profile (v1.1) [2008]).

The CAP profile document is defined as a set of additional requirements within the scope and conformation of basic CAP specification. These constraints establish rules and conventions to ensure that local requirements and alerting policies, as well as particular data requirements, are translated into a fully validated CAP message format. A CAP profile therefore defines a specific instantiation while ensuring that messages created and distributed by that instantiation remain CAP compliant and will "make at least basic sense to recipients that are unaware of the profile restrictions" (CAP Cookbook 2009). This last point is especially important to facilitate information sharing and growth of an alerting system across organizational and jurisdictional boundaries.

14.4.3 CAP Implementation for the RTBP Initiative

Within the RTBP initiative, alerts will be created using a message broker based on CAP v1.1. Message contents are contained in a CAP envelope that is transported using one or more transport protocols appropriate to the message distribution subsystem and end-user devices. Later stages of the RTBP project may include the addition of an EDXL envelope, which adds an additional layer of information using the EDXL Distribution Element. Table 14.1 shows the relationship between three types of end-user devices (long text, short text, and voice), CAP elements, and the contents of an alert message. The required alert attributes listed in the second column are described in more detail in the following section.

TABLE 14.1

RTBP Alert Messages Using CAP to Support Interoperability with Multiple End-User Devices

Message delivery type	Terminal device display attributes (expressed in CAP)	Presented content of the alert message
Long text	*<info.headline>*	Cholera outbreak is in effect Kurunegala District
	<area.areaDesc>	Health
	<info.category>	Disease outbreak
	<info.event>	Sarvodaya Suwadana Center
	<info.senderName>	suwacevo@sarvodaya.org
	<alert.sender>	200907240001
	<alert.incident>	suwacevo-200807240001001
	<alert.identifier>	2009-07-24T16:49:00+05:30
	<alert.sent>	Alert
	<alert.msgType>	Exercise
	<alert.status>	Restricted
	<alert.scope>	This message is for registered health care workers
	< alert.restriction>	English
	<info.language>	Priority
	<info.value>	High
	<info.valueName>	Expected
	<info.urgency>	Moderate
	<info.severity>	Observed
	<info.certainty>	This message is for an *Exercise* event, repeat this message is for an *Exercise* event. A *high priority cholera outbreak is in affect* for the *Kurunegala District*. The *Health* alert for the *disease outbreak* was issued at *4:49 pm on 24th day of July 2009* by the *Sarvodaya Suwadana Center*. For further instructions visit the Web site at http://www.sarvodaya.org/healthalert/ or call *+9411255566* . This message is for an *Exercise*, repeat this message is for an *Exercise* event.
	<info.description>	
	<info.web>	
	<info.contact>	
		http://www.sarvodaya.org/healthalert/
		+9411255566

(Continued)

TABLE 14.1 (CONTINUED)

RTBP Alert Messages Using CAP to Support Interoperability with Multiple End-User Devices

Message delivery type	Terminal device display attributes (expressed in CAP)	Presented content of the alert message
Short text	*<info.headline>*	Cholera outbreak is in effect
	<area.areaDesc>	Kurunegala District
	<info.value>	Priority
	<info.valueName>	High
	<info.category>	Health
	<info.event>	Disease outbreak
	<info.senderName>	Sarvodaya Suwadana Center
	<alert.identifier>	sarvodaya-rtbp-2255
	<alert.sent>	2009-07-24T16:49:00+05:30
	< alert.msgType >	Alert
	< alert.status>	Exercise
	<info.web>	http://www.sarvodaya.org/healthalert/
	<info.contact>	+9411255566
Voice text	*<info.headline>*	Cholera outbreak is in effect
	<info.description>	This message is for an *Exercise* event, repeat this message is for an *Exercise* event - A *high priority Cholera outbreak is in affect* for the *Kurunegala District*. The *Health* alert for the *disease outbreak* was issued by the *Sarvodaya Suwadana Center*. For further instructions visit the *Suwadana Center Health Alert* Web site or call *their hotline number +9411255566* - This message is for an *Exercise*, repeat this message is for an *Exercise* event.

14.5 Message Attributes

One method of creating a CAP profile is to identify a set of high-level message attributes to support semantic compatibility across systems. These attributes are then mapped to CAP sub-elements, followed by specification of values and usage conventions. Along these lines, the RTBP initiative has adapted the CDC PHIN PCA approach (U.S. Centers for Disease Control and Prevention 2008) and identified a set of standardized message attributes for health alerting. In this case, these efforts have been done to support notification for a real-time biosurveillance program. These attributes provide a framework for shared vocabulary, predictable system response, and, more broadly, for identifying policy and procedural issues of interest for the research project.

Each RTBP alert message entering the message distribution subsystem must include the following nine attributes:

- Identity of the agency that issued the alert {*agencyIdentifier*}
- Message identifier for tracking purposes {*alertIdentifier*}
- Time and date that the message was sent from the issuing agency {*sendTime*}
- Indication of whether it is an actual alert, exercise or test {*status*}
- Indication of whether it is an original alert, update, or cancellation of a previous alert {*msgType*}
- Indication of the scope of distribution for the alert (i.e., public, restricted, or private) {*scope*}
- The priority of the message (i.e., urgent, high, or low) {*priority*}
- Indication of the event or incident type {*event*}
- Contents of the alert message {*message*}

14.5.1 Message Attribute {*agencyIdentifier*}

Each message must include a unique identifier for the agency that issued the alert. PHIN PCA Guide v1.0 refers to an Object Identifier (OID) of the originating agency and the future creation of an OID and ebXML (Electronic Business using eXtensible Markup Language) registry for PHIN. CAP v1.1 specifies this attribute as a required sub-element within the alert block as *<alert.sender>*. CAP v1.1 further specifies that it must identify "the originator of this alert. Guaranteed by assigner to be unique globally; e.g., may be based on an Internet domain name" and "MUST NOT include spaces, commas or restricted characters (< and &)."

14.5.1.1 CAP Profile Considerations for RTBP Project

Based on CAP v1.1 requirements, the research team has recommended that every person, organization, and agency authorized to issue alerts within the RTBP project be assigned a unique "object identifier" (OID) based on a valid and appropriate Internet domain name (e.g., RTBP@lirneasia.org). In some cases, discussion was needed to ensure that each organization was willing and able to meet this requirement.

In addition, the research team also identified a need to establish and maintain a registry of object identifiers associated with persons, organizations, and agencies authorized to issue alerts for the RTBP project. In the case of RTBP initiative, the number of authorized issuers consists of a relatively small number of authorized users; but, as the project grows in size and possibly extends across jurisdictions, it is expected that identifying ways to effectively manage this registry will become increasingly important.

14.5.2 Message Attribute {*alertIdentifier*}

Each message must be assigned a unique identifier. The CDC-PHIN PCA Guide v1.0 does not specify an encoding requirement for this attribute. However, it notes that "every alerting program must have a unique namespace and its own protocol for generating unique alert identifiers." CAP v1.1 specifies this as a required sub-element within the alert element as *<alert.identifer>*. CAP v1.1 further specifies that it must be "a number or string uniquely identifying this message, assigned by the sender" and "MUST NOT include spaces, commas or restricted characters (< and &)."

14.5.2.1 CAP Profile Considerations for RTBP Project

Based on these considerations, the research team recommended that RTBP establish a convention for generating and assigning the attribute {*alertIdentifier*}. This must conform to CAP v1.1. Participants and authorized issuers should be encouraged to adopt that convention when issuing alerts over the system.

14.5.3 Message Attribute {*sendTime*}

Each RTBP message must include the time and date that it was first issued. PHIN-PCA Guide v1.0 specifies that this attribute is to be encoded using ISO 8601 format, which corresponds with CAP v1.1 requirement. CAP v1.1 specifies this as a required sub-element within the alert element as *<alert.sent>*. CAP v1.1 further specifies that it must be "represented in [dateTime] format (e.g., "2002-05-24T16:49:00-07:00" for 24 May 2002 at 16:49 PDT)" and that "Alphabetic timezone indicators such as 'Z' MUST NOT be used. The time zone indicator for UTC MUST be represented as '−00:00' or '+00:00.'"

14.5.3.1 CAP Profile Considerations for RTBP Project

The research team recommended that RTBP adopt the ISO 8601 dateTime standard format, taking into account any other considerations related to the W3C form for XML dateTime. Furthermore, it was recommended that the ISO 8601 format be embedded in the message creation subsystem software to eliminate need for individuals to enter this data themselves.

It was also recommended that assignment of the {*sendTime*} attribute should be done automatically by the message creation subsystem only at the moment the message is sent to the distribution sub-system. The {*sendTime*} attribute should NOT be assigned at the time the message is drafted in order to avoid confusion in situations where a message is created and then stored as a standby template.

Looking ahead to potential expansion of a regionwide biosurveillance program, there is a need to examine potential issues with time zone coordination and to identify a reliable, common source for the dateTime data feed.

14.5.4 Message Attribute {*status*}

Each RTBP alert message must indicate whether it is an actual alert, exercise, or test. PHIN PCA specifies enumeration values of "Actual" (referring to a live event), "Exercise" (indicates that designated recipients must respond to the alert as part of an exercise), "Test" (indicates that the message is related to a technical system test and should be disregarded by recipients). CAP v1.1 specifies this as a required sub-element within the alert element as *<alert.status>*. CAP v1.1 further specifies that it is to be represented as one of five designated code values, each with specific meaning and intent:

- "Actual"—actionable by all targeted recipients
- "Exercise"—actionable only by designated exercise participants
- "System"—for messages that support alert network internal functions
- "Test"—technical testing only; all recipients disregard
- "Draft"—a preliminary template or draft, not actionable in its current form

CAP v1.1 recommends that *<alert.note>* sub-element be used to provide an exercise identifier when message is assigned "Exercise" status.

14.5.4.1 CAP Profile Considerations for RTBP Project

The research team recommended that RTBP adopt the full CAP v1.1 code values and definitions for the {status} attribute to provide maximum flexibility in terms of accommodating future requirements of the biosurveillance program. It was also recommended that message creation software provide a menu choice "Draft" in addition to the other status values to enable the creation of preliminary templates that can be saved for use when needed. Importantly, however, the research team recommended that message creation software be designed to prevent messages with "Draft" status from being sent to the distribution subsystem. This would help to reduce incidents of accidental alerts sent when drafting templates.

Other considerations identified by the research team included the need to consider establishing unique identifiers for messages that refer to exercises and simulations as distinct from those that refer to actual alerts. This would provide users and system administrators with an additional degree of redundancy in the event that the {status} attribute failed to be displayed on an end-user device. Furthermore, there is a need to establish clear specifications and rules for using the values "System" and "Test" within the scope of the RTBP project to ensure that issuers and recipients are aware of when and how these are to be assigned.

14.5.5 Message Attribute {*msgType*}

Each RTBP message must indicate whether it is an original alert, update, or cancellation of a previous alert. PHIN PCA specifies enumeration values "Alert" (to indicate an original alert), "Update" (to indicate that a prior alert has been update and superseded), "Cancel" (to indicate that a prior alert has been cancelled), or "Error" (to indicate that a prior alert has been retracted).

If {*msgType*} is "Update," "Cancel," or "Error," then the message attribute {*reference*} must be included in the message to provide a unique identifier of the message being updated, cancelled, or issued in error. CAP v1.1 specifies this as a required sub-element within the alert element as *<alert.msgType>*. CAP v1.1 further specifies that it is to be represented as one of five designated code values, each with specific meaning and intent:

- "Alert"—initial information requiring attention by targeted recipients
- "Update"—updates and supersedes the earlier message(s) identified in <references>
- "Cancel"—cancels the earlier message(s) identified in <references>
- "Ack"—acknowledges receipt and acceptance of the message(s) identified in <references>
- "Error"—indicates rejection of the message(s) identified in <references>

CAP v1.1 requires that <alert.references> sub-element be used to provide an unique message identifier when message type is "Update," "Cancel," "Ack," or "Error." CAP v1.1 suggests that <alert.note> sub-element be used to provide an explanation when message type is "Error."

14.5.5.1 CAP Profile Considerations for RTBP Project

It was recommended that RTBP adopt the CAP v1.1 code values and definitions for <alert.msgType> within the CAP envelope. The research team also suggested that RTBP adopt EDXL Distribution Element v1.0 code values and definitions for message distribution, mapped appropriately to the CAP v1.1 values for the EDXL envelope (e.g., "Alert" is equivalent to "Report"; "Update is equivalent to "Update). It was suggested that it is not necessary for RTBP to implement the code values "Request," "Response," and "Dispatch" at this time, as these do not apply to the aims or activities of the biosurveillance program. The research team also identified the need to establish a procedure and associated rules for issuing various message types, with particular guidelines for updates, cancellations, and errors. There is a need to establish a method for generating and assigning <alert. reference> when required.

14.5.6 Message Attribute {*scope*}

Each RTBP message must indicate the scope of distribution for the alert (i.e., public, restricted, private). PHIN PCA Guide v1.0 specifies that "PHIN alerting systems should always use the value 'Restricted,' meaning 'for dissemination only to users with a known operational requirement.'" This is not a required attribute in PHIN-PCA Guide v1.0, but it is acknowledged that the attribute must be included to produce valid XML messages conforming to CAP. CAP v1.1 specifies this as a required sub-element within the alert element as <alert.scope>. CAP v1.1 further specifies that it is to be represented as one of three designated code values, each with specific meaning and intent:

- "Public"—for general dissemination to unrestricted audiences
- "Restricted"—for dissemination only to users with a known operational requirement
- "Private"—for dissemination only to specific addresses

CAP v1.1 requires that sub-element <alert.restriction> be used when the scope value is "Restricted." The <alert.restriction> sub-element is therefore conditional, and contains "text describing the rule for limiting distribution of the restricted alert message." CAP v1.1 requires that sub-element <alert. addresses> be used when the scope value is "Private." The <alert.addresses> element is therefore conditional, and contains "the group listing of intended recipients of the private alert message." CAP v1.1 specifies certain rules for this sub-element: "each recipient SHALL be identified by an identifier or address"; "multiple space-delimited addresses MAY be included. Addresses including white space MUST be enclosed in double-quotes."

14.5.6.1 CAP Profile Considerations for the RTBP Project

It was recommended that RTBP adopt the CAP v1.1 code values and definitions for <alert.scope> within the CAP envelope. However, it was noted by the research team that, since the RTBP was a testbed project, it should adopt a rule whereby all messages issued within the scope of the project be designated as "Restricted" or "Private." This would ensure that CAP messages that might be distributed beyond the confines of the system would not inadvertently be sent to members of the public or those not authorized by the RTBP.

In terms of message creation, it was recommended that the RTBP software interface provide menu options only for "Restricted" or "Private" messages, but with future provision for "Public" messages should this become an option at some point in time. The use of restricted or private messages introduces a number of administrative duties to ensure appropriate and effective distribution of alert messages. For example, when using the "Restricted" value, system designers must assign text to describe the rule for limiting distribution of those messages, ensuring that it conforms to CAP v1.1 sub-element <alert.restricted>. When assigning messages the "Private" value, there is also a need to establish a registry of addresses for specific recipients that are designated to receive such messages. This registry must be capable of expressing the designated recipients in a format that conforms to requirements defined in CAP v1.1 sub-element <alert.addressess>.

14.5.7 Message Attribute {*priority*}

Each RTBP message must indicate the priority level of the alert. PHIN PCA Guide v1.0 does not specify an equivalent message attribute {*priority*}, but includes three related message attributes: *severity, urgency,* and *certainty.* Of these, *severity* is the only required attribute. Code values for these attributes are to follow CAP v1.1 enumeration values for corresponding CAP sub-elements. CAP v1.1 establishes message priority with the info element using three required sub-elements: <info.urgency>, <info.severity>, <info.certainty>. All three elements must be included to produce a valid CAP-XML document.

CAP v1.1 specifies the following code values for the sub-element <info.urgency>:

- "Immediate"—responsive action should be taken immediately
- "Expected"—responsive action should be taken soon (within next hour)
- "Future"—responsive action should be taken in the near future
- "Past"—responsive action is no longer required
- "Unknown"—urgency not known

CAP v1.1 specifies the following code values for the sub-element <info. severity>:

- "Extreme"—extraordinary threat to life or property
- "Severe"—significant threat to life or property
- "Moderate"—possible threat to life or property
- "Minor"—minimal threat to life or property
- "Unknown"—severity unknown

CAP v1.1 specifies the following code values for the sub-element <info. certainty>:

- "Observed"—determined to have occurred or to be ongoing
- "Likely"—likely (p > ~50%)
- "Possible"—possible but not likely (p <= ~50%)
- "Unlikely"—not expected to occur (p ~ 0)
- "Unknown"—certainty unknown

A potential drawback to the CAP v1.1 approach to message prioritization is complexity. While the three sub-elements of urgency, severity, and certainty permit a high degree of precision in defining the nature of an alert, it also makes it more difficult to establish consensus as to how any particular incident should be defined according to the three variables. As a result, both issuers and recipients may find it difficult to quickly ascertain the nature of an alert and the action required.

To address this problem of potential ambiguity, previous efforts adapting CAP v1.1 for a hazard alerting project in Sri Lanka resulted in a simplified message prioritization scheme by adopting a bundled approach (Gow 2007). This approach uses pre-assigned code values for each of the CAP sub-elements noted above. The issuer selects from a menu one of three priority levels—low, high, urgent—and the software interface automatically populates the CAP sub-elements with preset values mapped to an optional CAP sub-element <info. value>, designated as "Priority." This sub-element is then further specified by the sub-element <info.valueName> "Urgent," "High," or "Low," depending on the combination of urgency, severity, certainty sub-elements. Required actions are based on the assigned priority level: low priority (information only); high priority (prepare to take action; standby); urgent priority (take action immediately).

14.5.7.1 CAP Profile Considerations for the RTBP Project

The research team recommended that RTBP adapt the simplified message prioritization scheme and ensure that message creation software provide users with a limited menu of choices based on this message prioritization scheme to enhance reliability and simplicity. It was also noted by the research team that issuers and recipients would benefit from a clear understanding of conditions by which priority levels are to be assigned to alert messages, as well as corresponding actions.

14.5.8 Message Attribute {*event*}

Each RTBP message must indicate the event or incident type. PHIN PCA Guide v1.0 does not specify a message attribute {event} but includes two related message attributes: *alertProgram* and *category*. Of these, only *alertProgram* is a required message attribute and is specified using CAP v1.1 required sub-element <info.event>. Enumeration values for this attribute refer to specific PHIN alerting programs (e.g., Health Alert Network (HAN) (Epidemic Information Exchange (Epi-X)).

The attribute *category* is specified using the CAP v1.1 required sub-element <info.category> and is always enumerated as "Health." CAP v1.1 specifies that all messages contain sub-elements <info.category> and <info.event>. Sub-element <info.category> denotes the general category of the subject event of the alert message and must correspond to a range code values specified in CAP v1.1 standard. For the RTBP project, the code value "Health" is appropriate. The code value for sub-element <info.event> is to provide "the text denoting the type of the subject event of the alert message" and is intended to be more specific than the <info.category> sub-element. CAP v1.1 does not provide specific code values.

14.5.8.1 CAP Profile Considerations for the RTBP Project:

Given the limited scope of the project to biosurveillance, it was recommended that CAP v1.1 sub-element <info.category> be specified as "Health" for all RTBP alert messages. As such, message creation software developed for the project should automatically assign all RTBP alerts as "Health" messages using CAP v1.1 <info.category>. It was also recommended, in contrast to the PHIN PCA Guide, that CAP v1.1 sub-element <info.event> be included in all RTBP alert messages to ensure CAP-XML compliance going forward. With this consideration, the team recommended that RTBP message creation software provide a list of one or more RTBP-designated events corresponding to the foreseeable subject events of potential alert messages. There is a corresponding need to develop an event list and registry suited to the needs of a biosurveillance project.

14.5.9 Message Attribute {*message*}

Each RTBP alert message must include a description of the alert. PHIN PCA Guide v1.0 refers to this as "the main message text" and specifies CAP v1.1 required sub-element <info.description> to convey this information. It is a required attribute in PHIN PCA Guide v1.0. CAP v1.1 does NOT require messages to include the info sub-element <info.description>. The element is specified as "an extended human readable description of the hazard or event that occasioned this message." CAP v1.1 also includes an optional info sub-element <info.headline> that provides "a brief human-readable headline … that SHOULD be made as direct and actionable as possible while remaining short. A useful target for headline length MAY be 160 characters."

In addition, CAP v1.1 includes an optional info sub-element <info.instructions> that provides "extended human readable instructions to targeted recipients" and describes "recommended action to be taken by recipients of the alert message." PHIN PCA Guide v1.0 specifies this sub-element for the optional message attribute *dissemination* intended to provide instructions for sharing message information beyond the initial intended recipient.

14.5.9.1 CAP Profile Considerations for the RTBP Project

It was recommended that RTBP adopt CAP v1.1 info sub-element <info.description> to convey a human readable description of the event that occasioned the alert message. Recognizing the need for a brief description of the alert, especially with respect to the use of small screen devices like mobile phones, it was also recommended that RTBP adopt CAP v1.1 info sub-element <headline> to convey a brief human readable message under 160 characters describing the event that occasioned the alert message.

It was also recommended that RTBP include consideration of CAP v1.1 info sub-element <info.instructions> for future implementation, when issuers might wish to provide recipients with specific directions in terms of responding to an alert message. There is a need to develop procedures and guidelines for message texts pertaining to various alerts that will be issued during the RTBP project. There is a need to ensure that message delivery software will correctly and reliably render message contents from <info.description> and <info.headline> sub-elements to correspond with long text, short text, and voice messages.

14.6 Conclusions

As noted above, experts in the field of biosurveillance and health informatics have argued that improvements in disease detection and notification can be achieved by introducing more efficient means of gathering, analyzing, and reporting on data from multiple locations. Alerting and notification is vital to "close the loop" within a biosurveillance project because it provides timely information to health officials necessary to prepare them to take appropriate action. Information technology standards play a key role in ensuring interoperability across various elements of a biosurveillance system, including the alerting sub-systems of message creation, distribution, and delivery. Adoption of Common Alerting Protocol (CAP v1.1) provides a standards-based approach to biosurveillance alerting that supports data interchange across platforms and enables new end-user devices to be introduced with minimum disruption to the system overall.

This chapter has described the initial steps taken toward an implementation of CAP v1.1 as an alerting protocol for the Real-Time Biosurveillance Program (RTBP) initiative. The first step in such a process is the creation of a reference document that defines a required set of alert attributes, as well as vocabulary and valid value sets for a local instantiation of CAP. The RTBP implementation is an adaptation based on pioneering work done by the CDC-PHIN and released in 2008 under its PHIN-PCA Guide. The aim here has been to illustrate an instantiation of CAP as derived from the PHIN-PCA Guide, highlighting a number of specific issues and considerations associated with health alerting for a biosurveillance project in a developing country.

References

Botterell, A., and R. Addams-Moring. 2007. Public warning in the networked age: Open standards to the rescue. *Communications of the ACM* 50 (3):59–60.

CAP Cookbook. 2009. *CAP Fact Sheet*, January 14, 2009 [cited April 2009]. Available from http://www.incident.com/cookbook/index.php/CAP_Fact_Sheet.

Common Alerting Protocol Canadian Profile (v1.1) 2009. Industry Canada, May 8, 2008 [cited April 2009]. Available from http://www.ic.gc.ca/eic/site/et-tdu.nsf/vwapj/CAPCPv1.1_May_8_2008_E.pdf/$FILE/CAPCPv1.1_May_8_2008_E. pdf.

Creating CAP Applications, January 19, 2009 [cited April 2009]. Available from http://www.incident.com/cookbook/index.php/Creating_CAP_Applications.

Evaluating Last-Mile Hazard Information Dissemination (HazInfo) 2009. LIRNEasia 2007 [cited April 2009]. Available from http://lirneasia.net/projects/2006-07/evaluating-last-mile-hazard-information-dissemination-hazinfo/.

Gow, Gordon A. 2007. Implementing common alerting protocol for hazard warning in Sri Lanka. *Journal of Emergency Management* 5 (2):50–56.

Hogan, W. R., and M. Wagner. 2006. Information technology standards in biosurveillance. In *Handbook of Biosurveillance*, edited by M. Wagner, A. Moore, and R. Aryel. London: Elsevier Academic Press.

Organization for the Advancement of Structured Information Standards (OASIS). 2008. *Common Alerting Protocol v1.1 (CAP -V1.1)* 2005 [cited May 2008]. Available from http://www.oasis-open.org/committees/download.php/15135/emergency-CAPv1.1-Corrected_DOM.pdf.

Sahana. 2008. *Sahana—Free and Open Source Disaster Management System*. Lanka Software Foundation 2008 [cited November 2008]. Available from http://www.sahana.lk/.

U.S. Centers for Disease Control and Prevention. 2008. *Public Health Information Network Communication and Alerting Guide (Version 1.0)*. Public Health Information Network (PHIN)—Guides, August 21 2008 [cited Sept. 2008]. Available from http://www.cdc.gov/phin/library/documents/pdf/PCA_Guide_V1.pdf.

Wagner, M. 2006. The challenge of biosurveillance: Introduction. In *Handbook of Biosurveillance*, edited by M. Wagner, A. Moore, and R. Aryel. London: Elsevier Academic Press.

15

Navigating the Information Storm: Web-Based Global Health Surveillance in BioCaster

Nigel Collier
National Institute of Informatics
Tokyo, Japan
and
PRESTO
Japan Science and Technology (JST) Corporation
Tokyo, Japan

Son Doan
Vanderbilt University Medical Center
Nashville, USA

Reiko Matsuda Goodwin
Fordham University
New York, USA

John McCrae
CITEC, University of Bielefeld
Bielefeld, Germany

Mike Conway
University of Pittsburgh
Pittsburgh, USA

Mika Shigematsu
National Institute of Infectious Diseases
Tokyo, Japan

Ai Kawazoe
Tsuda College
Tokyo, Japan

CONTENTS

15.1 Introduction

On April 21, 2009, the U.S. Centers for Disease Control and Prevention (CDC) issued a report informing physicians about two cases of swine influenza in Southern California (Cohen and Enserink 2009; Centers for Disease Control and Prevention 2009). BioCaster, a publicly available global health surveillance system (GHIS) based in Tokyo, picked this story up on the first day it was reported in the English-speaking media (Associated Press 2009). Four days later, with cases of a novel influenza A (H1N1) influenza centered on Mexico, Southern California, and Texas, the World Health Organization (WHO) convened its first Emergency Committee and declared a public health emergency of international concern.

With only a few confirmed cases, national and international agencies struggled to analyze the virus and accumulate enough data to assess the transmissibility and virulence of the new virus, as well as the population groups at risk. Meanwhile, media coverage and public concern increased with reports of exported cases in Canada, several European Union countries, and New Zealand (Figure 15.1). By April 29, the WHO had confirmed 148 officially

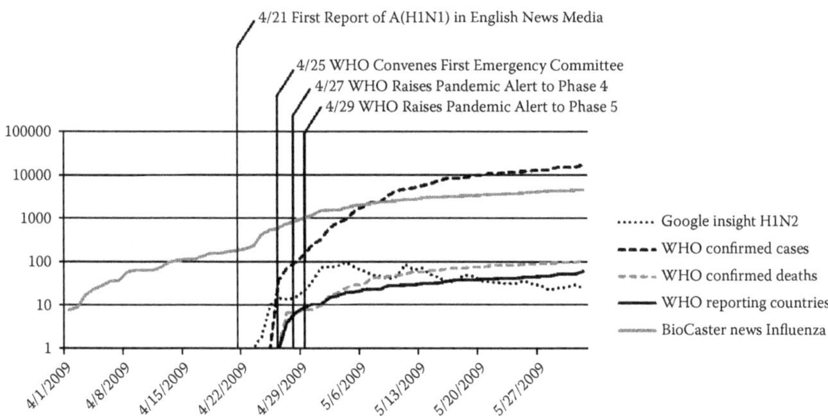

FIGURE 15.1
Log10 scale plots for April 1, 2009, to June 1, 2009, showing (a) Normalized Google Insights search volume for the term "H1N1" from Google Insight, (b) WHO laboratory confirmed cases for influenza A (H1N1) (n = 17,410 on June 1, 2009), (c) WHO laboratory confirmed deaths for A(H1N1) (n = 115 on June 1, 2009), (d) WHO countries reporting A(H1N1) cases (n = 62 on June 1, 2009), (e) cumulative frequency of positively identified news reports found by BioCaster for the term "Influenza" (n = 4609 on June 1, 2009). WHO data sourced from Epidemic and Pandemic Alert and Response situation reports for Influenza A (H1N1).

reported human cases of a novel influenza A (H1N1) outbreak centered on Mexico in seven countries. Subsequently, the WHO formally requested all countries to activate pandemic preparedness plans and to remain on high alert for unusual outbreaks of influenza-like illness. The WHO increased its pandemic threat level for swine influenza to "Phase 5" as reports of multiple fatalities in Mexico emerged. At the same time, general concern around the world rose and the information storm in the media moved from reports on the level of hundreds to the level of thousands. Against this background, automatic gathering of event-based health intelligence from open media sources began to take on increased importance as the number of reports increased rapidly to fill the public's demand for information.

The overall goal of event-based GHISs is to find linguistic signals in unstructured Web reports for the purposes of near-real-time detection, quantification, and reporting of public health events to the appropriate authorities. As we show in this chapter, public health organizations are increasingly considering automatic analysis of natural language data from the Web as well as search engine data so as to extend traditional indicator-based methods (e.g., notifiable disease reporting and over-the-counter [OTC] sales monitoring [Ginsberg et al. 2008]). The rationale for this decision is driven by the need to build global surveillance capacity. The abundant and near-real-time nature of online news makes it a cost-effective means of early detection and tracking of health events on a global scale. Open media sources can bridge the gap between national and international surveillance as well as provide timely access to sources on the ground.

At the same time, we must keep in sight the limitations with using media reports, which can sometimes be misinformed, are often prediagnostic, and tend to be written by nonexperts—sometimes with inbuilt distribution biases. There are also the concerns of the public in such areas as privacy. We do, however, consider that *rumor-based information* may be of particular value in helping (a) extend international coverage to areas where traditional surveillance system infrastructure is absent, and (b) strengthen the early detection capacity of existing systems, particularly at the local level. GHISs should properly be considered a part of a range of solutions for enabling a timely and appropriate public health response.

In this chapter, we briefly survey several extant GHISs being utilized by national agencies before detailing BioCaster, a freely available nongovernmental system developed by our team at the National Institute of Informatics in collaboration with a group of partners in Japan, Vietnam, Thailand, and the United States (Figure 15.2; Collier et al. 2008). Although BioCaster's coverage of health threats is global, it aims to enhance existing surveillance efforts by prioritizing languages within the Asia-Pacific region. With the incorporation of a multilingual ontology of 11 languages, BioCaster contains a single high-throughput system with advanced text mining and inference capabilities for the detection of linguistic signals for severe events of international significance,

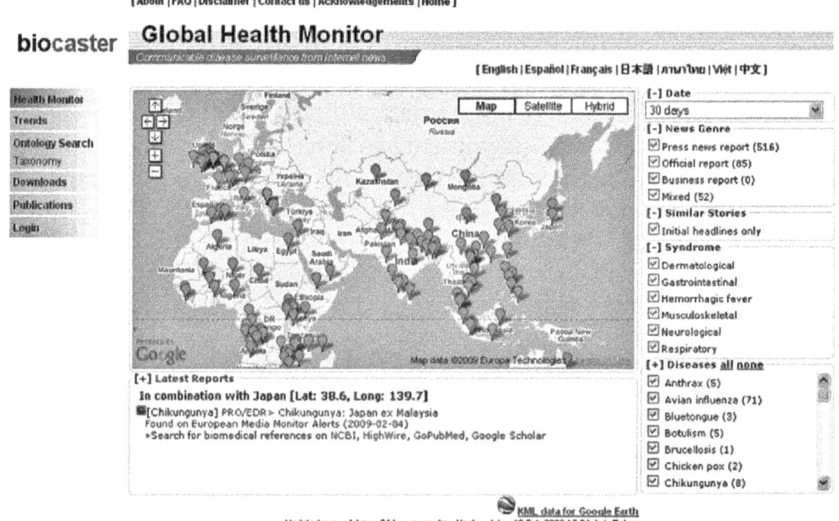

FIGURE 15.2
Screenshot of BioCaster's Global Health Monitor. News reports that are positively identified as disease outbreaks are processed to detect country, province, and disease terms before being plotted on a biogeographic Google map. The map allows users to filter the previous 30 days of news reports by time, document type, syndrome, or disease, as well as linking to the BioCaster ontology and external reference sources such as GoPubMed or HighWire.

such as international transmission or accidental release of agents. We explore the rationale, methodology, and user interface within the BioCaster system.

15.2 Existing Global Health Information Systems: An Overview

Our early discussions with domain experts in the public health community revealed that timely information is especially important on the following: (1) outbreak of newly emerging diseases such as novel pandemic influenza, (2) the moment of transition from animal-to-human and sustained human-to-human transmission, (3) the importation of exotic diseases across international borders, and (4) accidental or deliberate release of biological, chemical, radiological, or nuclear agents. Such are a precise reflection of the concerns addressed in the WHO's revised International Health Regulations (IHR) (Gostin 2004). Given the practical barriers to compliance that many countries face due to competing economic pressures, GHISs using open media sources have a special role to play in helping make health threats more transparent to the world public health community, thereby contributing to the ongoing capacity building required to implement the revised IHR.

The challenges in developing automated GHISs able to understand events in news reports should not be underestimated. Traditional keyword searches and page rankings are now a generic technology; however, these may not be precise enough to locate the customized and detailed information required for disease surveillance. Despite the advances made in tracking user health queries about influenza, Internet penetration is still lacking in many regions of the world that are most at-risk for emerging and reemerging diseases (Ginsberg et al. 2008). Having the timeliest information clearly requires human experts to have access to rare localized reports in the early epidemic stages; often, these are only available in local languages. Finding such reports requires sophisticated automatic natural language processing (NLP) to detect the weak initial signal of an epidemic's "storm front" and help control efforts during a pandemic surge. It is also necessary to consider the need for interdisciplinary collaboration—effective GHISs require a combination of expertise at the technological and domain levels that takes time and resources to develop.

In this section, we provide the results of a brief survey of several rapidly developing GHISs. The findings here are a result of an early 2009 investigation conducted for the Japanese Ministry of Health in collaboration with Global Health Security Action Group (GHSAG) member systems (Collier et al. 2009). We briefly examine the similarities and differences of news sources, domain knowledge, processing, and the dissemination of reports. Integration of manual and automated analyses is also given consideration. Given time and space limitations, the survey was intended only to be indicative of current technology trends without claiming to be comprehensive. A number of other systems that perform similar functions, as well as sites that specialize in reporting natural disaster information—such as the United Nation's Global Disaster Alert Coordinating System[1] (GDACS)—also exist. Of particular note are human network systems. ProMED-mail is an outstanding example that is used as a source by several of the systems we survey here (Madoff 2004). To provide a technological context to the following discussion, we briefly detail the basic methodological processes that a prototypical system will need to employ below:

1. Data ingestion is the first stage of processing, with sources that originate from a variety of document types such as e-mails, newswire reports, business reports and blogs (Web logs). Contents can be formatted in standard syntaxes, including: HTML (HyperText Markup Language), RSS (Really Simple Syndication) feeds, and PDF (Portable Document Format) documents.
2. Data cleansing is a technologically mundane process; however, it is vital in practice to both remove unwanted noise from the text (e.g., advertisements or links to unrelated news stories) as well as join together broken sentences.
3. Data triage is applied after the first two stages, and is the stage during which the more-or-less clean text is grouped into topic categories for either trashing or subsequent processing using detailed fact extraction. Trashing is necessary in the case of documents found that are clearly outside the task definition. At this stage, redundant information (e.g., multiple reports of the same event) is usually detected through document clustering.
4. Machine translation of the source text may be required during the data triage stage if the system does not have a native fact extraction capability in the source language.
5. Fact extraction is used to obtain structured information about an event—such as the name of the condition, the type of agent, the number of victims, and the time and the location where an event happened. In other words, this is the *who, what, where, when,* and *how* of an event.
6. Significance scores are calculated using results from available data. This could be from the data triage stage alone, or may result in conjunction with fact extraction. High-end systems will use sophisticated statistical analysis to assign an alerting level to each detected event.
7. Human judgment is key throughout these processes. It is almost always needed to understand what is abnormal, to discover rare events that

the system may have missed, to make the final decision about vague reports, and to link together disparate events. Processes 1 through 6 make human judgments quicker, cheaper, and more reliable through data search and visualization of the database of mined facts.

8. Feedback and improvement is the last of the processes. After deployment, text mining systems require maintenance and updates in order to keep up-to-date on new vocabulary, document types, and sources of information, as well as to correct for misunderstandings.

15.2.1 GPHIN (Public Health Canada)

The Global Public Health Intelligence Network (GPHIN) is a secure, continuously accessible (24 hours a day, 7 days a week) public health surveillance system focused on civil emergency detection, risk assessment, and response (Mawudeku et al. 2007). The system combines both automated and manual detection methods, and is run from within the Centre for Emergency Preparedness and Response (CEPR) under the Public Health Agency of Canada (PHAC). In operation 11 years, GPHIN has expertise in both the technical and managerial aspects of emergency response, offering practical support for Canadian provincial and central government agencies in the area of first response and public health security. Since its beginnings in the mid-1990s, GPHIN has developed a close partnership with the WHO to evaluate unsubstantiated news reports of public health significance (Mykhalovskiy and Weir 2006).

Language coverage in GHPIN aims to maximize global media coverage, and includes the six official working languages of the United Nations—Arabic, Simplified Chinese, English, French, Russian, and Spanish, in addition to traditional Chinese, Portuguese, and Farsi. In terms of health threat coverage, GPHIN takes an all risks approach and has taxonomic coverage for most human and animal diseases.

Data sourcing comes from two major commercial aggregators: Factiva (most languages) and Al Bawaba (for Arabic). Additionally, Farsi is sourced manually from the Web by human analysts. GPHIN analysts also review output from MedISys and the EMM (Europe Media Monitor) in the European Union regularly.

The GPHIN system combines both automatic and human analyses with input from approximately 14 analysts whose backgrounds cover a range of disciplines (e.g., the life sciences, journalism, and economics). The automatic component incorporates a highly developed, multilingual taxonomic classification system that performs document filtering and ranking. Human analysts rank news items according to their domain expertise and understanding of the regions they cover, as well as source additional news sources and edit machine translation system output when quality falls below standard thresholds. Output to the end user is provided by a secure Internet portal in the form of alerts, biogeographic maps, and a searchable list of ranked news articles.

15.2.2 Project Argus (Georgetown University)

Since 2004, Project Argus, based at Georgetown University Medical Center, has been working in the detection and tracking of biological events outside of the United States. Project Argus is a mixed-mode system with an automatic analysis component and a large team of approximately 40 human analysts. The U.S. Centers for Disease Control and Prevention (CDC) and other federal agencies oversee health surveillance within the United States (Wilson 2007). A novel feature of Project Argus has been its pioneering use of early warning indicators. Approximately 200 have been identified and incorporated into a staging model analogous to the U.S. National Weather Service's. Categories exist for unifocal events, multifocal events, severe infrastructure strain, social collapse, and recovery.

Project Argus covers approximately 40 languages, 29 of which are automatically indexed by the article retrieval system, and 13 of which are machine translated. The languages were chosen based on the availability of source texts and regional analysts. Coverage of diseases is focused on approximately 150 fast-spreading diseases that affect humans, animals, and plants.

The system's automatic component ingests news directly from the Web using a set of constantly maintained wrappers. Documents are initially selected based on weighted keywords within an indicator and warning ontology. A score is generated that reflects its public health severity. Human analysts have access to both the automatic alerts as well as output from their own standing searches on the news database. Working in regional teams, the automated component identifies significant stories that are synthesized into daily reports for the population of users.

15.2.3 MedISys (Joint Research Centre, Italy)

The European Commission's Medical Information System (MedISys) is a fully automatic GHIS developed and run by the Joint Research Centre (JRC) in Ipsa, Italy (Steinberger et al. 2008). Working in close collaboration with the Health Threats Unit at the Directorate General for Health and Consumer Protection in the European Commission (DG SANCO), MedISys offers early warning of infectious disease, chemical, radiological, and nuclear health threats to EU institutions and member state organizations. Since 2007, MedISys has been working in collaboration with the University of Helsinki's Pattern-Based Understanding and Learning System (PULS), which we describe in the next section. PULS performs precise linguistic analysis on document contents. Results from both systems appear together on a common portal site run by MedISys.

In total, approximately 40 languages are covered by MedISys, including all European Union languages. News reports in 26 of these languages are made available on the MedISys Web portal. An extensive range of public health threats is covered by the system and categorized into approximately 300 health-related categories in a multilingual ontology. Geographically,

MedISys covers the world, with geographic information contained in a multilingual gazetteer (Atkinson et al. 2008). Data sourcing comes from Web-crawling on 4,000 news sites in 43 languages, as well as on ProMED-mail. Additionally, news from commercial aggregators such as Lexis Nexis is also ingested.

As noted above, MedISys is fully automatic. It is characterized by language-independent algorithms that employ a range of keyword classification methods and statistical analysis of trends by threat and country. MedISys uses a clustering algorithm with an 8-hour window to detect and flag duplicate stories. After clustering, positive articles are selected based on a set of Boolean queries. Both standing queries and user-defined queries are used. Automatic threat alerting is accomplished by searching for anomalies across aggregated information within the previous week's news reports. Output to the end user is provided in several formats, including biogeographic mapping, aggregated graphs, alerting statistics, and a news search interface.

15.2.4 PULS (Helsinki University)

PULS is a non-governmental, working research prototype GHIS operated by Helsinki University (Steinberger et al. 2008). The system became operational in 2006, but its origins go farther back to work that was conducted at New York University (Grishman et al. 2003). In 2007, a close collaboration was formed between PULS and the MedISys group. This relationship was based on a loose integration of the two systems over the Internet; PULS provided relatively high-end language understanding and MedISys provided document sourcing and early stage topic filtering. Currently, PULS operates only on English-language news; although, there are plans to incorporate French- and Spanish-language news sources in the near future. In addition to MedISys, PULS also makes its output available to a variety of other EU organizations, such as the European Center for Disease Control and Prevention (ECDC) and the National Public Health Institute in Finland (KTL).

The PULS ontology focuses mainly on agents and conditions with an extensive terminology harvested and verified from publicly available health news collections such as ProMED-mail. The total number of agent concepts is estimated at 1000. Similarly, geographic terms are harvested from online resources (e.g., CIA World Factbook) that allow global coverage to very fine levels of granularity for the United States (Central Intelligence Agency 2008).

PULS is predominantly an automatic system that uses a range of language technologies to extract structured frames of information from news articles. The structured information is made available to users through a searchable database table. One unique feature of PULS is its ability to incorporate a confidence score into the events that it extracts. This is done by measuring how many candidates could have filled an informational slot (such as for country/location of event or disease condition) in the event frame. When a large number of candidates could have been applied, the confidence level for the event is reduced.

15.2.5 HealthMap (Harvard–MIT)

Since beginning operation in September 2006, the HealthMap project provides a free and openly available automated surveillance tool run from the Children's Hospital Informatics Program at the Harvard Medical School Division of Health Sciences and Technologies (Brownstein et al. 2008; Freifeld et al. 2008). The system combines both an automatic and a manual detection component with an emphasis on providing an integrated view of disease outbreak information. Since 2007, HealthMap has been closely associated with ProMED-mail. HealthMap benefits from ProMED reports, and, in turn, ProMED makes HealthMap output available to subscribers via report submissions on the mailing list.

Currently, the HealthMap system monitors news in six major world languages (English, Chinese, French, Portuguese, Russian, and Spanish) and has approximately 170 human, animal, and plant diseases under surveillance. Additionally, HealthMap monitors conditions for early warning indicators of outbreaks, such as poisoning, environmental disaster, and conflict. Terminology is contained within large structured dictionaries that have been derived from a variety of publicly available sources. Dictionary lists themselves are integrated into a large number of language-dependent patterns for determining the name and location of the outbreak in actual news texts.

The automatic component within HealthMap performs several levels of analyses on each document. The first stage identifies country and disease using patterns described above. The next stage utilizes Bayesian methods to classify news reports into the categories of breaking news, warning, context, old news, and nondisease news. The final stage detects and removes redundant information. Alert detection focuses on high-impact news using statistics that determine the recency of an event as well as the reliability of the news source. Dissemination is made through a variety of formats available from HealthMap's Web page, including biogeographic maps, links to external sources, and mailing lists.

15.3 Development of BioCaster

We now turn to a structured discussion of the technical characteristics of the BioCaster system, which began operation in 2006. BioCaster was an early adopter of high-throughput cluster technology to minimize the time between data sourcing and distribution to users. News is gathered on a 30-minute cycle, which can be shortened as necessary during health emergencies.

15.3.1 Data Sources

In order to simplify news collection, BioCaster ingests data in RSS format. This provides low maintenance access to frequently updated Web feeds, such as news or blogs. BioCaster ingests approximately 1700 feeds from a large variety of sites, including Google News, ProMED-mail, the European Media Monitor, WHO outbreak reports, and news reported by international, national, and local providers. From 2009, the BioCaster group has outsourced part of its news collection to a private media monitoring company, allowing access to more than 90,000 news providers in approximately 110 countries. However, because of copyright restrictions, links to these reports will be made available to login users only. The BioCaster group expects the number of detected reports to increase as the system extends operational coverage of languages to Chinese, French, Russian, Spanish, and Portuguese.

15.3.2 Selection and Encoding of Diseases

The central knowledge resource within BioCaster is a multilingual application ontology (BCO) that was developed by engaging an interdisciplinary team of experts with skills ranging from the areas of computational linguistics, national public health, genetics, and anthropology (Collier et al. 2007). Formal concept analysis was used to organize the BCO around a backbone of Suggested Upper Merged Ontology (SUMO) upper-level taxonomy (Kawazoe et al. 2006; Kawazoe et al. 2008). Domain entity classes such as "Disease," "Country," "Province," "Symptom," and "Chemical" were carefully grafted onto this taxonomy (Niles and Pease, 2001). Root terms (the key concepts that play roles in events) appear as instances of the domain entity classes. The selection of terms was centered on diseases selected from various country's notifiable disease lists and ranked for public health impact. The resulting ontology is made available for browsing on the BioCaster portal site,[2] and also as a free and downloadable OWL (Web Ontology Language) file. The third version of the ontology, released in 2009, encodes multilingual equivalences between eleven languages: Chinese, English, French, Indonesian, Japanese, Korean, Malay, Spanish, Russian, Thai, and Vietnamese. Cross-language term equivalents are handled as multilingual synonym sets in a manner similar to that used in EuroWordNet (Vossen 1998). The new version of the system will contain more than 300 human and animal diseases, representing an increase of nearly 200 from the second version released in April 2008.

15.3.3 Automated Analysis

As shown in Figure 15.3, the initial stages of automatic analysis begin with data ingestion and cleansing, followed by machine translation (MT). Although BioCaster has native-named entity and event extraction

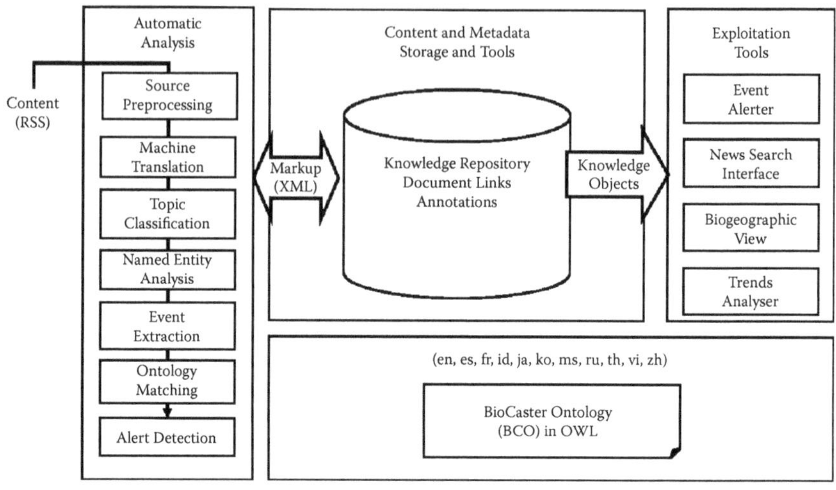

FIGURE 15.3
Data pathway through the BioCaster system.

modules for some languages (English, Japanese, Thai, and Vietnamese), MT is a cost-effective option for when dedicated modules do not exist. Use of MT allows the English rule book to be applied. The resulting target text inevitably loses signal (e.g., "swine influenza" can appear as the less preferable "pig influenza" when translated), but in practice, it can often be understood after further processing in the later stages due to redundancy of information in the news report. A small amount of tailoring in pattern rules has been made to accommodate nonstandard terminology such as "pig influenza."

After the step of machine translation, the process of topic classification follows (Doan et al. 2009). In practice, at this stage, the content examined could concern almost any topic; it is important, then, that the "gatekeeper" be aware of both major and subtle differences between topics. For example, it should be relatively easy to spot the vocabulary differences between a report on a soccer team winning a match and one on an outbreak of dengue fever. But, this task is not always straightforward when met with reports about chronic diseases, polio prevention campaigns, and/or developments in vaccines. For the BioCaster group, it was first necessary to construct an objective case definition for the topics that the system would allow. This was done in collaboration between a linguist and a public health expert. In practice, guidelines were heavily influenced by the WHO IHR annex 2 decision tree, and more detail was added to address potential ambiguities that might arise in practice. The guidelines were then used to hand-annotate a gold standard media corpus containing approximately 1000 classified texts; of these, one-third were positive on the topic of infectious disease outbreaks, and two-thirds on nonrelevant topics, such as business, politics, technology, sport, and entertainment.

An important feature of the topic classification task is the need for high recall so as not to reject any true positives. Posting side-by-side comparisons with other learning algorithms, the BioCaster group selected a support vector machine model able to help achieve a classification accuracy over 93.5% (F-score = 91.2). However, a small proportion of false positives still remained—for example, when the condition is unclassified or vague, when the outbreak is hypothetical, or when the outbreak is historical or negative. More subtle borderline cases frequently occur in stories that discuss disease outbreak reports, but not as their main topical contribution, such as in prevention and control campaigns. Later stages of processing are designed to detect and, if necessary, reject such reports.

For named entity analysis and event extraction, the BioCaster group developed Simple Rule Language,[3] a freely available, regular expression pattern-matching language. SRL is designed to allow users without a background in computer science to quickly build up rule books. Although this is laborious in general, the BioCaster group has tried to make the task easier by developing a freely available graphical user interface (McCrae et al. 2009). SRL has influences from earlier pattern-based languages, such as Declarative Information Analysis Language (DIAL), and incorporates a capability to match string literals, named entity classes, skipwords, and word lists (Feldman 2003). The general SRL syntax is a label followed by a head expression and a body expression. The head expression is output if the regular expression in the body matches to the text. Examples of these follow:

- Ex 1. "D1: name(disease) { list(%disease) }" matches to any phrase in the list "disease" and outputs a named entity of type "disease."
- Ex 2. "L2: name(location) { list(@cardinal_directions) list(@country) }" matches to any country name preceded by a cardinal direction such as "northeastern" and outputs the whole phrase as a named entity of type "location."
- Ex 3. "IT1:international_travel("true") :- "recently" "traveled" "to" words(,2) name(location,L) { list(@country) }" matches to the phrase "recently traveled to" followed by up to two words and a location name and outputs the fact that "international travel" is true.

As shown in the examples above, lists and named entities are used to encode semantically related terms such as disease names, country names, victim expressions, verbs of infection, and so on with several of the lists coming from the BCO. The advantage of this approach is that it can be easily used by nonexperts in software engineering, can be quickly changed to accommodate new terms or events, and is not limited to any particular language. SRL is therefore well suited to resource-poor languages, but can easily be extended to incorporate lexical level features such as parts of speech or orthographic labels (if greater rule generality is required and resources exist). The limitation of the language is in the modeling of long-distance syntactic relations, but in practice, we have not found this to be a problem in news reports.

The English SRL rule book for biohazard events incorporates approximately 110 rules for entity detection, 12 major word lists containing 870 terms, and more than 2800 template rules for detecting direct signals (e.g., international travel, zoonosis, category A agents, novel diseases, and malformed blood products), as well as indirect signals (distal indicators, e.g., infrastructure strain in social services). Template rules are also used to detect temporal aspects of events such as the historical or hypothetical. One important point to note is that much of the biohazard rule book, such as lists of countries or victim expressions, can be reused in a modular fashion for the detection of other public health events planned for future development in BioCaster.

After extracting the basic event frame, objects still require disambiguation. It is often the case that country names are not given explicitly within the article. Instead, this information can be inferred at times from role titles or organization names. For example, "Victoria chief health officer" could potentially imply countries such as Canada, Australia, or the Seychelles. Country, province, disease, and agent names are disambiguated statistically, and then geopositioned to a latitude and longitude using lookup in the BCO. The final event frame is then stored in the knowledge base for exploitation tools to access.

15.3.4 Data Dissemination

BioCaster provides output in a variety of forms. The open access public portal provides users with 30 days of access to the Global Health Monitor, a news collection site with biogeographic mapping capability based on Google Maps[4] (Figure 15.2). News articles can be searched by time, text type, syndrome, or disease, and further sources of information can be found through dynamically generated links to existing biomedical ontologies and academic database. News headlines are ranked on the site according to an algorithm that calculates the novelty of the disease and location based on the previous 30 day's data, with special provision for potentially fast-spreading events and highly stressed health systems.

A login-restricted alerting interface is used by a small test community at the Ministry of Health in Japan and the Health Protection Agency in the United Kingdom. Here, users can define targeted rules that let them receive e-mail alerts whenever news comes into the system on topics of interest. For example, a user could define a rule asking to be alerted on the topic of novel influenza in Europe involving a case of international travel. More advanced news search and analytics are also incorporated into the login site allowing users access to aggregated data on events. It is expected that this service will soon be opened up to more users within the global public health community.

As noted above, the multilingual ontology is made available for browsing on the Web portal and also for download as a Web Ontology Language (OWL) file. Users can lookup unfamiliar terms, identify causal agents, find synonyms in different languages, and link to external resources such as Unified Medical Language Service (UMLS), SNOMED CT, and ICD-10 (Lindberg et al. 1993, Stearns et al. 2001, World Health Organization 2001). A recent innovation has been the use of micro-blogging to disseminate BioCaster reports. During the influenza A H1N1 outbreak in May 2009, human analysts submitted more than 400 micro-blogs to Twitter.[5] This helped to reach out to a new community of users and also reduced the user load on our server during the surge period.

15.4 Results

The BioCaster Web portal currently receives on average between 2000 and 3000 unique user accesses per month from 30 to 50 countries with the majority coming from United States, South Korea, Japan, China, the United Kingdom, Germany, and Thailand. Partnership networks are also crucial for disseminating data directly to key user groups. For example, since the start of the influenza A (H1N1) epidemic, BioCaster has collaborated with InSTEDD (Innovative Support to Emergencies Diseases and Disasters) Evolve to make geo-located reports available via RSS feed (Kass-Hout and Tada 2008). It follows that Evolve amalgamates BioCaster as one of its data sources, and adds a new layer of collaborative filtering. The second version of the open access multilingual ontology is widely accessed online and has been downloaded by more than 73 academic, industrial, and public health groups worldwide, including the WHO and other groups located in North America (25 groups), Asia (32 groups), Europe (14 groups), and Oceania (1 group).

In 2008, an average of 68 positive reports were collected each day for English-language news covering 150 countries and 88 infectious diseases in humans and animals. Normalized frequencies are shown for the top 31 most frequent countries and diseases in Figures 15.4 and 15.5. Although, there is a clear bias toward English-speaking countries, the graph indicates the key importance of the Asia Pacific region with significant numbers of reports from China, Indonesia, Japan, Philippines, Thailand, and Vietnam.

Returning to Figure 15.1, several characteristics of how the recent influenza A (H1N1) epidemic was reported and queried on the Web can be clearly seen. First, it is clear from the BioCaster data that the number of news reports is not related in a simple way to the real-world frequencies of cases or deaths from the outbreak. Editorial control, country bias, user interest, media distribution capacity, and so on all play a part in determining how news is reported. Second, we see a small but significant lead in the reporting and querying of news about

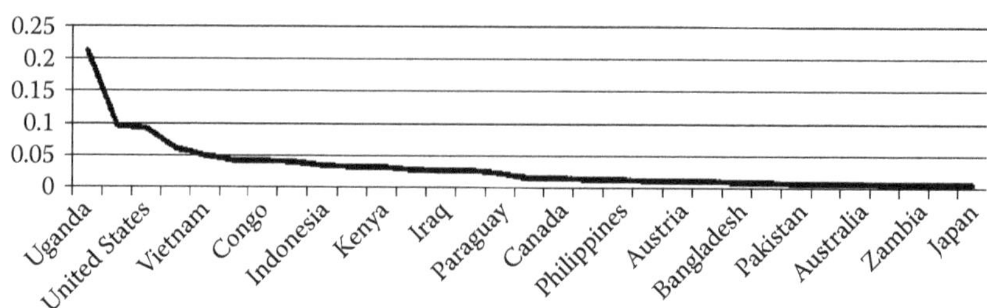

FIGURE 15.4
Number of outbreak reports by country in the open media for January 1, 2008, to December 31, 2008. The curve represents the distribution of news in the top 31 most frequently mentioned countries divided by the total number of news reports for all 31 countries.

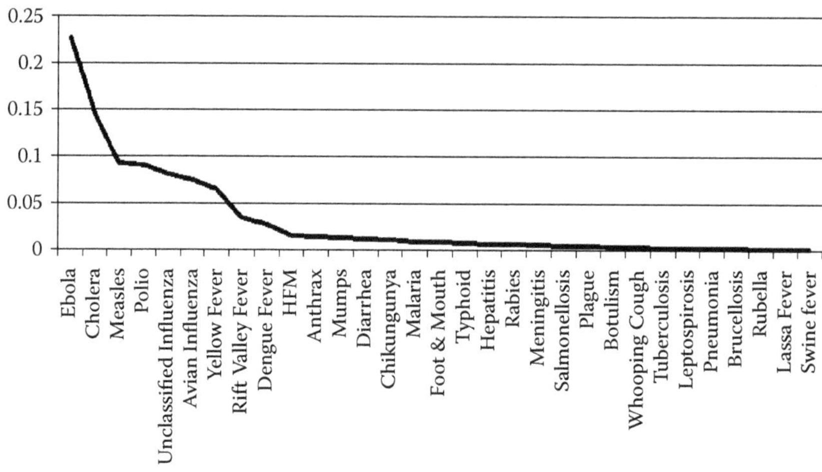

FIGURE 15.5
Distribution of outbreak reports by disease in the open media for January 1, 2008 to December 31, 2008. The curve represents the distribution of news in the top 31 most frequently mentioned diseases divided by the total number of news reports for all 31 diseases.

H1N1 and influenza before WHO made its first official announcement. Given the delays in setting up laboratory tests for a novel virus, this supports previous observations in the literature that news rumors can support advanced warning of international events. It is important to remember though, that the results we present here are for English-language news only. Spanish-language news would probably show an even greater lead in time. Third, it can be seen that, after around May 12, despite the increasing number of disease cases, the rate of increase in news reporting did not keep pace. Moreover, user interest as represented by news queries to Google News actually decreased.

15.5 Future Work

Now that the world has past the initial stages of the A (H1N1) epidemic, people have begun asking, "Given the current state of preparedness, why didn't [we] detect it earlier?" Mexican authorities detected the epidemic as early as March 18, but considered it to be late season influenza (Wikipedia 2009). Moreover, a May 11 study in the journal *Science* estimated that there could have potentially been as many as 23,000 suspected cases in Mexico before the 23rd of April, with possibilities of concession possibly beginning as early as mid-February 2009. The linguistic signals before April 21, 2009, need careful examination, but are most likely to be found in the Spanish-language media, which BioCaster, unfortunately, did not cover at the time. The clear lesson (Figure 15.6) is the advantage of having multilingual coverage. Work in BioCaster has already begun to expand its language sources to several major world languages, including Chinese, English, French, Russian, Spanish, and Portuguese.

Electronic publication has removed the physical space limits that previously existed in newspapers; modern newswire reports circulate widely and are republished in many different forms. The disparity between real-world frequencies of events and news frequencies needs to be handled to allow for better situation awareness. How to normalize the frequency and volume of news so as to reduce the effects of reporting bias also requires further study.

Understanding location and time are key foundations to effective GHIS. Although studies have taken place in the area of temporal understanding (e.g., TimeML[6]), few guidelines or resources exist for geolocating events outside of the English language. The GeoNames database[7] is one example

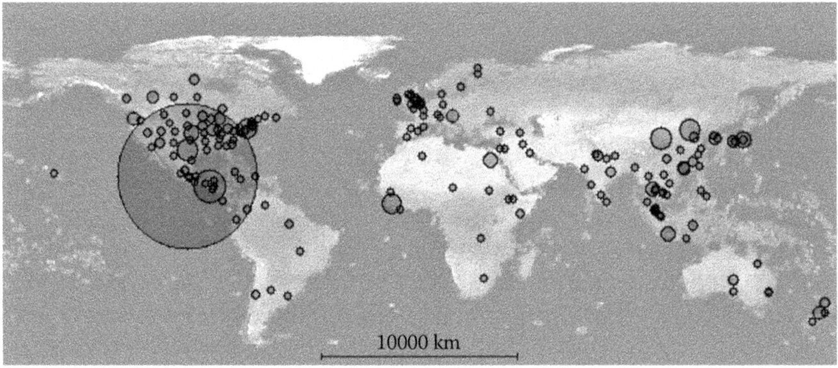

FIGURE 15.6
Distribution of influenza reports found by BioCaster in the open media for April 21, 2009, to June 1, 2009 ($1 \leq n \leq 1176$). In comparison to WHO situation report case count totals for June 1, the plot indicates under-reporting in South America, several false positives in Western Africa, and under-reporting in Spain and South America and over-reporting in India and Western Africa. Outbreaks of A (H5N1) occurring simultaneously were also sometimes not easily differentiated from A (H1N1) as seen in the Egypt cluster. Maps are generated by GPSVisualizer

of an extensive location resource for English as is the Yahoo! Geocode API (Application Programming Interface). To the best of our knowledge though, no open resource exists that encodes population frequencies by province; this is the minimum level necessary for the determination of at-risk populations. The BioCaster group is now working toward expanding the system's location ontology to include this information.

At the user level, it is important for BioCaster developers to more closely engage the public health community in countries with both strong and weak health systems to explain the benefits of news media sources. This two-way dialogue is particularly important for BioCaster as, currently, the group lacks the human resources to carry out a full-time manual check on system output. In the future, the BioCaster group envisages that it will be crucial to engage user understanding of the technology, and involve users in extending the reporting and checking of outbreak reports.

In the future, it should be possible to solicit even more timely news sources, such as blogs and microblogs (Twitter feeds), from social networks, and also monitor social semantic metadata such as Hashtags.[8] The time to publication for these reports is extremely short; anyone with SMS capabilities can post a microblog to Twitter almost instantaneously. However, one limitation with this method is a high signal-to-noise ratio due to lack of editorial control and the limited context each message provides. Other challenges include the highly informal language used on blogs, as well as their often subjective nature. Making practical use of these resources is a current research area and will require much stronger filtering than we currently employ, including perhaps novel techniques to model trust in a report.

15.6 Conclusions

BioCaster is one of a range of systems for international disease monitoring. The benefits, limitations, and successes of the Web as a near real-time means for collecting and distributing data about public health events have been highlighted in this chapter. Based on advanced text mining technology, we have been providing a freely available service to the global public health community since 2006. The BioCaster group is continually working to improve the system by (a) increasing accessibility and better integration with public health users by conducting a usability survey, (b) developing qualitative metrics to measure and improve detection rates, (c) extending coverage to new languages and health threats, (d) collaborating with other system developers and user groups to enhance data sharing and interchange standards, and (e) continuously improving the quality of linguistic signals that indicate unusual events.

Access to BioCaster can be requested by public health organizations from the first author.

Acknowledgments

BioCaster is supported by grant-in-aid monies from the Japan Science and Technology (JST) Corporation's PRESTO program. Funding for the survey of systems was from a Japanese Ministry of Health, Labour, and Welfare (MHLW) grant-in-aid. The authors would like to express their gratitude to the system owners who participated in the MHLW survey: Dr. Noele Nelson (Project Argus, Georgetown University), Dr. Abla Mawudeku (GPHIN, PHAC), Dr. John Brownstein (HealthMap at MIT–Harvard), Dr. Ralf Steinberger (MedISys, JRC), and Dr. Roman Yangarber (PULS, University of Helsinki) as well as BioCaster partners for their support: Dr. Asanee Kawtrakul (Kasetsart University), Dr. Koichi Takeuchi (Okayama University), Dr. Kiyosu Taniguchi (National Institute of Infectious Diseases), Dr. Yoshio Tateno (the National Institute of Genetics), and Dr. Dinh Dien (Vietnam National University).

References

Associated Press. 2009. CDC warns doctors about swine flu. WJZ. April 21, http://wjz.com/health/swine.flu.CDC.2.990540.html (accessed June 3, 2009).

Atkinson, M., Piskorski, J., Pouliquen, B., Steinberger, R., Tanev, H., and Zavarella, V. 2008. Online-monitoring of security-related events. Paper presented at COLING 2008: Companion Volume—Posters and Demonstrations, pp. 145–148, Manchester, U.K.

Brownstein, J., Freifeld, C., Reis, B., and Mandl, K. 2008. Surveillance san frontières: Internet-based emerging infectious disease intelligence and the HealthMap project. *PLOS Medicine* 5(7): 1019–1024.

Centers for Disease Control and Prevention (CDC). 2009. Swine influenza A(H1N1) infection in two children—Southern California, March–April 2009. *Morbidity and Mortality Weekly Report*, April 24.

Central Intelligence Agency. 2008. The World Factbook. https://www.cia.gov/library/publications/the-world-factbook/ (accessed January 29, 2009).

Cohen, J. and Enserink, M. 2009. As swine flu circles globe, scientists grapple with basic questions. *Science* 324: 572–573.

Collier, N., Doan, S., Kawazoe, A., Matsuda Goodwin, R., Conway, M., Tateno, Y., et al. 2008. BioCaster: Detecting public health rumors with a Web-based text mining system. *Bioinformatics* 24(24): 2940–2941.

Collier, N., Kawazoe, A., Jin, L., Shigematsu, M., Dien, D. Barrero, R., Takeuchi , K., and Kawtrakul, A. 2007. A multilingual ontology for infectious disease surveillance: rationale, design and challenges. Language Resources and Evaluation, DOI: 10.1007/s10579-007-9019-7: 405–413.

Collier, N., Shigematsu, M., Doan, S., Takeuchi, K., and Taniguchi, K. 2009. A survey of Web-based global health intelligence systems—methodology recommendations on a future Japanese national system design. Final report to the Japanese

Ministry of Health, Labour and Welfare Grant in Aid for Scientific Research Promotion, March 9.

Doan, S., Kawazoe, A., Conway, M., and Collier, N. 2009. Towards role-based filtering of disease outbreak reports. *Journal of Biomedical Informatics*, DOI: 10.1016/j.jbi.2008.12.009.

Feldman, R. 2003. Mining text data. In *The Handbook of Data Mining*, ed. Nong Ye, 481–517. Lawrence Erlbaum Associates.

Fraser, C., et al. 2009. Pandemic Potential of a Strain of Influenza A(H1N1): Early Findings. Science DOI: 10.1126/science.1176062.

Ginsberg, J., Mohebbi, M., Patel, R., Brammer, L., Smolinski, M., and Brilliant, L. 2008. Detecting influenza epidemics using search engine query data. Nature, doi:10.1038/nature07634, http://www.nature.com/nature/journal/vaop/ncurrent/suppinfo/nature07634_S1.html (accessed January 30, 2009).

Gostin, L. O. 2004. International infectious disease law—Revision of the World Health Organization's International Health Regulations. *J. American Medical Association (JAMA)* 291(21): 2623–2627.

Grishman, R., Huttunen, S., and Yangarber, R. 2003. Information extraction for enhanced access to disease outbreak reports. *J. Biomedical Informatics* 35: 236–246.

Kass-Hout, T. and di Tada, N. 2008. International system for total early disease detection (InSTEDD) platform. *Advances in Disease Surveillance* 5(2): 108.

Kawazoe, A., Jin, L., Shigematsu, M. Barerro, R., Taniguchi, K., and Collier, N. 2006. The development of a schema for the annotation of terms in the BioCaster disease detection/tracking system. Paper presented at the International Workshop on Biomedical Ontology in Action (KR-MED 2006), Baltimore, Maryland, November 8, pp. 77–85.

Madoff, L. 2004. ProMED-mail: An early warning system for emerging diseases. *Clinical Infectious Diseases* 39(2): 227–232.

Mawudeku, A., Lemay, R., Werker, D., Andraghetti, R., and St. John, R. 2007. The global public health intelligence network. In *Infectious Disease Surveillance*, ed. M'ikantha, N., Lynfield, R., Van Beneden, C. and de Valk, H., 304–317. Blackwell Publishing.

Mykhalovskiy, E. and Weir, L. 2006. The Global Public Health Intelligence Network and early warning outbreak detection: A Canadian contribution to global public health. *Canadian Journal of Public Health* 97(1): 42–44.

Niles, I. and Pease, A. 2001. Origins of the standard upper merged ontology. Paper presented at the IJCAI-2001 Workshop on the IEEE Standard Upper Ontology, Seattle, Washington, USA.

Stearns, M. Q., Price, C., Spackman, K., and Wang, A. 2001. Clinical terms: overview of the development process and project status. Paper presented at the American Medical Informatics Association (AMIA) Symposium. pp. 662–666.

Vossen, P. 1998. Introduction to EuroWordNet. *Computers and the Humanities* 32: 73–89.

Wikipedia. 2009. Swine Flu Outbreak, http://en.wikipedia.org/wiki/2009_swine_flu_outbreak (accessed June 3, 2009).

Wilson, J. 2007. Argus: A global detection and tracking system for biological events. *Advances in Disease Surveillance* 4: 21.

Wilson, J., Polyak, M., Blake, J., and Collmann, J. 2008. A heuristic indication and warning staging model for detection and assessment of biological events. *Journal of American Medical Informatics Association* 15: 158–171.

World Health Organization (WHO). 2004. ICD-10, International Statistical Classification of Diseases and Related Health Problems, 10th Revision, http://apps.who.int/classifications/apps/icd/icd10online/ (accessed June 11, 2009).

Endnotes

1 GDACS is available from http://www.gdacs.org/ (last accessed June 12, 2009).
2 BioCaster is available from http://www.biocaster.org.
3 The SRL editor is available from http://code.google.com/p/srl-editor/ (last accessed June 12, 2009).
4 Google Maps is available from http://maps.google.com (last accessed June 12, 2009).
5 BioCaster Twitter is available from http://twitter.com/biocaster (last accessed June 12, 2009).
6 TimeML specification is available from http://www.timeml.org (last accessed June 12, 2009).
7 Geonames database is available from www.geonames.org (last accessed June 12, 2009).
8 HashTags is available from http://hashtags.org (last accessed June 12, 2009).

16

A Snapshot of Situation Awareness: Using the NC DETECT System to Monitor the 2007 Heat Wave

David B. Rein
RTI International
Atlanta, Georgia

CONTENTS

16.1 Introduction

Given its location in the southeastern United States, North Carolina has historically experienced high summertime temperatures. A certain degree of heat is expected in the South and has been dealt with architecturally—through the use of vaulted ceilings, east-to-west ventilation patterns, and covered outdoor porches—and culturally—through the slower pace of society. Over the latter half of the 20th century, in-migration from other areas of the United States and immigration from other parts of the world have changed these traditional patterns of living and added vast tracks of suburbia in key urban areas of the state. Since 1980, North Carolina's population has increased by more than 3 million people, or 55% (North Carolina Rural Economic Development Center 2005; U.S. Census Bureau 1995). Over this time, North Carolina has grown more densely populated and more urban, and residents of North Carolina are increasingly transplants from other parts of the United States (North Carolina Rural Economic Development Center 2005). Given the faster pace of modern society, many of the newer generation of transplanted North Carolinians might lack the protective cultural habits of older generations, such as slowing down and seeking shelter when the weather is oppressively hot.

In addition to population changes, changes in North Carolina's built environment have led many areas of North Carolina to feel hotter today than they had in past decades. Since the late 1950s, suburban development had led to the development of many formerly wild or agricultural spaces replacing fields and forests with asphalt roads and housing developments. As a result, many areas of North Carolina have developed a so-called heat island effect because darkened asphalt and concrete buildings absorb more of the sun's heat than the rural pine forests and farmlands they replaced. In addition, urbanization likely resulted in urban spaces that feel hotter because they lack the shade offered by natural settings or mature urban areas. According to the National Aeronautics and Space Administration's "Common Sense Heat Index," which measures the extent to which climatic warming trends can be perceived by the average individual, all of the major population centers of North Carolina have grown increasingly warmer since the 1960s (although the 1930s through the 1950s felt roughly as warm as today) (Hansen 2005; Hansen et al. 1998).

Still, the summer of 2007 was hot even by southern standards, and the relentless heat of August 2007 was some of the worst on record in North Carolina history. According to the National Oceanic and Atmospheric Administration, the summer of 2007 was the sixth warmest summer on record, and August was its warmest month. Throughout August, the extreme heat contributed to several gaudy weather records. On August 9, Charlotte reached its all-time high temperature of 104°F. On August 21, Raleigh-Durham equaled its all-time high temperature of 105°F. The heat was sustained and extreme, with a duration and severity not seen in North Carolina since the heat waves of 1983 and 1954 (NOAA 2007). Fayetteville, North Carolina, experienced 6 consecutive days with high temperatures above 102°F. Just over the border in South Carolina, Columbia experienced 14 days in August when temperatures exceeded 100°F.

By the mid-2000s, several major events had raised public health officials' awareness of the potentially catastrophic dangers of extreme heat. In 1995, a severe heat wave in the city of Chicago resulted in widespread power outages and other disruptions of city services along with nearly 600 deaths (Dematte et al. 1998; Klineberg 2002). In 2003, a heat wave in Western Europe led to approximately 33,000 deaths across the continent (Kosatsky 2005).

Whether because of changes in society, warming of the climate, or simply increasing awareness that periods of extreme heat can have profound public health consequences, in the summer of 2007, North Carolina public health officials were nervous about the heat. This anxiety only increased as the summer, already unusually hot, grew historically so in the first weeks of August. Officials wanted to protect the population from the extreme effects of heat seen in the recent past, but they needed information to do so. Fortunately, by 2007, North Carolina had a new information system in place that could help them monitor and respond to the problem.

16.2 What Is Syndromic Surveillance?

Syndromic surveillance (see Introduction chapter) refers to data from any nontraditional source that are delivered repeatedly over a timely interval (usually daily) and analyzed to identify and track emerging trends in injuries, accidents, or diseases that traditional surveillance could potentially miss. The term "syndromic" refers to the monitoring of patterns or collections of symptoms or events that taken together may indicate an underlying health condition. In public health, surveillance refers to the monitoring or tracking of disease conditions.

Traditional health surveillance systems typically focus on identifying and confirming diagnoses of specific disorders. Traditional surveillance data are generally collected through direct physician reporting, diagnostic lab reporting, and probabilistic surveys. Although not always the case, traditional surveillance systems usually emphasize accuracy, completeness of reporting, and the ability to infer results to the population of interest over timeliness of reporting. For example, a traditional influenza surveillance program might test all patients with influenza-like illnesses (ILI) who seek health care at specific sentinel sites for flu and report those cases that are diagnostically confirmed.

In contrast, syndromic surveillance is far more concerned with the timely detection of events and the ability to identify and monitor trends. Syndromic surveillance systems generally assume that certain conditions will result in behaviors that produce records and then compare and evaluate those records to detect disease trends in terms of deviations from historical norms. A typical syndromic surveillance system for influenza might evaluate all chief complaint records from emergency departments across a state and look for spikes in complaints of ILI itself, whether those patients test positive for influenza or not. The underlying assumption of syndromic surveillance is that detecting a spike in ILI provides nearly as much information as detecting a spike in actual diagnoses of influenza, but that the information can be obtained more quickly and potentially at a lower cost.

Since the mid-1990s, states, counties, and municipalities have implemented a number of types of syndromic surveillance systems. Most commonly, areas collect emergency department (ED) chief complaint data. These ED systems involve daily reporting of the reasons patients seek emergency services to a centralized public health department located in the city, the county, or the state (e.g., the International Society for Disease Surveillance (ISDS) Distribute Project (ED ILI Syndromic Aggregation) http://isdsdistribute.org). Other types of syndromic surveillance systems track over-the-counter pharmacy sales data (usually in cooperation with a major credit card company), hospital, or public health clinic admissions, or electronic diagnostic lab records, or obtain data from emergency services or

911 call centers, poison control centers, or information on school attendance (Lesesne et al., working paper). Following the Al Qaeda terrorist attacks and the subsequent anthrax exposures in the fall of 2001, the federal government vastly enhanced the amount of funding available to support syndromic surveillance systems. As of 2008, approximately 54 states, counties, or municipalities had implemented some form of syndromic surveillance system (Lesesne et al., working paper).

Syndromic surveillance systems were originally envisioned as early warning systems to detect bioterrorist attacks, acts of sabotage, emerging infections such as pandemic influenza, or contamination of the food or water supply. Policy makers feared that traditional surveillance systems—which often rely on weekly, monthly, or even quarterly reports from participating surveillance sites—would be too slow to detect rapidly emerging health trends. In theory, by monitoring near- to real-time syndromic information, health threats could be detected earlier, and this additional time could be used to contain the damage of the health threat.

However, early warning represents only one possible use for syndromic surveillance systems and traditional surveillance systems may be just as timely as syndromic surveillance systems in detecting extreme health events because providers are motivated to report these events to health departments. Even when syndromic surveillance systems provide early detection, these signals may be missed or misinterpreted. For example, the Google Flu Trends system could have provided early detection of the Mexican swine flu outbreak in the spring of 2009, except that it was not focused on Mexico (Madrigal, 2009). Furthermore, it is unclear whether early syndromic detection could be translated into appropriately vigorous policy action, given the difficulties in motivating appropriate outbreak responses even in the face of existing traditional surveillance information. In practice, the information from syndromic surveillance systems is far more often used to enhance the day-to-day situation awareness of public health professionals than to provide early warning of previously undetected health threats.

Situation awareness (see Chapter 3) refers to the mental ability to comprehend the dynamics of a situation within a finite area of space and time. Situation awareness has been subdivided into three basic concepts: (1) perception of the basic problem or challenge, (2) comprehension or understanding of the mechanisms underlying the problem, and (3) projection of information or the ability to forecast future events or changes (Endsley 2000). Syndromic surveillance systems are potentially most valuable in enhancing comprehension of how a health threat is manifesting itself in a specific context over time and in helping to predict where the health threat is most likely to spread in the future.

16.3 The North Carolina Disease Event Tracking and Epidemiological Collection Tool

The monitoring of the 2007 heat wave by the North Carolina Division of Public Health and the response it enabled represents an archetypical example of using syndromic surveillance to enhance situation awareness of an emerging crisis. The North Carolina Disease Event Tracking and Epidemiological Collection Tool (NC DETECT) is among the nation's leading syndromic surveillance information systems. According to Dr. Jean-Marie Maillard, Director of the Communicable Disease Branch in the North Carolina Division of Public Health, prior to NC DETECT, public health data in North Carolina had not changed much since the Centers for Disease Control and Prevention (CDC) installed Epi Info™ in the health department offices in 1987. Before NC DETECT, North Carolina's Division of Public Health relied on traditional surveillance methodologies, such as physician and lab reports of nationally notifiable diseases as mandated by state law, sentinel influenza reporting, and national annual surveys for chronic conditions such as diabetes. These data were often incomplete and weeks to months old by the time they reached the health department and failed to track the vast majority of health conditions and injuries. State health officials had long wanted a better surveillance system for North Carolina, but the funds to support such a system were out of reach.

Following the terrorist attacks of 2001, Washington, DC, grew increasingly interested in surveillance and funded the development of systems that could provide early warning and detection of future attacks. Dr. Leah Devlin, then the state health director, and others at the division viewed the new source of funding as an opportunity to develop the type of comprehensive monitoring and surveillance system they had long thought North Carolina needed. Health officials decided to use the newly available surveillance monies to vastly expand a small pilot project run by the University of North Carolina at Chapel Hill. Led by Dr. Anna Waller, that project was attempting to get hospital admission data reported back to the University on a daily basis, and Waller was interested in the greater reach and funding her project could obtain through collaboration with the state. Together, State Health Department officials, the North Carolina Hospital Association, Waller, and her team of researchers envisioned a system that would take chief complaint information and other admission notes entered into a computerized ED record system from EDs across the state and route that information to the health department on a daily basis. Real-time reports of these data could then be generated twice daily for the health department to use to track health impacts regionally and among specific population groups.

Initially, most of the work in developing the system involved convincing new EDs to launch the system. In 2003, approximately 1 year after initiating NC DETECT, only about 12% of all ED visits were covered by the system. For the system to be truly useful to health officials, more EDs had to participate. In 2004, in a major breakthrough, the North Carolina General Assembly enacted a bill mandating that all state EDs report their data to the NC DETECT system (North Carolina General Assembly 2004). As of 2009, North Carolina remained the only U.S. state with such a reporting mandate on the books. Following passage of the bill, ED coverage increased from 25% of all ED visits in 2004 to nearly 97% of visits by 2007. NC DETECT system grew in other ways over that time period as well, incorporating information from the Carolinas Poison Center, the emergency medical system, and the Piedmont Wildlife Center (a regional center located in the center of the state).

Although the justification for the NC DETECT system had always been to provide early warning and thus information to protect against bioterrorist attacks or emerging infections,* between 2001 and 2003 the NC DETECT system was being used to enhance situation awareness of known threats. For example, in 2003, the system was actively monitored to try to detect imported cases of severe acute respiratory syndrome (SARS) although only one case of SARS was diagnosed in North Carolina. In an attempt to demonstrate the value of a system like NC Detect, in 2003 the Division of Public Health attempted to replicate the data gained from the system from nonparticipating emergency departments in order to monitor the health effects of Hurricane Isabel. The manual collection of data demonstrated the value of the NC DETECT system since the manual collection of data was very time consuming and costly. By 2007, with record heat scorching North Carolina, the NC DETECT system was fully in place and ready to monitor a public health situation across the state in real time.

16.4 "Exactly What You Go to School For"

In the summer of 2007, Rhonda Roberts, a 27-year-old with a master's degree in epidemiology and biostatistics from the University of South Carolina, was an employee of the North Carolina Division of Public Health. Roberts was an example of the many Americans who had moved to North Carolina from other parts of the United States since the early 1990s. Like many of these

* The mandate states that the purpose of the system is to track "threats that may result from (i) a terrorist incident using nuclear, biological, or chemical agents or (ii) an epidemic or infectious, communicable, or other disease."

transplants, Roberts did not mind the heat, having moved from her native Michigan to escape the winter cold. "I knew it was hot because everyone was complaining, and you know, the air conditioning isn't working right, but for me the heat just meant more time in the pool," Roberts told me when I spoke with her.

On August 8, 2007, with the temperature in downtown Raleigh reaching nearly 103°F, officials at the Division Public Health, including the future N.C. State Health Director, Dr. Jeffrey Engel, the Department's Public Information Officer at the time, Debbie Crane, and Dr. Jean-Marie Maillard decided to use the NC DETECT system to track the impacts of the heat. Dr. Maillard e-mailed Roberts and asked her to query the system regarding the heat, although at first, neither Maillard nor Roberts were exactly sure what they were looking for. The NC DETECT system provided a lot of data, but it had never been used to track a heat wave before, and it was unclear whether the effects of heat would be seen in emergency department visit records. At the division's request, Amy Ising and Clifton Barnett of Anna Waller's University of North Carolina team built a filter or record selection algorithm to select patient records in the NC DETECT database that had information that might indicate a heat-related hospital visit. Roberts then ran that filter on the data and searched through the free text portion of those records to get a sense of why people were being admitted for heat-related reasons.

The system's functionality allowed Roberts to analyze records of patients who visited emergency departments for obvious indicators of heat distress, such as chief complaints of dehydration or heat exhaustion, as well as for less obvious indicators of heat-related distress, such as "passed out on the football field" or "felt dizzy when gardening." Roberts was not sure whether she would find anything as she methodically plotted the chief complaint data, but once she organized her data into graphs, she knew she was looking at something important.

"I thought something went wrong," Roberts recalled, "because they [the heat admissions and the temperature trends] were so right together. It was like a perfect epidemiological story." Her figures indicated that the hottest days of the summer were associated with the highest peaks in cases. She shared the graphs with Dr. Maillard who suggested she plot the number of cases directly against the daily high temperature reported at Raleigh Durham Airport (Figure 16.1). Again, the results, reported back to Maillard a few days later, were striking. From August 3 to August 11, North Carolina experienced a dramatic surge in heat-related emergency department visits, peaking at between 150 and 160 admissions per day on August 8 and 9. Although heat-related admissions were lower before and after the worst days of the heat, looking back over the summer, each temperature increase was accompanied by a corresponding increase in heat-related admissions. Roberts was excited; as she recalled, "This was exactly what you go to school for in epidemiology. You look at that graph and anyone can see that pattern."

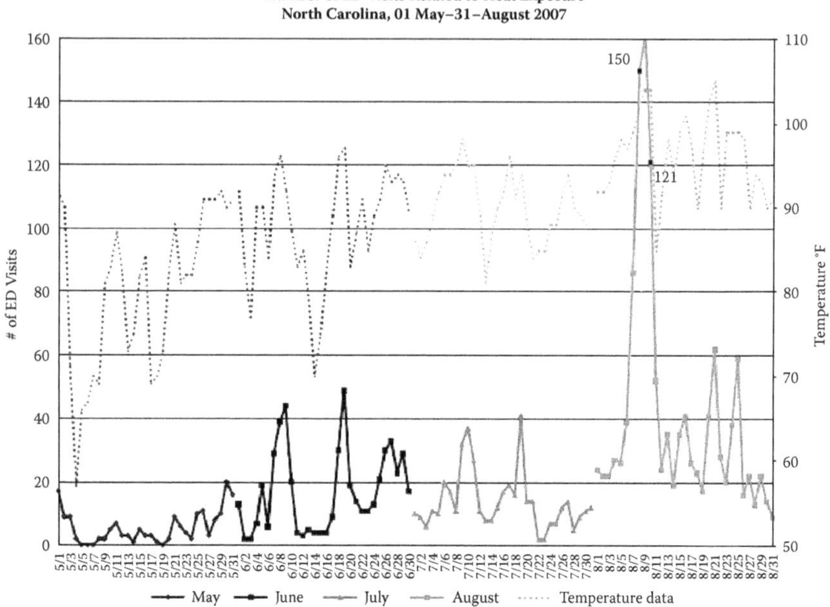

FIGURE16.1
A snapshot of situation awareness: final version of North Carolina Division of Public Health's graphic plotting heat-related admissions by date.

Still, it's not exactly revelatory to learn that emergency department visits for heat exhaustion increase when it is hot. The fact that the NC DETECT system picked up surges in heat-related admissions when it was supposed to indicated that it was working as designed. It remained to be seen whether this information could be translated into effective programmatic changes.

At Dr. Maillard's suggestion, Roberts began to analyze the characteristics of the patients being admitted for heat-related illnesses. Based on the past extreme heat episodes, such as those in Chicago and Europe, conventional wisdom at the time held that the elderly and small children were at the greatest risk from the heat. For example, CDC's standard media advisory defines children under 4, persons aged 65 and older, or other older people who are overweight as being at highest risk of heat-related illness (CDC Office of Enterprise Communications 2009). As of June 30, 2007, North Carolina's heat recommendations mirrored those of CDC.

> "Children, the elderly, people with chronic illnesses, and people on certain medications like tranquilizers or diuretics are especially at risk from high summer temperatures. So are older people who live in homes or apartments without air conditioning or good air-flow, and people who don't drink enough water. Hot weather also adds to ozone levels, making those with respiratory illness more vulnerable (NC DHHS Public Affairs 2007)."

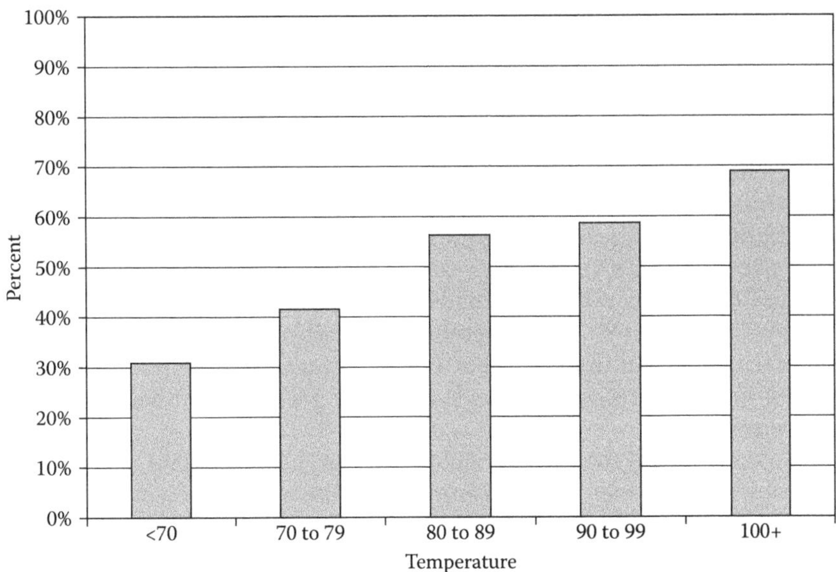

FIGURE 16.2
Percentage of heat-related emergency department admissions identified in the NC DETECT data among men aged 18 to 64 by temperature, January 1, 2006, to August 29, 2007.

However, when Roberts looked at it, the NC DETECT data told a different story. Rather than seeing a spike in the number of children and the elderly succumbing to the heat, the data revealed that working-age men were most at risk.

In 2007, men aged 18 to 64 comprised approximately 28% of the North Carolina population. If men in this age category were really at normal or lower risk of heat-related injuries, then it would follow that they would comprise a smaller percentage of the heat-related ED admissions than their proportion of the population, but that was not what the NC DETECT data indicated. In August 2007, men aged 18 to 64 were responsible for more than 62% of ED visits for heat, more than double the amount expected if they were at normal risk (U.S. Census Bureau 2009a, 2009b). In contrast, the groups thought to be at the highest risk for heat-related illness were in fact disproportionately underrepresented. Children aged 0 to 4 comprised 7% of North Carolina's population but contributed only 1.5% of the heat-related admissions in August. Similarly, adults aged 65 and older comprised 12% of North Carolina's population but contributed only 9% of the heat-related admissions.

The NC DETECT data also indicated a dose response between the heat and the risk for working-age men; as the temperatures grew warmer, the risk among working-age men grew more extreme (Figure 16.2). Between January 1, 2006, and August 29, 2007, excluding fire-related injuries, an estimated 727 ED visits for heat-related causes were reported to the NC DETECT system.

Of these, approximately 2% occurred when the maximum temperature recorded at Raleigh Durham Airport was lower than 70°F, 3% when the temperature was between 70° and 79°F, 23% when the temperature was between 80° and 89°F, 48% when the temperature was between 90° and 99°F, and 24% when the temperature was 100°F or greater.

When the temperature was less than 70°F, men aged 18 to 64 comprised approximately 31% of the total heat-related ED visits, a percentage that was statistically indistinguishable from the percentage of males aged 18 to 64 in the population (28%). However, as the temperature increased, so did the share of ED visits by men aged 18 to 64; from 42% at a temperature between 70° and 79°F up to 69% at temperatures exceeding 100°F. In contrast, at no temperature did children aged 0 to 4 or adults aged 65 and older comprise a share of total heat cases that was statistically greater than their proportion of the population.

Roberts evaluated the free text field of the NC DETECT data to get a better sense of why adult men were succumbing to the heat at such disproportionate numbers. Based on information supplied by the patients and contained in NC DETECT, she categorized male heat-related ED visits into those that occurred at work, home, or during recreational activities; those that were related to excessive alcohol consumption; and those among the homeless (Figure 16.3). The majority of heat-related admissions among men were work related, followed by a small surge among high school–aged boys who played sports. Admissions related to other causes contributed only a small degree to the surge of admissions seen in August 2007.

When Dr. Maillard received this information and shared it with other senior staff at the Division of Public Health, they quickly realized that their strategy to mitigate the impacts of heat waves was missing a key demographic group. Rather than children and the elderly exhibiting the greatest observable impact from the heat, as had been the pattern in Chicago and Western Europe in previous heat waves, North Carolina was experiencing a surge in heat-related injuries among healthy working-age men. What was different in North Carolina, and how could this information be put to use?

Health department staff speculated that farm laborers and construction workers might be responsible for the bulk of the surge in admissions. Although not noticed at the time, the NC DETECT data reveal that 20.8% of heat-related admissions in August occurred in the rural areas of Raleigh and Kinston, North Carolina, where the bulk of the state's tobacco farming takes place (U.S. Census Bureau 2009a). A 2008 CDC report supports the anecdotal evidence from NC DETECT that farm-workers in general and tobacco farmers in particular are at a highly elevated risk of heat-related illness because of their need to wear thick protective clothing to avoid tobacco poisoning while harvesting (CDC 2008).

Some observers speculated that the building boom of the mid-2000s might also be contributing to the surge in emergency room admissions. In August 2007, North Carolina had issued more than 28,500 building permits over

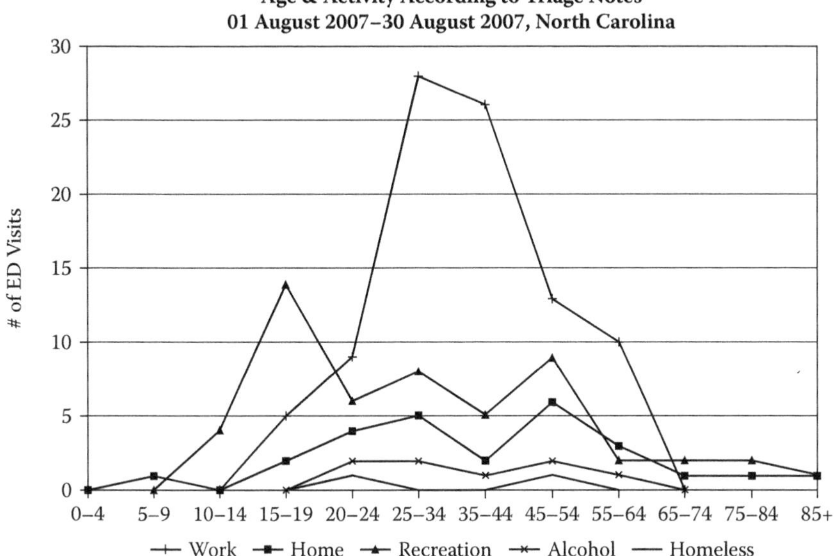

FIGURE 16.3
North Carolina Division of Public Health's August 2007 Analysis of the Causes of Heat-Related Emergency Department Admissions Among Men.

the past 6 months with a declared value of $5.6 billion. Although this was slightly lower than the summer of 2006, it was still far higher than historical norms. With the rush to construct so many buildings so quickly, it was possible that workers were being pushed to work longer hours in the hot sun than they would have been if construction demands had been lower.

Whatever the cause, by mid-August 2007, it was clear to health department staff that outdoor workers were the primary victims of the record heat and that the state had done little to that point to target public education activities to them. Even in mid-August 2007, halfway through one of the most extensive periods of extreme heat in the state's history, North Carolina's heat advisories were still directed primarily toward children and the elderly. Dr. Maillard and others revised the heat advisory and circulated it around the health department for comments and prepared a press release to get the word out. By August 28, with temperatures again climbing near 95°F in many parts of the state, and less than 3 weeks after Rhonda Roberts first queried the NC DETECT system, the state officially changed its heat advisory and disseminated a press release to the public, which resulted in a flurry of news reports.

State health director Leah Devlin was quoted by multiple print and TV sources as saying, "We need to talk to those people [adult males] and tell them they can become sick as a result of excessive heat. In particular, they need to watch their exertion level and remain hydrated. In the future we'll be talking to those people." New warnings to adult men who work outside were carried by the WRAL evening news in Raleigh. The *Raleigh News and Observer* ran the story on August 28 and 29. In the excitement and rush to get the message out, records were not kept on each press report; however, Roberts, Maillard, and Devlin all report that information about changes in the heat recommendations were carried widely over English- and Spanish-language radio following the press release. The health department staff were exhilarated with the results. As Roberts said, "It was a lot of fun. We discovered something novel. Newspapers published the information, and things got done."

16.5 Conclusions

It is difficult to determine the extent to which the news advisories resulted in direct health benefits making it difficult to quantify the impact of the NC DETECT on health benefits. Theoretically, targeting health bulletins to those at highest risk as opposed to those at relatively lower risk intuitively makes a lot of sense. Preliminary statistical evidence suggests that North Carolina experienced fewer heat-related admissions in September of 2007 than on days of similar temperatures that occurred earlier in the summer and that working age men were responsible for this decrease (Rein et al., working paper). However, these statistical analyses are as yet unpublished and merely show an association between the time period following the announcement and lower heat admissions as opposed to a causal relationship. Still, this use of the NC DETECT serves as a case study, demonstrating the value of syndromic surveillance to track public health events in real time.

Syndromic surveillance represents a new technology that uses administrative records to identify and track emerging trends in public health. Although first envisioned as an early warning system, syndromic surveillance is potentially more useful as a tool for enhancing situation awareness of public health events. The story of using North Carolina's NC DETECT system to monitor the 2007 summer heat wave provides some important lessons in both the possible uses of syndromic surveillance and the contextual details that facilitate its use. The comprehensiveness of the systems statewide coverage and the systems flexibility greatly enhanced the systems utility in shaping real-time changes in health policy. NC DETECT's high coverage levels were achieved through a statewide mandate requiring the participation of all emergency rooms across the state, a situation unique to North Carolina as of 2009. Much of the systems flexibility resulted from the strong partnership developed between the North Carolina Division of Public Health and the University of North Carolina. This longstanding collaboration allowed policy makers to quickly translate their needs to academics and programmers who could develop the appropriate filter to investigate heat admissions.

The story illustrates how emerging syndromic surveillance systems represent complimentary enhancements of the traditional surveillance systems and methods. Syndromic surveillance is inaccurately envisioned by many as a cold and automated system designed to provide early detection of anticipated threats using specially developed computerized algorithms. While syndromic surveillance systems can play this role, the story of the NC DETECT system's use to track the heat wave of 2007 demonstrates that these systems are living systems that could be integrated into public health practice, used to challenge conventional wisdom, and ask new questions.

References

Centers for Disease Control and Prevention (CDC), Office of Enterprise Communications. 2009. Media advisory: Tips on managing heat. http://www.cdc.gov/media/pressrel/a980722.htm (accessed August 10, 2009).

Centers for Disease Control and Prevention (CDC). 2008. Heat-related deaths among crop workers—United States, 1992–2006. *MMWR Morbidity Mortality Weekly Report*; 57:649–53.

Das, D., K. Metzger, R. Heffernan, S. Balter, D. Weiss, and F. Mostashari. 2005. Monitoring over-the-counter medication sales for early detection of disease outbreaks—New York City. *MMWR Morbidity and Mortality Weekly Report* 54 Suppl: 41–46.

Dematte, J. E., K. O'Mara, J. Buescher, C. G. Whitney, S. Forsythe, T. McNamee, R. B. Adiga, and I. M. Ndukwu. 1998. Near-fatal heat stroke during the 1995 heat wave in Chicago. *Annals of Internal Medicine* 129 (3): 173–81.

Endsley, M. R. 2000. Theoretical underpinnings of situation awareness: A critical review. In *Situation analysis and measurement*, ed. M. R. Endley and D. J. Garland. Mahwah, NJ: Lawrence Erlbaum and Associates.

Ginsberg, J., M. H. Mohebbi, R. S. Patel, L. Brammer, M. S. Smolinski, and L. Brilliant. 2009. Detecting influenza epidemics using search engine query data. *Nature* 457 (7232): 1012–14.

Hansen, J. E. 2009. Common sense climate index, climate index for individual stations. Goddard Institute for Space Studies 2005. http://data.giss.nasa.gov/csci/stations/ (accessed August 5, 2009).

Hansen, J. E., M. Sato, J. Glascoe, and R. Ruedy. 1998. A common-sense climate index: Is climate changing noticeably? *Proceedings of the National Academies of Science of the United States of America* 95 (8): 4113–20.

Klineberg, E. 2002. *Heat wave: A social autopsy of disaster in Chicago*. Chicago: Chicago University Press.

Kosatsky, T. 2005. The 2003 European heat waves. *Eurosurveillance* 10 (7): 148–49.

Lesesne, S. B., P. J. Leese, L. Rojas-Smith, and D. B. Rein. 2008. Working paper. Characteristics and geographic dispersion of syndromic surveillance systems in the United States in 2008.

Madrigal, A. 2009. Google could have caught swine flu early. Wired. Condé Nast Digital. http://www.wired.com/wiredscience/2009/04/google-could-have-caught-swine-flu-early/ (accessed August 5, 2009).

NC DHHS Public Affairs. 2009. N.C. Public Health tips for beating the heat. North Carolina Division of Public Health and Human Services 2007. http://www.dhhs.state.nc.us/pressrel/2008/2008-6-30-tips-heat.htm (accessed August 10, 2009).

NOAA. 2007. Warm summer in U.S. ends with record heat in South, widespread drought continues in Southeast, West. NOAA 2007-049. Washington, DC: NOAA.

North Carolina General Assembly. 2004. Emergency department data reporting 130A-480.

North Carolina Rural Economic Development Center, Inc. 2009. Rural data bank: Population in North Carolina 2005. http://www.ncruralcenter.org/databank/trendpage_Population.asp (accessed July 28, 2009).

Rein, D. B., S. B. Lesesne, L. Rojas-Smith. Working paper. The impact of heat advisories on heat-related emergency department admissions in North Carolina in 2007.

U.S. Census Bureau. 1995. Urban and rural population: 1900 to 1990. http://www.census.gov/population/www/censusdata/files/urpop0090.txt.

U.S. Census Bureau. 2009a. North Carolina state and county quick facts. http://quickfacts.census.gov/qfd/states/37000.html (accessed August 11, 2009).

U.S. Census Bureau. 2009b. Projections of the population, by age and sex, of states: 1995 to 2025. http://www.census.gov/population/projections/state/stpjage.txt (accessed August 11, 2009).

17

Linking Detection to Effective Response

Scott F. Wetterhall, MD, MPH
RTI International
Atlanta, Georgia

Taha A. Kass-Hout, MD, MS
Atlanta, Georgia

David L. Buckeridge, MD, PhD
McGill Clinical and Health Informatics
McGill University
Montreal, Quebec, Canada

CONTENTS

17.1 Current Operation of the Public Health Response System

Biosurveillance serves as a cornerstone of epidemiology in public health practice, while epidemiology—the study of the distribution of diseases and their determinants in populations—provides the framework for designing and shaping effective responses to current and emerging health threats that menace society. To successfully link the activities and outputs of detection systems to effective responses, one must understand the origins and operations of the current public health system.

In the United States, legal responsibility for public health largely developed as a local phenomenon, with temporary entities initially created to address acute threats from epidemics of infectious diseases. In the 1850s, for example, in New Orleans, officials appointed a Sanitary Commission to investigate the yellow fever outbreak of 1853 in this thriving seaport enriched by international commerce; the commission dissolved after the epidemic threat had passed (Freedman 1951). Attempts to create a federal presence in public health, the National Board of Health, were short-lived, lasting only 4 years, after which Congress refused its reauthorization (Smillie 1943). In ensuing decades, as additional local and state health departments became established on a more permanent basis, the collection and reporting of information on persons with infectious diseases became more standardized and systematic (Koo and Wetterhall 1996). During the first half of the 20th century, the duties of state and local health departments continued to grow, with outreach into broader fields, such as those of maternal and child health and environmental health (e.g., milk pasteurization) (Parran 1945). Concomitantly, the role of the federal public health authorities continued to expand, both as a recipient of surveillance information as well as through growth in other activities of the Public Health Service, which provided consultative and technical assistance to many state and local health authorities.

During the latter half of the 20th century, with the creation of the Centers for Disease Control and Prevention (CDC), the federal role in public health continued to grow, both in providing direct financial support to state and local health departments, as well as in providing scientific leadership in designing and implementing public health surveillance systems (Etheridge 1992). In the aftermath of the anthrax outbreak of 2001, which some considered a period of infamy for medical and public health response (Gersky 2003), there followed an unparalleled surge in resources to bolster public health preparedness and response. With a flurry of activity, the federal government provided unprecedented amounts of money ($918 million and $125 million in fiscal year 2002 in cooperative agreements with CDC and HRSA, respectively) to hire staff and create systems, at all levels of public health—local, state, and federal—for early detection and response to emerging health threats (U.S. Government Accountability Office [GAO] 2004).

This flurry of new activity has been undertaken within a diverse public health system, one whose complexity reflects its incremental development, varied local origins, and differing legal authorities, sources of fiscal support, and diverse stakeholders. Currently, there are approximately more than 2,500 local health departments in the United States. These vary considerably by staffing and size. Some, such as those in large metropolitan areas like New York City, boast large staffs of professionals, many of whom have advanced degrees in public health. Most local health departments, however, are quite small; nationally, the median full-time staff size of local health departments is 20 (range 1 to 21,700), and the majority serve jurisdictions with fewer than 50,000 population (Fraser 1998). In some rural areas, the local health department office may comprise a clerical staff member and an itinerant public health nurse. The legal organization of local health departments varies, from a centralized state health department with no independent local health department jurisdictions to a fully decentralized system with relatively autonomous local entities. The focus on individual patient care varies from jurisdictions in which delivery to underserved populations is the paramount mission and highest priority to those that provide no clinical services (and thus rely upon other aspects of the health care sector to make these provisions). Not surprisingly, some local health departments function as a key component in a well-integrated local system of community governance that includes other agencies (e.g., hospitals, emergency medical services, and emergency management) that would be called upon to respond to a disaster, whereas other health departments have limited connectivity and interaction with these response sectors.

Public health surveillance has been concisely characterized by CDC as "the ongoing, systematic collection, analysis, and interpretation of health data essential to the planning, implementation, and evaluation of public health practice." (CDC 1988). Despite nuanced attempts to refine this definition over the years, this 1988 definition still holds, as does the old saw that, "all surveillance is local," a perspicacious phrase inspired by Tip O'Neill's prescient commentary on our political system. Surveillance is locally grounded primarily because the first inkling that something may be amiss typically arises in proximity to its initial occurrence. Public health surveillance is also best characterized as cyclical (Buckeridge and Cadieux 2007), with steps ranging from identifying individual cases to detecting population patterns to conveying information for action (Figure 17.1).

With such a local focus and emphasis on actionable intelligence, the infection control practitioner at the community hospital will call the local health department's communicable disease nurse after a patient who was seen in the emergency department is belatedly diagnosed with measles. Or the local child care operator will call the health department seeking information after one of her staff members is diagnosed with a shigella infection. Or an astute physician will suspect foul play when a blood culture comes back positive for *B. anthracis*, the causative organism of anthrax (CDC 2001).

Detection signals may emerge from a variety of sources—telephone calls from astute observers (e.g., the local infectious disease physician), clinical laboratory reports, local newspaper articles on increased school absenteeism, and alerts generated by syndromic surveillance systems that are automatically combing through electronic records from emergency departments. Regardless of the source of the signal, the public health profession, largely through the leadership of the CDC, has developed and adopted a robust

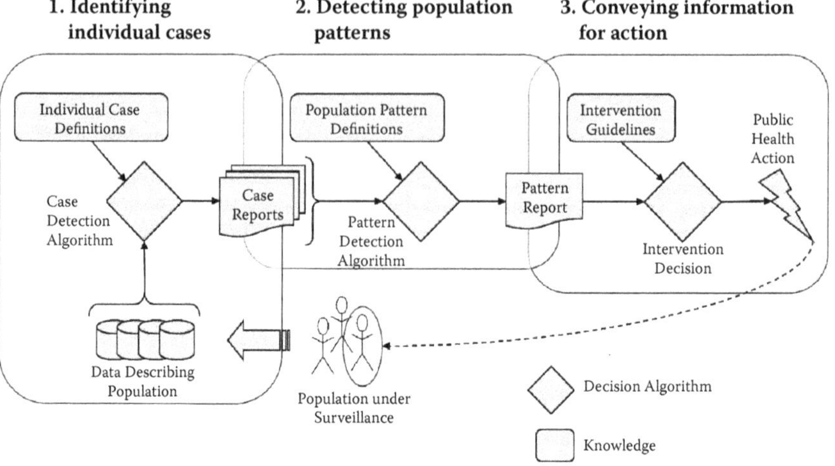

FIGURE 17.1
Public health surveillance cycle. (From Buckeridge, D. and Cadieux, G. 2007. Surveillance for newly emerging viruses. In *Emerging Viruses in Human Populations,* Vol. 16, ed. Edward Tabor, The Netherlands: Elsevier, 325–343. With permission.)

process for systematically assessing and responding to acute public health problems. For decades, the systematic steps of the epidemiologic field investigation have repeatedly been used to successfully identify the cause and guide the response to a public health emergency (Goodman 1990). The first three steps in the process are to

1. Confirm the diagnosis
2. Establish that an outbreak is occurring
3. Identify additional cases

These initial steps, which frequently are undertaken concurrently rather than sequentially, are those that are most germane to the discussion of linking detection to effective response. Confirming the diagnosis involves establishing that the signal that has been detected is a "true" signal. For example, the child with a cough, conjunctivitis, and a runny nose may be suspected of having measles, but before taking additional public health actions (such as recommending use of gamma globulin for exposed pregnant women), one would typically wait for disease confirmation with a positive laboratory test for measles. Establishing that an outbreak is occurring may require referencing historical data, as well as examining other sources of information. For example, a sudden uptake in school absenteeism in a rural county's high school in Virginia in early October one year was suspected by the newly hired local health officer to be a harbinger of a respiratory outbreak, perhaps a novel H1N1 infection. His concerns were dispelled only after his communicable disease nurse, a long-term resident of the community, pointed out that the opening of deer season coincided with the increase in absenteeism. Once an outbreak has been confirmed, however, efforts typically focus on identifying additional cases. In the typical parlance of biosurveillance, this phase of the investigation focuses on "situation awareness." Such awareness provides public health officials and others with a sense of the magnitude of the problem, helping them to craft and temper their response. Equally important, however, is the need to find additional cases whose experiences may shed light on the nature and route of exposure, and, thus, direct selection of the appropriate public health interventions.

17.2 Current Strengths and Weaknesses of the Public Health Detection and Response System

17.2.1 Physical and Electronic Connectivity

One of the most dramatic transformations that public health system has undergone in strengthening its capacity to detect and respond to acute and emerging health threats has been the improved connectedness that now characterizes its communications operations on a global basis. Not too many decades ago, state and local health departments used to rely primarily upon written communications—notifiable disease forms or, during circumstances that warranted greater urgency, a telephone call, from a physician to a local or state health agency (Koo and Wetterhall, 1996). The growth of the Internet and other technological advances has dramatically altered how health officials both learn of disease outbreaks as well as implement their control measures.

A variety of systems have been developed to accelerate the discovery of outbreaks of known and emerging pathogens. Examples include ProMED-mail, an Internet-based system sponsored by the International Society for Infectious Diseases. ProMED-mail uses reports from members and media reports to identify acute infectious disease outbreaks in humans, animals, and plants. It has grown from a small private e-mail list of interested scientists to a fully moderated Listserv that currently connects more than 30,000 e-mail recipients in 180 countries (Madoff and Woodall 2005). The global Public Health Intelligence Network is a subscription-based system operated by Health Canada that scans thousands of electronic media reports using data mining methodologies. The Global Emerging Infectious Surveillance and Response System (GEIS) is operated by the U.S. Department of Defense and utilizes overseas medical research laboratories to conduct clinical and laboratory surveillance. GEIS shares information with the World Health Organization (WHO), CDC, and other government agencies (Hitchcock et al. 2007). Operating since September 2006, HealthMap brings together disparate data sources to achieve a unified and comprehensive view of the current global state of infectious diseases and their effect on human and animal health (Brownstein et al. 2008). Data sources of varying reliability range from news sources (such as Google News) to curated personal accounts (such as ProMED-mail) to validated official alerts (such as WHO). Through an automated text processing system, the data is aggregated by disease and displayed on a freely available Web site (http://www.healthmap.org) by location for user-friendly access to the original alert. In parallel to these automated efforts, HealthMap has built a community component, whereby site users are able to contribute to and curate data.

In addition to enhancing early detection of threats, new technologies and management approaches have facilitated the targeting and guiding of intervention efforts. A number of medical journals have modified the so-called Inglefinger rule to prepublish electronic versions of articles of significant importance. The CDC's MMWR has, over the past decade, accelerated its editorial process to allow electronic publication of information and guidance for important breaking events (dispatches). The anthrax outbreak of 2001 illustrated the need for timely provision of guidance to public health officials, medical providers, and the public during a complex and rapidly evolving situation. At the time, CDC was subjected to criticism for its inability to provide timely and definitive answers to a host of novel challenges and unique circumstances (Gursky 2003). More recently, in contrast, in responding to the threats posed by pandemic influenza, the U.S. government created a Web site, www.flu.gov, that is described as "one-stop access to U.S. government H1N1, avian, and pandemic flu information." The site is populated with transcripts of press conferences and recommendations created by CDC and its partners to address a variety of circumstances in the home, school, and workplace. It also provides answers to frequently asked questions and other relevant information.

Member states of the WHO are bound by the International Health Regulations, which mandates reporting of a small group of specified communicable diseases; prior to their revision in 2005, for other diseases, including newly emerging ones, WHO had to rely upon voluntary reporting from member states (Tucker 2005). The Chinese government delayed reporting the initial outbreak of severe acute respiratory syndrome (SARS) to the WHO when it first emerged in Guangdong Province in late 2002. This failure to report the outbreak resulted in SARS spreading to other countries via international travel and impeded the initial response efforts (WHO 2003).

Countries may choose to suppress notification of disease outbreaks within their borders for a variety of reasons: The outbreak may represent an accidental release of an offensive biological or chemical weapon, as in the anthrax outbreak in Sverdlovsk in 1979 (Meselson et al. 1994). A sovereign state may not wish to publicize the event because it may be a source of embarrassment, exposing inadequate infrastructure (the medical care system, or the system for overseeing food and water safety). A nation may also view itself as "at risk" for becoming stigmatized, as with the recent emergence of novel influenza A (H1N1) in Mexico City (with some U.S. talk show hosts then referring to the illness as "Mexican flu"). Or, perhaps most commonly, a state will wish to minimize any negative economic consequences—the loss of tourism, the prohibition of travel by persons from the affected country, or the outright ban imposed on a country's agricultural products or other critical commodities (Heyman 2006).

Systems such as ProMed-mail, GEIS, and other public health surveillance efforts have illustrated their utility in detecting new and emerging health threats in a highly connected world where the 24-hour news cycle, blogs, Twitter notifications (Tweets), and other forms of near instantaneous communications now reign. One public health official attests that the majority of information about new outbreaks comes from these alternative sources—the Internet and other forms of electronic communications—rather than from voluntary submissions by member states. At the same time, SARS, and more recently novel influenza A (H1N1), can spread rapidly throughout the world, posing new challenges that derive from our enhanced physical connectivity.

17.2.2 Collaboration across Sectors

Despite the availability of accurate and timely information from one of the best and most technologically advanced detection systems in our country, that is, those reports and images from the National Weather Service's National Hurricane Center, the botched preparedness and response to Hurricane Katrina will endure as a historically unprecedented uncoupling of detection and response. The absence of inter-sectoral collaboration has been documented in numerous investigative reports issued by multiple branches and agencies of the government. These documents have described the fundamental failings of multiple governmental agencies at the local, state, and federal level to integrate command structures, share information, communicate effectively with the public, and provide emergency supplies and other forms of relief (Select Bipartisan Committee 2006; U.S. GAO 2007a). Many of the critiques of the government's response to Katrina have emphasized the need for improved situation assessment and awareness, and enhanced emergency communications.

The federal government has committed significant resources in its attempt to improve the coordination of disease detection and situation awareness. Following the issuance of Homeland Security Presidential Directives 9 and 10, the Department of Homeland Security was tasked with creation of the National Biosurveillance Integration Center (NBIC) (Smith 2007). The purpose of the NBIC is to combine information from multiple federal agencies, as well as open source information, to support a timely response to an attack with biological weapons. The NBIC components include a powerful management information system that can sift through massive quantities of data, as well as a bevy of subject matter experts from a range of disciplines who can interpret and provide context for any suspicious patterns that may be detected. CDC, as the nation's lead public health agency, participates as a federal partner in the NBIC. In 2003, CDC initiated its BioSense program, which was initially designed using syndromic (or prediagnostic) data from patients treated at facilities operated by the Departments of Defense and Veterans Affairs, and now, more recently has relied upon obtaining data from existing, state-based syndromic surveillance systems.

Similarly, inter-sectoral collaboration to manage response efforts has improved since Katrina. During the past decade, the federal government has placed a priority on protecting the nation's critical infrastructure (e.g., the 17 sectors: food and agriculture, water, transportation, energy, and others) against disruption from natural and man-made catastrophic events (U.S. GAO 2007b). Each of the critical sectors contains a unique interface between the public and private sectors where policies and actions must be coordinated. To address these challenges, the federal government has developed cross-sector councils that interact with private sector, as well as governmental coordinating councils that coordinate strategies, activities, and policies within a particular sector. In the past few years, as concerns grew about preparations for a possible influenza pandemic, the federal government has worked with the private sector to develop guidance documents, such as checklists for continuity of operations, as well as conducting preparedness drills, workshops, and preparations.

Although the above efforts appear to reflect some progress in coordinating efforts across the various federal sectors, the key measure of our capacity to detect and respond to health threats still resides at the community level. Preparedness and response is a collective effort that involves all community participants—individuals, medical providers, the business sector, the school system, local government agencies and elected officials, and public health officials. Local communities vary in their capacity, as well as commitment, to ensuring their preparedness. The more robust and better prepared communities, compared with those that are less prepared, are typically characterized by having a local health agency that is led by a strong public health official with an appreciation for a population-based perspective on health. The public official is a recognized spokesperson in the local media and a respected arbiter at town hall meetings on matters of health. The lines of authority among the health official, elected officials, and other key stakeholders—the school superintendent, the hospital administrator, and the local emergency manager—are well-understood, respected, and maintained. Key groups, such as operators of child care facilities, as well as those who serve vulnerable populations (including clients of community health centers, residents of long-term care facilities, persons with mental health needs, those who receive home health care, and other recipients of social services) actively participate in planning efforts and all preparedness exercises. Community preparedness is an ongoing process that requires sustained commitment and leadership, qualities that can be found in some, but not all, locales.

17.2.3 Laboratory Capacity for Rapid Diagnosis

During the past decade, growth in laboratory diagnostic capability at all levels of the public health system has been a rare and consistently bright spot on the spectrum of emergency preparedness. In 1998, a survey by the Association of Public Health Laboratories (ASPL) found that only a handful of state laboratories had Biosafety Level 3 (BSL-3) capability (CDC 2007). BSL-3 laboratories have the requisite safety features for processing and testing most infectious agents that can cause serious public health harm, such as highly infectious influenza viruses or anthrax bacteria. Why were there so few of these laboratories available? The general sense at the turn of the 21st century was that the public health infrastructure was woefully inadequate to respond to any emerging infectious disease threats. Years of budget cuts and lack of investment, fueled by ignorance and insufficient advocacy, had taken their toll.

The 1999 Department of Health and Human Services (DHHS) Budget Initiative for Bioterrorism Preparedness, when appropriated into law, became a landmark in reinvigorating the infrastructure of public health, including that of state public health laboratories. Congress provided multiple DHHS agencies—the National Institutes of Health (NIH), the U.S. Food and Drug Administration (FDA), the Agency for Healthcare Research and Quality (AHRQ), and CDC—with funding. CDC's $121 million allocation was used to create the newly minted Bioterrorism Preparedness and Response Program, whose mission was to "upgrade infrastructure and capacity to respond to a large-scale epidemic, regardless of whether it … [was] … the result of a bioterrorist attack or a naturally occurring infectious disease outbreak" (U.S. GAO 2001).

The Laboratory Response Network (LRN), an offspring of the initial bioterrorism budget initiative, was cofounded by the CDC, the Association of Public Health Laboratories (APHL), the Federal Bureau of Investigation (FBI), and the U.S. Army Medical Research Institute of Infectious Diseases (USAMRIID) (Gilchrist 2000). The purpose of the LRN was to create a linkage of local, state, and federal diagnostic laboratories that could be mobilized to provide diagnostic support for any biological threats to humans, both naturally occurring (and emerging) as well as those considered intentional. CDC provided support to the LRN by supplying funding, training, and technical assistance in diagnostic methodology. The number of LRN laboratories has continued to grow each year.

Meanwhile, CDC has invested in its own infrastructure, both reflected in an accelerated construction of new laboratory facilities on its main Atlanta campus, as well as in individual laboratory programs within its centers. Neighborhoods adjacent to the Clifton Road facility were purchased and razed to make room for the expansion. While training provided through the LRN has been credited with facilitating recognition of the 2001 anthrax outbreak in Florida, the same epidemic also forced the creation of new

CDC-based processing entities for handling surges of human specimens. CDC's creation of this processing unit reflects its more general efforts to develop additional rapid diagnostic tests for use by the constituents of the LRN.

The SARS outbreak that began in China in late 2002 served as an unparalleled example of collaboration between the laboratory and epidemiologic sciences. Multidisciplinary CDC and WHO teams descended on sites where cases of SARS first emerged in Hong Kong and Southeast Asia, with (1) early epidemiologic confirmation that the mystery disease was being transmitted from person to person and (2) the suggestion that a single infectious person may be a point source for the outbreak.

Armed with these key parameters, CDC and other labs tested specimens from multiple persons diagnosed with SARS for a variety of plausible pathogens. Their inquiry was bounded by a search for those infectious agents that may be plausibly transmitted person-to-person and may cause upper and lower respiratory illness—the clinical and epidemiologic characteristics of the outbreak at that point. The laboratory assessment proceeded systematically, with initial culture of the putative virus (after select bacterial pathogens had been ruled out), followed by morphologic characterization, and then molecular confirmation that SARS represented a novel infection with a heretofore unrecognized coronavirus. Within weeks of this discovery, member labs of the LRN, as well as other diagnostic labs worldwide, were provided with the molecular primers and other reagents to permit widespread testing for this novel and emergent virus (Ksiazek 2003).

The emergence of novel influenza A (H1N1) in the spring of 2009 heralded another opportunity for CDC and the LRN to demonstrate its diagnostic prowess. In April 2009, CDC diagnosed two patients from California (who were not epidemiologically linked) with infection from a novel influenza A (H1N1) of swine origin. In a matter of months, this novel influenza A virus became pandemic, causing thousands of cases in countries worldwide (Dawood 2009). In June 2007, human infection from novel influenza A virus became a nationally notifiable disease. State health laboratories typically forward influenza isolates that cannot be subtyped using the commonly available subtyping reagents. In 2005, CDC first identified a human case of infection with a triple-reassortant swine influenza A (H1) virus. Triple reassortant viruses contain genetic material from human, swine, and avian influenza strains. In subsequent years, an additional 11 cases of human infection from triple reassortant swine influenza A were detected, and epidemiologic investigations found that a majority of these ill persons had had close or proximate contact with pigs by participating or visiting agricultural fairs (Shinde 2009). CDC developed an FDA-approved real-time RT-PCR test to subtype these swine-origin viruses. When the novel influenza A (H1N1) strains emerged in the two patients from California in April 2009, CDC was able to modify the PCR test to detect this emergent strain and distribute to all the members of the LRN an FDA-approved (under its Emergency Use Authorization) within a matter of days. The rapidity with which this test for this emerging infectious disease arrived in the hands of state public health laboratories (Dawood 2009) was unprecedented.

17.2.4 Workforce Capacity

Public health workers are a diverse group, comprising nurses, physicians, health educators, sanitarians, epidemiologists, and those with other skill sets. In many ways the public health workforce believes in and reflects an enduring faith in the transformative power of social capital. A trained and competent public health workforce is a foundational requirement for ensuring an adequate response to public health threats, regardless of their cause. Recent interest, and concern, about the viability of the public health infrastructure was first prompted by a 2002 Institute of Medicine report that highlighted the fragility of the public health professional workforce (IOM 2002). Others have claimed that workforce shortages in public health are just over the horizon, as an aging population approaches retirement eligibility or seeks opportunity elsewhere. During the past decade, we have seen the size of the public health workforce subjected to larger market forces, with parallel gains realized with rising anxiety about dread diseases and the intentional use of microbes as terrorist weapons, as well as losses accrued in the face of mounting state and local government budget shortfalls.

Prompted, in part, by President Clinton's interest in bioterrorism, which was allegedly sparked by his reading of Richard Preston's *The Cobra Event* (Preston 1997), the Department of Health and Human Services submitted a Fiscal Year 1999 budget initiative to Congress, and Congress allocated $120.8 million to create CDC's Bioterrorism Preparedness and Response Program (U.S. GAO 2001; Nash 2002). In fiscal year 2000, Congress allocated $56.9 million to award to the states and major metropolitan areas. State and local public health agencies used this unexpected but welcome largesse to hire additional personnel, particularly those staff with desirable skills in disciplines such as epidemiology and emergency preparedness. Following 9/11 and the anthrax outbreak, federal outlays to state and large metropolitan health departments grew rapidly and peaked in 2005 (Trust for America's Health 2008). As a result, between 2001 and 2006, the number of epidemiologists employed in state and local public health grew by 40%, according to a series of surveys conducted by the Council of State and Territorial Epidemiologists (CSTE) (Boulton et al. 2009). At the same time, various other measures of preparedness, such as the number of states participating in LRN, showed similar positive gains.

These advances, although quite laudable, may be obscuring some developments that will have serious long-term impact upon the capacity and resiliency of the public health system. While federal dollars were pouring into state coffers to support bioterrorism preparedness, many observers with firsthand knowledge believed that state and local governments were shifting their staff onto positions in these newly funded programs (Gebbie and Turnock 2006). The CSTE survey found that in most states their support for epidemiology programs did not increase between 2001 and 2006, suggesting that federal funds may have supplanted funds that had previously been supported with state and local funds. By 2006, federal funding for state epidemiology programs had increased 9% to 71%. Since 2001, state funding for epidemiology had declined 13% to an average of 23% (Boulton et al. 2009). In 2008, during a period of serious economic decline, at the beginning of what has been called "The Great Recession," a survey of local health departments (LHDs) found that a majority of LHDs had frozen hiring or reduced staff, representing an estimated 7,000 local public health workers nationwide (National Association of County and City Health Officials [NACCHO], 2009).

Thus, in both upward and downward economic times, the federal government has been gaining "market share" as financier of the last resort for public health. However, this societal function—protecting the health and welfare of the public—has traditionally and constitutionally been viewed as a domain of the state and not the federal government. Despite this historical perspective that all public health—and certainly all public health surveillance—is local, public health advocacy groups typically promote an even larger role for the federal government as the solution for the looming crisis facing the public health workforce (Perlino 2006). Suggested solutions include federally funded public health workforce scholarships, additional funding for Health Resources and Services Administration (HRSA) programs, federally funded leadership development programs, and internships and fellowships at agencies such as CDC and NIH. This is not to say that such recommendations lack value; many of them do strive to address important needs. Rather, the cautionary analogy is from an economic market perspective; whenever there is an overreliance within a multi-tiered sector upon one supplier of a critical commodity, that sector can experience significant volatility during both up and down markets. Since 2005, federal support to states for bioterrorism preparedness has begun to decline (Trust for America's Health 2008). We do not yet know what the long-term effects of this will be (perhaps influenza funding will serve as a bridge loan, at least while the current pandemic smolders); but, thus far, state and local governments do not seem to be stepping up to meet their fiscal responsibilities to perform their role in protecting the public's health.

17.3 Maximizing Linkage between Detection and Response

The key to maximizing the linkage between detection and response is dependent upon two critical factors. First, the public health surveillance (or detection) system must have clear objectives, and these objectives must reign paramount in shaping the design of the system. Second, emerging health threats, whether natural or man-made, typically evolve through a series of phases, such as those of pre-impact, impact, and post-impact characteristics of a natural disaster. This has been illustrated by our experiences with Hurricanes Katrina and Rita. Information needs, as well as methods of data collection and analysis, will vary by phase.

17.3.1 System Objectives Should Drive Design

The evolution of syndromic surveillance over the past decade illustrates the importance of setting clear objectives in designing any surveillance system. Initial bioterrorism funds to CDC during 1999–2000 were designed to build "multi-purpose" public health infrastructures for preparedness and response, and, thus, lacked specific directives regarding surveillance activities. Following the anthrax attacks in late 2001, however, CDC and its state and local public health partners began to emphasize the need for early detection of health threats. This is not surprising, considering that the United States felt under siege after the opening of spore-laden letters in the offices of a national news organization and within the Senate mail room. The series of sneak attacks heralded an unprecedented period of uncertainty and anxious dread for health officials and the general public.

Methods for early detection of outbreaks caused by bioterrorist attacks rose to paramount value in the months following 9/11, as concerns about weapons of mass destruction flooded the media during the build up to the 2003 invasion of Iraq (Weiner 2007). Aerial photographs of Saddam Hussein's mobile laboratories for generating stockpiles of offensive biological weapons circulated first in the intelligence community, and then in the mainstream media, providing additional justification for the military buildup to the impending conflict in the Gulf. In December 2002, the president announced a national program to vaccinate health care workers against smallpox. Although some experts in public health viewed this sudden announcement of a national program to vaccinate 50,000 health care workers with skepticism, citing the opaque uncertainty about the likelihood of such an attack, others supported these initiatives and began developing local vaccination strategies for their health care workers. All things considered, these concerns were scientifically credible; a widely cited hypothetical model of an aerosolized anthrax outbreak published in 1997 (Kaufman et al. 1997) clearly demonstrated the value of early detection, particularly in terms of lives saved and economic costs averted.

During the unsettling times between 9/11 and the start of the Gulf II conflict, the CDC states, academic researchers, and the military responded by creating numerous new systems specifically for bioterrorism surveillance. Fueling this growth in surveillance systems was the increasing availability of electronic patient-based data, as well as new methods for analyzing and displaying data (Bravata 2004). Very early detection of disease outbreaks was revered as an "emerging science" (Wagner et al. 2001). Concerned public health professionals formed a Society for International Disease Surveillance (Mandl et al. 2004) dedicated to improving the science basis of early event detection. CDC began to support extramural, peer-reviewed research to improve early event detection while creating a framework for evaluating the capacity of surveillance systems to rapidly detect outbreaks (CDC Working Group 2004).

The development of the BioSense program illustrates the importance of using the objectives of a surveillance system to drive its design. The initial objective of the federally funded BioSense program was to create a national system for early detection of disease outbreaks (Buehler et al. 2009; Eban 2007). CDC initially used DOD and VA data, and hired contractors to build a vast data mining system where detection algorithms would identify potential disease spikes. CDC would oversee the analysis of data and send out alerts to state health departments. A series of false alarms resulted in states being skeptical and prompted concerns that the system being designed and implemented would not and could not meet its overarching object of providing an early warning system (Eban 2009). Critics pointed out that syndromic surveillance systems such as BioSense could only be expected to detect outbreaks of a certain size; the anthrax outbreak of 2001, for example, was simply too small and geographically dispersed to be picked up by a centralized data mining operation at a distant federal facility (Reingold 2003). And, if an outbreak had to have a certain critical numerical mass, could the data mining operation be expected to be more timely than other, more localized efforts led by astute clinicians and local public health officials? Finally, the opportunity costs associated with responding to these externally generated false signals—because the natural consequence of increasing the sensitivity of the system is to decrease specificity and diminish predictive value positive–became too much for resource-strapped state and local health departments to bear.

As a result, the objective of the BioSense system changed from that of early detection to one of providing situation awareness (Eban 2007; Buehler et al. 2009). Situation awareness is the current catchword for public health officials' ability to quickly scan the health service delivery environment to gauge how widespread—or not—a particular health threat might be. For example, reports of influenza-like-illness that typically do not have laboratory confirmation may give a reasonably accurate picture of how widespread influenza activity is within a given locale, particularly when combined with data, including laboratory results, from other sources.

With the infusion of federal preparedness funds, state and local jurisdictions have developed a variety of syndromic surveillance systems, and, in many locales, officials have used these systems to successfully supplement information from other sources. Typically, these local systems have been found to be useful in characterizing situations in which the health threats are widespread, such as those associated with influenza or certain environmental disasters, such as wildfires with smoke exposure (Buehler et al. 2009). Despite a significant investment in the BioSense program, estimated at $184 million by 2008 (U.S. GAO 2008), many state and local health officials viewed the data from the CDC program as less useful than that from their own systems. The common refrain among many local officials was that their input and needs were not considered when the BioSense program was being developed. This lesson for system design is telling. Officials assumed that the objective of the BioSense surveillance system was to design a federally operated and centralized operation first to provide enhanced capability for "early detection," and later—once this objective could not be achieved—to provide "situation awareness." The point that was missed, however, was that the overall objective in designing the BioSense program needed to be guided by appropriate and continuous input from key stakeholders such as state and local health officials. The objective of the BioSense program should have been to create a system that enhanced the capacity of these stakeholders to perform their jobs within their own jurisdictions, not simply to provide data feeds to a federal agency that lacked capacity and clear vision to amplify their utility.

17.3.2 Conducting Surveillance for Emerging Threats

When a public health official is tasked with responding to a novel health threat, his or her institution typically dispatches personnel to gather clinical, observational, laboratory, and environmental information as well as samples. Conducting surveillance for emerging threats is a particularly vexing issue, with many unforeseen challenges (Wetterhall 1996), but monitoring and investigating these threats can be made more effective and efficient by considering the following three tenets:

1. Focus the investigation on the basis of usual routes of exposure for a known pathogen:

   In the ideal world of public health, the practicing epidemiologist in the local health department facing an outbreak of disease in the community will have at his or her disposal a diagnostic laboratory test with perfect attributes—100% sensitivity (to detect true "cases") and 100% specificity (thus not allowing any false positives to blur his or her perception of the epidemic's boundaries). Armed with the certitude afforded by such a gold standard test, the epidemiologist's ability to predict which ill persons are cases and which are not (the test's predictive value positive and negative) would be fail-safe, particularly if she had an inkling as to the route of exposure. Thus, if the putative cause of the outbreak is known—for example, the cluster of schoolchildren in his or her county has been diagnosed with viral hepatitis A—the epidemiologist then merely needs to query the ill persons (and suitable controls) about their recent likely exposures to the virus. A cluster of illness with hepatitis A in schoolchildren would prompt the epidemiologist to ask questions about the sources of food, water, and bodily fluids (perhaps from close, intimate contact with an ill person) that may have occurred during the suspected period of exposure. Oftentimes, such a methodical approach, which is founded on having a reliable laboratory test and familiarity with the organism's likely routes of exposure, can produce results—including detection of foodborne outbreaks of international origin—in a remarkably efficient and timely manner (CDC 1997).

2. Let the epidemiologic investigation refine your understanding of potentially new and plausible routes of exposure:

   Unfortunately, we do not live in the ideal. More so, the norm in first responding to a putative disease outbreak is fragmentary and incomplete knowledge of both the cause of the epidemic, as well as likely routes of exposure. In the anthrax outbreak of 2001, laboratory diagnosis (supported by training of personnel under the LRN efforts) of systemic anthrax infection signaled the initial appearance of the disease cluster. With well-understood familiarity with how humans become ill from *B. anthracis* exposure, initial efforts to identify the source of illness in the index case-patient had teams scouring the recent travel routes in North Carolina for any possible contact with infectious livestock. Once environmental samples from the mailroom of a building in South Florida tested positive, the route of exposure became clearer, and efforts began in earnest to better understand how the U.S. postal system distributed mail (Dewan 2002). Thus, a new mode of exposure of a known pathogen was established. Meanwhile, other public health investigators fanned out over Florida and other places where subsequent laboratory-confirmed cases emerged to seek additional cases. In such circumstances, these investigators, engaging in what later become known as "situation awareness," used a very broad, and hence sensitive, but not very specific, case definition.

3. Support and maintain the laboratory capacity to develop rapid diagnostic tests for novel sources of infection and illness:

   We have already illustrated important examples of having the laboratory capacity to develop new diagnostic tests for previously unrecognized pathogens, both with our international experience with SARS and, more recently, novel influenza A (H1N1) pandemic. The importance of a strong linkage between a well-trained workforce versed in outbreak investigation and control and the capacity to systematically develop and distribute new, reliable diagnostic tests cannot be overestimated. The marriage between shoe-leather epidemiology and state-of-the-art diagnostic capabilities will continue to serve as our strongest bulwark in addressing all of the new threats to health that will surface and gain foothold in the upcoming century. The threats will be new, but the well-regarded, tested paradigm is the same.

4. Future challenges and research needs:

   The specific modifications, refinements, enhancements, and even novel approaches that will improve our ability to detect and respond to public health threats are far too numerous to be enumerated in the space here. Some of these are ably characterized in the ensuing chapters of this book. Rather, we will point out here some larger themes that will need to be addressed, regardless of which specific endeavor or nuanced "tweak" is promoted and adopted. A few of the paramount challenges that need to be addressed in the future are as follows; we need to:

- Refine and continually recommit the process to develop public health surveillance and other detection systems on the basis of *user needs.* This requires full comprehension of the complex operations of the public health system, as well as recognition that, in rapidly developing situations, the information needs—and the means of satisfying them—may be evolving at a similarly brisk pace.
- Develop the political will at all levels of government, not simply the federal level, to support a viable and stable workforce that is well-positioned and committed to facing the dynamic public health challenges in the 21st century—those of emerging infectious diseases, changes in the environment, and other novel threats that will no doubt arise as the world population grows in a setting in which global resources are ultimately finite.
- Continue to support the capacity to develop and deploy novel rapid diagnostic tests. The laboratory plays a critical role in effective response by characterizing the nature of the threat, proving a sense of the distribution and scope of the health threat, and in guiding the choice and implementation of treatment and preventive measures.

17.5 Conclusions

Designing and operating a public health surveillance system is a rather straightforward exercise, almost menu-like in some regards, especially for those experienced in addressing operational issues in a complex and often politically charged environment. Creating a successful one is much more challenging. Be clear, first and foremost, about the intent or purpose of the detection system that you wish to build. Consult with all the key stakeholders who will use or be affected by your surveillance system. Only when you are confident that you can succinctly articulate what their needs and concerns are, and how this system will meet and fulfill their objectives at an acceptable cost, should you proceed. It is not the technology that provides cohesion; only the collective vision of the stakeholders, and their supportive relationships, can provide that.

References

Boulton, M. L., Lemmings, J., and Beck, A. J. 2009. Assessment of epidemiologic capacity in state health departments, 2001–2006. *Journal of Public Health Management and Practice* 15:328–336.

Bravata, D. M., McDonald, K. M., Smith, W. M. et al. 2004. Systematic review: Surveillance systems for early detection of bioterrorism-related diseases. *Annals of Internal Medicine* 140:910–922.

Brownstein, John S., Freifeld, Clark C., Reis, Ben Y., and Mandl. Kenneth D., 2008. Surveillance Sans Frontiers: Internet-based emerging infectious disease intelligence and the HealthMap project. *PLoS Med* 5 (7):6.

Buckeridge, D. and Cadieux, G. 2007. Surveillance for newly emerging viruses. In *Emerging Viruses in Human Populations*, Vol. 16, ed. Edward Tabor, The Netherlands: Elsevier, 325–343.

Buehler, J. W., Whitney, E. A., Smith, D., Prietula, M. J., Stanton, S. H., and Isakov, A. P. 2009. Situational uses of syndromic surveillance. *Biosecurity and Bioterrorism* 7:165–177.

CDC. 1997. Hepatitis A associated with consumption of frozen strawberries—Michigan, March 1997. *Morbidity Mortality Weekly Report (MMWR)* 46:288–297.

CDC. Improving the public health laboratory infrastructure. http://www.bt.cdc.gov/lrn/infrastructure.asp (accessed October 6, 2009).

CDC. 2001. Notice to readers: Ongoing investigation of anthrax—Florida, October 2001. *Morbidity Mortality Weekly Report (MMWR)* 50:877.

CDC. 2009. 2009 Pandemic influenza A (H1N1) virus infections—Chicago, Illinois, April–July 2009. *Morbidity Mortality Weekly Report (MMWR)* 58:913–918.

CDC Working Group. 2004. Framework for evaluating public health surveillance systems for early detection of outbreaks. *MMWR Recommendations and Reports* 53:1–11.

Centers for Disease Control and Prevention. 1988. *CDC Surveillance Update*. Atlanta, GA: CDC.

Chapin, C. V. 1916. *A Report on State Public Health Work*. American Medical Association, Chicago, IL. Reprint published 1977, Arno Press, New York.

Dawood, F. S., Jain, S., Finelli, L. et al., 2009. Emergence of a novel swine-origin influenza A (H1N1) virus in humans. *New England Journal of Medicine* 360:2605–2615.

Dewan, P. K., Fry, A. M., Laserson, K., Tierney, B. C., Quinn, C. P., Hayslett, J. A., et al. 2001. Inhalational anthrax outbreak among postal workers, Washington, D.C., *Emerging Infectious Diseases* 8, no. 10, (October 2002), http://www.cdc.gov/ncidod/EID/vol8no10/02-0330.htm.

Eban, K. 2007. BioSense or Biononsense? *The Scientist* 21:32–39.

Etheridge, E. W. 1992. *Sentinel for Health: A History of the Centers for Disease Control.* Berkeley University of California Press.

Fraser, M. 1998. Preliminary results from the 1997 profile of U.S. local health departments. National Association of County and City Health Officials Research Brief, September 1998, no.1, http://www.naccho.org/topics/infrastructure/research/upload/1997-Research_Brief_1.pdf (accessed September 25, 2009).

Freedman, B. 1951. The Louisiana State Board of Health established 1855. *American Journal of Public Health* 41:1279–1285.

Gebbie, K. M. and Turnock, B. J. 2006. The public health workforce, 2006: New challenges. *Health Affairs* 25:923–933.

Gersky, E., Inglesby, T., and O'Toole, T. 2003. Anthrax 2001: Observations on the medical and public health response. *Biosecurity and Bioterrorism* 1:97–110.

Gilchrist, M. J. R. 2000. A national laboratory network for bioterrorism: Evolution from a prototype network of laboratories routine surveillance. *Military Medicine* 156 (Suppl.):28–34.

Goodman, R. A., Buehler, J. W., and Koplan, J. P. 1990. The epidemiologic field investigation: Science and judgment in public health practice. *American Journal of Epidemiology* 132:9–16.

Heyman, D. L. 2006. SARS and emerging infectious diseases: A challenge to place global solidarity above national sovereignty. *Annals Academy of Medicine* 35:350–353.

Hitchcock, P., Chamberlain, A., Van Wagone, M., Inglesby, T. V., and O'Toole, T. 2007. Challenges to global surveillance and response to infectious disease outbreaks of international importance. *Biosecurity and Bioterrorism* 5:2006–2227.

Institute of Medicine. 2002. *Who Will Keep the Public Healthy? Educating Public Health Professionals for the 21st Century.* Washington, D.C.: National Academies Press.

Kaufman, A. F., Meltzer, M. I., and Schmid, G. P. 1997. The economic impact of a bioterrorist attack: Are prevention and postattack intervention programs justifiable? *Emerging Infectious Diseases* 3:83–94.

Ksiazek, T. G., Erdman, D., Goldsmith, C. S., et al. 2003. A novel coronavirus associated with severe scute respiratory syndrome. *New England Journal of Medicine* 348:1953–1966.

Koo, D. and Wetterhall, S. F. 1996. History and current status of the National Notifiable Diseases Surveillance System. *Journal of Public Health Management Practice* 2:4–10.

Madoff, L. C. and Woodall, J. P. 2005. The Internet and the global monitoring of emerging diseases: Lessons from the first 10 years of ProMED-mail. *Archives of Medical Research* 36:724–730.

Mandl, K. D., Overhage, J. M., Wagner, M. M., Lober, W. B., Sebastiani, P., Mostashari, F., et al. 2004. Implementing syndromic surveillance: A practical guide informed by the early experience. *Journal of the American Medical Informatics Association* 11(2): 141–150.

Meselson, M., Guillemin, J., Hugh-Jones, M., Langmuir, A., Popora, I., Shelekov, A., et al. 1994. The Sverdlovsk anthrax outbreak of 1979. *Science* 266:1202–1208.

NACCHO. 2009. NACCHO survey of local health departments' budget cuts and workforce reductions (January 2009). National Association of County and City Health Officials. http://www.naccho.org (accessed October 4, 2009).

Nash, M. 2002. IN PERSON: Where terrorism meets optimism. *New York Times,* November 24, N.Y./Region section, Online edition, http://www.nytimes.com/2002/11/24/nyregion/in-person-where-terrorism-meets-optimism.html?scp=1&sq=richard%20preston%20cobra%20event%20clinton&st=cse&pagewanted=1 (accessed October 6, 2009).

Parran, T. 1945. Public health in the reconversion period. *American Journal of Public Health* 35:987–993.

Perlino, C. M. 2006. The public health workforce shortage: Left unchecked, will we be protected?. *American Public Health Association Issue brief,* September 2006, http://www.apha.org (accessed on October 4, 2009).

Preston, R. 1997. *The cobra event.* New York: Random House.

Reingold, A. 2003. If syndromic surveillance is the answer, what is the question? *Biosecurity and Bioterrorism* 1:77–81.

Select Bipartisan Committee to Investigate the Preparation for and Response to Hurricane Katrina. 2006. Congressional Reports: H. Rpt. 109-377—A Failure of Initiative: Final Report of the Select Bipartisan Committee to Investigate the Preparation for and Response to Hurricane Katrina. Washington, D.C.: U.S. Government Printing Office. http://www.gpoaccess.gov/serialset/creports/katrina.html (accessed on October 6, 2009).

Shinde, V., Bridges, C. B., Uyeki, T. M., et al. 2009. Triple-reassortant swine influenza A (H1) in humans in the United States, 2005–2009. *New England Journal of Medicine* 360:2616–2625.

Smillie, W. G. 1943. The National Board of Health 1879–1883. *American Journal of Public Health* 33:925–930.

Smith, K. 2007. Testimony of Dr. Kimothy Smith, Acting Director of the National Biosurveillance Integration Center before the Senate Homeland Security and Governmental Affairs, Subcommittee on Oversight of Governmental Management, the Federal Workforce, and the District of Columbia. Department of Homeland Security, (October 4, 2007), http://www.dhs.gov/xnews/testimony/testimony_1191608625983.shtm (accessed October 6, 2009).

Trust for America's Health. 2008. Issue report: Ready or not? 2008: Protecting the public's health from diseases, disasters, and bioterrorism. Robert Wood Johnson Foundation, December 2008. http://healthyamericans.org/reports/bioterror08/ (accessed October 6, 2009).

Tucker, J. B. 2005. Updating the international health regulations. *Biosecurity and Bioterrorism* 3:338–347.

U.S. Government Accountability Office (GAO) 2001. Bioterrorism: Federal research and preparedness activities (GAO-01-915). *United States General Accounting Office Report to Congressional Committees,* September 2001, www.gao.gov/new.items/d01915.pdf.

U.S. Government Accountability Office (GAO) 2008. Health information technology: More detailed plans needed for the Centers for Disease Control and Prevention's redesigned BioSense program (GAO-09-100). *United States General Accounting Office Report to Congressional Committees,* November 2008, www.gao.gov/new.items/d01900.pdf.

U.S. Government Accountability Office (GAO) 2004. HHS Bioterrorism Preparedness Programs: States reported progress but fell short of program goals for 2002 (GAO-04-360R). *United States General Accounting Office Briefing for Congressional Staff*, February 2004, http://www.gao.gov/new.items/d04360r.pdf (accessed September 25, 2009).

U.S. Government Accountability Office (GAO) 2007a. Homeland Security: Preparing for and responding to disasters (GAO-07-395T). *United States General Accounting Office Testimony before the Subcommittee on Homeland Security*, March 2007, www.gao.gov/new.items/d07395t.pdf.

U.S. Government Accountability Office (GAO) 2007b. Influenza pandemic: Opportunities exist to address critical infrastructure protection challenges that require federal and private sector coordination (GAO-08-36). *United States General Accounting Office Report to Congressional Requesters*, October 2007, www.gao.gov/new.items/d0836.pdf.

Wagner, M. M., Tsui, F., Espino, J. U. et al. 2001. The emerging science of very early detection of disease outbreaks. *Journal of Public Health Management Practice* 7:51–59.

Weiner, T. 2007. *Legacy of ashes: the history of the CIA.* New York: Doubleday.

Wetterhall, S. 1996. CDC Surveillance for unknown pathogens. In H. Bendixen, F. Manning, and L. Sparacino (Eds.), *Blood and Blood Products: Safety and Risk.* Washington, DC: Institute of Medicine, National Academy Press, 59-64.

World Health Organization. 2003. Update 95—SARS: Chronology of a serial killer. World Health Organization. http://www.who.int/csr/don/2003_07_04/en/ (accessed October 4, 2009).

Index

E

G

H

I

T

X

Z

Milton Keynes UK
Ingram Content Group UK Ltd.
UKHW020317111024
449327UK00040B/1348